AF753145

Pharmacognosy

Pharmacognosy

Current Herbal Medications and Natural Product Chemistry for a PharmD Curriculum

First Edition

Edited by Yan Zhang
Virginia Commonwealth University

cognella
SAN DIEGO

Bassim Hamadeh, CEO and Publisher
Tony Paese, Project Editor
Jess Estrella, Senior Graphic Designer
Stephanie Kohl, Licensing Associate
Natalie Piccotti, Director of Marketing
Kassie Graves, Vice President of Editorial
Jamie Giganti, Director of Academic Publishing

Copyright © 2021 by Cognella, Inc. All rights reserved. No part of this publication may be reprinted, reproduced, transmitted, or utilized in any form or by any electronic, mechanical, or other means, now known or hereafter invented, including photocopying, microfilming, and recording, or in any information retrieval system without the written permission of Cognella, Inc. For inquiries regarding permissions, translations, foreign rights, audio rights, and any other forms of reproduction, please contact the Cognella Licensing Department at rights@cognella.com.

Trademark Notice: Product or corporate names may be trademarks or registered trademarks and are used only for identification and explanation without intent to infringe.

Cover images:
Copyright © 2015 Depositphotos/Botamochy.
Copyright © 2016 Depositphotos/kchngtw.

9781516594573

cognella® | ACADEMIC PUBLISHING
3970 Sorrento Valley Blvd., Ste. 500, San Diego, CA 92121

Contents

Preface

Yan Zhang

PHARMACY EDUCATION HAS BEEN EVOLVING IN the United States continuously since the day of its formal introduction in this country. One of the motivations and impulses of such an evolution comes from the nonstop changing of pharmacy practice. Among all the medications managed by practicing pharmacists, herbal medications (including alternative and complementary treatments) and education on such topics have probably been the most dramatically changed over the past 50 years. More recently, attention from patients and their health care providers to these herbal products continues to increase, while the market value of herbal medications and alternative medicines has been growing magnificently in the past few decades. However, there is a paucity of literature on the current role of pharmacognosy in the doctor of pharmacy (PharmD) curriculum in the United States. Though pharmacognosy as a component of pharmacist education has been in the literature since 1947, there is little guidance and no consensus in the literature on its role in the modern PharmD curriculum. More particularly, few currently available textbooks on pharmacognosy seem to be concurrent in addressing the continuous evolution of this teaching topic and its practicum needs.

In the spring of 2009, we launched the course of Pharmacognosy in the School of Pharmacy at Virginia Commonwealth University. The course took about a year and a half to be formulated. During that process, all the lecturers, including the course coordinator (myself), struggled to identify a suitable textbook for the course. We certainly do not want to teach all the classic knowledge on herbs, as our current pharmacists are no longer handling the herbs directly due to improvements in formulation and commercialization by the pharmaceutical industry. Meanwhile, the major role of natural products utilized in the current pharmacy practice has shifted from direct medications to lead compounds. Facing this challenge, we decided to adopt several then-available textbooks as reference books while developing a contemporary course based on current pharmacy practice and drug discovery efforts in the field. Yet students are not fully satisfied, and neither are the lecturers teaching in the course.

After ten years of teaching practice, we all felt it was time to put together a new textbook to reflect our own efforts in the past dozen years of teaching in this course. Instead of presenting all the nomenclature and discussing different parts of the herbs, we focus on the regulation and practicum of herbal medications in the real world. By introducing natural products as lead compounds for drug design, discovery, and development, instead of focusing on the chemical features of them, we have tried to build a bridge between herbal medications and current Western medicines. To equip our students with tools and knowledge in order to deal with an unbelievable amount of information and data in this hot area generated on a daily basis, we put together a case study component as a training protocol and introduced it to the readers and potential users of this book. In other words, we have tried to present the outcome of our teaching efforts on such a classic topic by turning it into a contemporary melody.

Acknowledgments

Yan Zhang

THIS BOOK IS AN EXCELLENT EXAMPLE of teamwork. All contributors to the book worked so hard to finish their chapters, and they demonstrated an outstanding team spirit in this process. I was extremely impressed.

All the PharmD students in the School of Pharmacy, Virginia Commonwealth University, from the class of 2013 through the current class of 2023, are essential contributors of the book, though their names are not shown here. Without their patience and support, I do not believe our teaching practice and this textbook as one outcome from the practice would be successful. All the faculty members from the school should be recognized for their support, one way or another, during the past dozen years of our teaching practice. The support of our leadership in the school has always been there for us. We feel so lucky to have them to back us up.

The editors from Cognella—Tony, Clare, and others behind the scene—encouraged us and guided me throughout this whole process. I learned a lot from them. Their patience and expertise are the keys to this book.

Introduction

Yan Zhang

IN 2007, THE ACCREDITATION COUNCIL FOR Pharmacy Education (ACPE) Standards reinforced the offering of pharmacognosy, along with alternative and complementary treatments as specific curriculum topics, for schools and colleges of pharmacy in the United States to teach to professional standards as part of the science foundation for the PharmD curricula. To meet this requirement, we created a new pharmacognosy course as a venue to provide didactic and relevant early experiential education for our first-year PharmD students. After ten years of teaching practice, we believe our course has fulfilled the ACPE standards and simultaneously prepared our students for their following years' clinical therapeutics courses, as well as future practice. As a product from these years of teaching practice, we put together this textbook to summarize our strategic design of the course to reflect current pharmacy practice. The book is aimed to show our efforts to cover the unique and rich history of pharmacognosy in pharmacy practice and the critical role of it in the evolution of modern Western medicine. We wish to share this book with pharmacy students and our colleagues in the practice and to help them construct their course and fulfill the requirements of the ACPE.

There are four parts in this book. The first three parts are constructed to provide didactic teaching material in the classroom practice. With basic concepts and principles emphasized up front and homework/exam questions at the end, we believe the most essential topics of pharmacognosy are covered coherently and comprehensively. The fourth part of the book is unique, not only in its structure but also because of its contents. We intend to present the case studies we adopted in our teaching practice and share some useful ideas and results coming from our teaching effort.

Our approach to teaching this topic seems to be successful in preparing our PharmD students for their future learning and practice, and we hope this textbook will provide a platform for other colleagues around the country to share their thoughts and successes from their practice as well.

Part I

Overview

Chapter 1

History of Pharmacognosy

Yali Liu, Ling Zhang, and Glen E. Kellogg

Introduction

The use of plants by man dates back to the beginning of humankind, and probably even earlier. From that moment on, plants became an instrument of power, since they were regarded not only as a powerful source of nutrition but also as excellent remedies for the ills of the body and soul.

In the early period, primitive man went in search of food and randomly consumed plants or their parts, like tubers, fruits, leaves, and others. As no harmful effects were observed, he considered them as edible material and used them as food. If he observed other effects from eating, they were considered inedible, and according to the effects, he would potentially use them in treating symptoms or diseases. The knowledge was empirical and was obtained by trial and error.[1]

There are several competing historical indications that claim the ancient use of natural remedies to resolve primary health issues in different parts of the world.[2][3][4][5] The pollen grains of the valuable medicinal plants *Achillea* species, *Centaurea solstitialis*, *Senecio* species, *Muscari* species, *Ephedra altissima*, and *Althea* species reported from excavations of the 60,000 BC burial of Shanidar IV suggest the practice of using plants for medicinal purposes by Neanderthals in the Paleolithic Age.[6] The ancient Hindu, Chinese, Greek, Egyptian, Mesopotamian, and Biblical texts show the use of various herbs and minerals for medicinal purposes throughout the world since antiquity.[7][8][9][10][11]

In the history of mankind, there is almost no site on earth where plants have not been used experimentally when the opportunity arose. Medical herbalists of Babylonia, Assyria, Sumer, and Egypt were thoroughly convinced that their practices were created by the gods, who had instructed men on the healing properties of water, herbs, plants, and oils. For that very reason, man has attributed a sacred link to the divine to plants. This link persists today, as many plants are still used in religious ceremonies and funeral rites, as well as by many tribal groups as elements of magic, in almost every corner of the world.[12]

Pharmacognosy's historical account makes it clear that pharmacognosy in its entirety is not the work of just one or two continental areas but the overall outcome of the persistent work of many bygone civilizations like the Chinese, Egyptian, Indian, Persian, Babylonian, Assyrian, and others. In short, pharmacognosy is derived from empirical attempts to harness nature for enhancing life. Gradually, pharmacognosy formed its own sets of theories, investigations, and practices. Over time, the usage of plants and plant extracts for health applications has been refined and guided in *ad hoc* and formal clinical settings, with the best technologies available. As a result, the principles and theory of pharmacognosy have matured to its evolution as a distinct professional discipline.

The History of Herbal Medication in Different Areas

Asia

China

Traditional Chinese medicine (TCM) is considered one of the most ancient systems of medicine, with an almost 5,000-year history. TCM aims at restoring "energies" using a holistic approach that considers all aspects of an individual's life, including symptoms, family relations, season, and weather, and a complex diagnostic pattern using inspection, listening, smelling, palpation, and inquiry.[13]

TCM originated in the era of the legendary clan leader Fu Xi (2593 BC) and established its theoretical system between the late years of the Warring States period and the Chin and Han dynasties (475 BC–AD 220).[14] Chinese herbal medicine was first described by another legendary figure called Shen-Nong, who is said to have lived from 2737 BC to 2697 BC.[15][16] It is reported that Shen-Nong, by tasting hundreds of herbs on one day, found more than 70 herbs that had medicinal value, selected those that were suitable as remedies, and described their properties.[17] The *Shennong Herbal Classic*, the earliest known pharmacological text in China, was written by authors who lived during the period immediately following the fall of the Han dynasty (202 BC–AD 220). This work recorded 365 kinds of herbal medicines.[18]

During the Jin and Tang dynasties (AD 265–907), traditional Chinese medicine experienced significant and noteworthy development as it absorbed considerable medical information from the Arabian countries, Japan, and India.[19] During the Tang Dynasty, Sun Simiao, summarizing the previous experience of Chinese herbalists, compiled *Beiji Qianjin Yao Fang* (*Essential Formulas for Emergencies* [*Worth*] *a Thousand Pieces of Gold*) in AD 652, and in AD 682, he compiled its supplement, *Qianjin Yi Fang*. These texts and Simiao's other works have had a great impact on future generations of pharmacologists and physicians in China and beyond.

During the Song and Yuan dynasties (AD 960–1368), the invention of printing technology and further advances in papermaking caused TCM to spread widely and to be deeply researched. At that time, there were many compendiums written by government functionaries or by individuals such as Zheng-Lei-Ben-Cao, Tai-Ping-Sheng-Hui-Fang, and Kai-Bao-Ben-Cao.[19]

Later, during the Ming and Qing dynasties (AD 1368–1911), every part of TCM was enriched, and TCM spread as long-distance travel and emigration opportunities increased to the countries of Europe and the Americas. The "Compendium of Materia Medica" (AD 1578), compiled by Li Shizhen, a medical scientist of the Ming Dynasty, summarized the experience of medicine before the 16th century.[19] It was praised as the encyclopedia of China by foreign scholars and regarded by many as a singular scientific achievement of the Ming dynasty.

From the beginning of the Opium War in 1840, and through numerous other conflicts, China was continually defeated by outside forces. This led to a general cultural malaise, and as a result, some Chinese people developed a cultural inferiority complex that yielded a tide of complete opposition to their own culture. Western medicine took firm root, and Chinese traditional medicine went into a 100-year decline[19] (Figure 1.1).

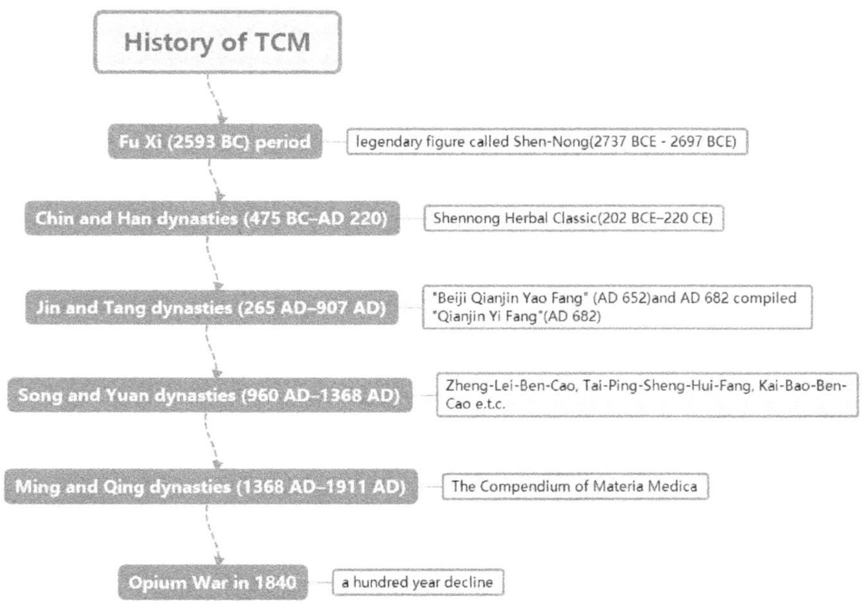

FIGURE 1.1

Japan

Traditional Japanese herbal medicine, known as Kampo medicine (*Kam* means Chinese, and *po* means method or prescription), was from its beginning highly influenced by ancient Chinese medicine, sharing some similar holistic medical theories.[20] However, the practice of Kampo treatments has evolved to better fulfill the indigenous needs of the Japanese people and medical practice. Ancient Chinese medicine traveled to Japan between the sixth and eighth centuries.[21] Its basic philosophy is the yin and yang of Taoism. In AD 984, Yasuyori Tamba compiled the Ishino, a vast compendium of Chinese medicine.[22] Between the 16th and 18th centuries, three Japanese schools of Kampo medicine were established, and until almost 150 years ago, the official medicine of Japan was Kampo. As the influences of Western culture and civilization grew, the practice of Kampo fell out of favor with the Japanese government, and Western medicine, practiced by doctors and taught in medical schools, became the official medicine of Japan during the Meiji Periods.[23] By the end of World War II, the traditional herbal practices of Kampo had almost completely vanished. However, as in the West, there has been renewed interest in Kampo medicine in recent decades. Patients and physicians have reevaluated the holistic and humane aspects of traditional medicine. Kampo medicine is increasingly recognized for its efficacy and safety. In fact, the cost of many treatments can be covered by medical insurance.

Although traditional systematic Japanese medicine did originate in China, many local herbs had been used for many centuries.[24] More than 50 Japanese-specific herbs are included in a book on ancient styles and earth that introduces unique natural products from all parts of Japan. In AD 808, *Daido Rui-ho*, the first Japanese pharmacopoeia book, collected information on 279 local herbs obtained from temples and famous clans, listing their Japanese names, origins, and methods of collection. This book was copied and disseminated and used as a medical textbook by Japanese physicians until the end of the Tokugawa period (1867), which is considered the final period of traditional Japan. During this latter era, new prescriptions were added and old and obviously irrational prescriptions were gradually eliminated from the Kampo canon. The completed and updated book was eventually published in 1827 (Figure 1.2).

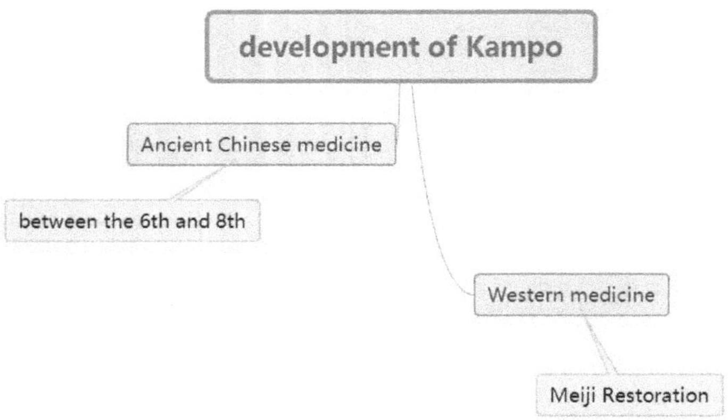

FIGURE 1.2

Korea

Chinese medicine passed into Korea more than ten centuries ago.[25] The Korean people had continued to develop their own medicine since the time they settled on the peninsula, but frequent interactions with the Chinese made Koreans dependent on the more advanced Chinese medicine.[26] Meanwhile, the Korean people made gradual efforts to embrace and adapt the advanced medical technologies of China to turn them into their own.

Around the tenth century AD, Korea introduced TCM in earnest. Moreover, the development of printing and paper production technologies expanded access to TCM concepts to the traditional medical sector of Korea. Combining this new knowledge with their own experiences, Korea's medical practitioners made extensive efforts to develop medicine of their own. Such efforts became more intense in the 13th century. In 1433, after 200 years of work, *Hyangyakjipseongbang*[27] was published; one of its most important features was a reconciliation of the official Korean names of herbs (Hyangyak) with those of Chinese herbs. Since that time, medicine could be practiced without depending on expensive medicines imported from China. The *Yixuerumen*[28] (*Introduction to Medicine*) (1575) contains a wide range of medical techniques that were accumulated during the 12th to 16th centuries. It, in turn, played a major role in the development of the later text *Dongeuibogam* (1613). This book (*The Precious Mirror of Oriental Medicine*) was written by the court physician Heo Jun and consolidated the latest medical knowledge of China and Korea of the 16th century while incorporating unique Korean viewpoints toward disease. Traditional Korean medicine took a different direction than TCM after the publication of *Dongeuibogam*. In particular, a distinctive school—constitutional medicine—was established in Korea[29][30][31][32][33] in the early 20th century. As traditional Korean medicine (TKM) has followed different routes from TCM, it is now totally different from TCM.[27]

The geomorphological characteristics of the Korean Peninsula focused its rich medicinal plant resources.[34] There are about 4,500 species of medicinal plants in Korea, including 3,400 species, 762 varieties, and 287 subtypes. More than 300 of these have been used as medicines. At present, the exact number of North Korean medicinal plant resources and sales are not known, but we can suspect that the Korean Peninsula has more herbal medicine resources than are currently accounted for (Figure 1.3).

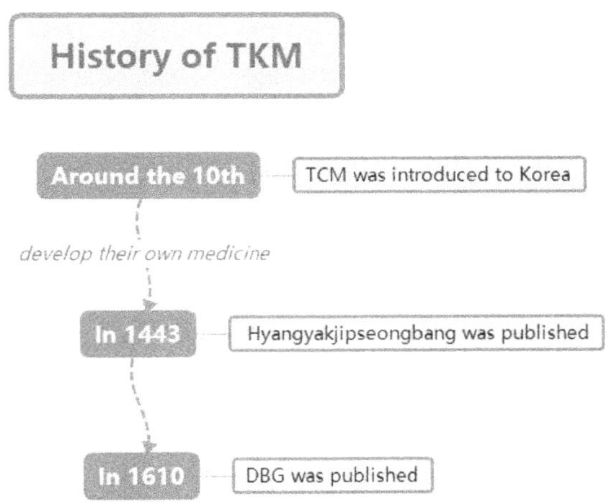

FIGURE 1.3

India

India has a rich history of traditional medicines (TIM) based on six systems. The Ayurveda system is the most ancient, the most widely accepted, and the most practiced.[35] The other systems of medicine are Siddha, Unani, Homeopathy, Yoga, and Naturopathy. Siddha medicine and Unani medicine are fundamentally very similar to Ayurveda in their approach to health and disease, but Siddha originated and is practiced more in southern India, whereas the Unani system is practiced more in the northern and western parts of India[36] (Figure 1.4).

Ayurveda, a major component of traditional Indian medicines, developed around 1500 BC. *Ayus* means the conjunction of body, sense organs, mind, and self and is known by the synonyms *dhari*, *jivita*, *nityaga*, and *annubandha*.[37] Ayurveda defines life as the combination of *Shareera* (body), *Indriya* (sense organs), *Satwa* (mind), and *Atma* (soul). Ayurveda belongs to the traditional health care and longevity systems. Because the belief that "everything can be a drug" is deeply rooted in Indian culture, Ayurvedic physicians made use of an extensive collection of medications, herbs/plants, and even the urine of animals in their studies and described their effects meticulously.[38]

In India, the history of using plant resources for treating diseases can be dated back to 6000–4000 BC (i.e., the Buddhist period). The earliest references to such plants, minerals, and animal products with their usage for medical purposes are found in the *Rig veda* (2000 BC), an ancient Indian sacred collection of Vedic Sanskrit hymns, which described 67 Ayurvedic medicines. The *Atharva veda* (1200–1000 BC) the fourth and last Veda of Hindu literature, recorded 290 Indian herbal medicines.[39]

The *Yajurveda* (1200–1000 BC) recorded 87 Indian herbal medicines. The *Charaka Samhita* (400 BC–AD 200) is the first recorded treatise fully devoted to the concepts and practice of Ayurveda, with a primary focus on therapeutics. The *Charaka Samhita* listed 526 Indian herbal medicines.[40] The next landmark in Ayurvedic literature is the *Sushruta Samhita* (c. 600 BC), and edited through circa AD 600. Although the text places special emphasis on surgery, it also describes 395 medicinal plants, 57 drugs of animal origin, and 64 minerals

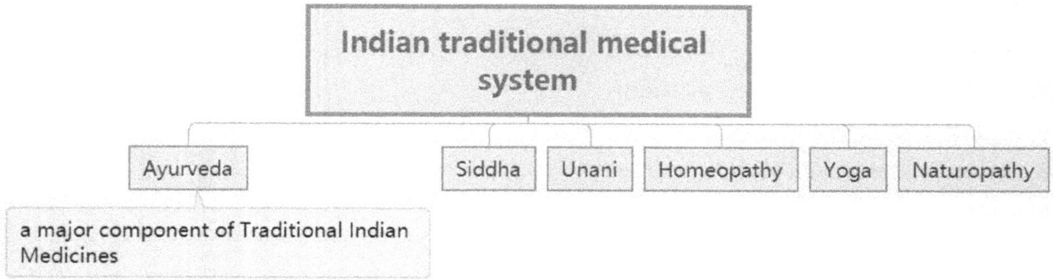

FIGURE 1.4

or metals as therapeutic agents.[41] *Bhava Prakasha* (1550), written by Bhava-Mishra, is the most important historical text on herbs/plants and is held in high esteem by modern Ayurvedic practitioners in its description of 470 Indian herbal medicines[42][43][44] (Figure 1.5).

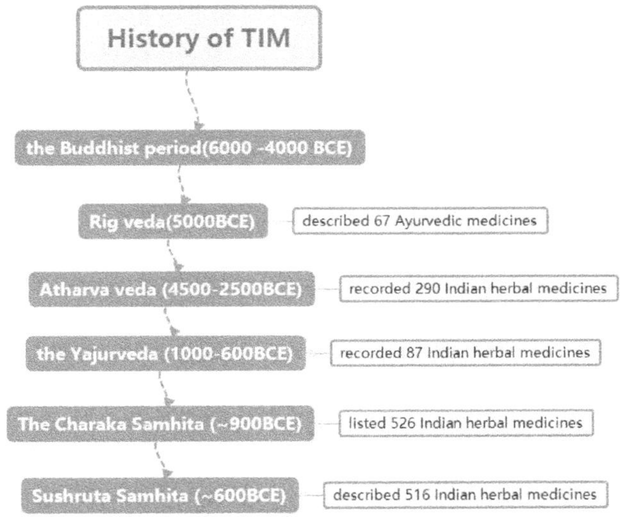

FIGURE 1.5

Southeast Asia

The nations of Southeast Asia have historically, culturally, and ethnographically been influenced by their neighbors to the north and west, China and India, respectively. The same is true for much of their practices of traditional medicine.

Singapore, a city-state island country, is situated on the southern tip of the Malay Peninsula. It is highly urbanized and has the third-highest per capita income in the world.[45] Singapore's primary health care system is based on allopathic medicine, so traditional herbal medicine is often termed "complementary and alternative medicine (CAM)." There are patients in Singapore who choose herbal medicine for health promotion or for the treatment of diseases, but these are largely ethnically based. For example, the local Chinese use TCM, the Malays use *Jamu* medicine, and the Indians use Ayurvedic medicine to complement the allopathic medicine. Most herbs are used or consumed in dried forms imported from the countries of origin where these therapeutic systems are established. Alternatively, because of the urbanization of Singapore, some herbal medicines are sold as finished products. However, some locals still resort to using fresh medicinal plants using herbal folk knowledge handed down verbally from the older generations who used to reside in many Kampong villages of Singapore and the neighboring country of Malaysia.

Traditional Malaysian medicine existed long before the development and spread of Western (European) medicine. Traditional Chinese medicine is one of the traditional and complementary medicines commonly used by the Malaysian population.[46][47] It is believed that TCM was introduced into Malaysia by Chinese migrants working in the tin mines,[48] who brought herbal medicines, acupuncture, and other forms of TCM treatments with them. The most commonly practiced forms of TCM are herbal medicine and acupuncture.[49]

A study conducted by Loh among Singaporean children regarding the use of TCM showed that herbal medicine was the most common TCM modality being used,[50] with 84.3 percent (253) of children using herbs.[51]

The development of traditional Thai medicine experienced four periods in Thai history: the ancient period of the Mongol Empire (1182–1186), Sukotai period (1238–1377), Ayutuoye period (1350–1767), and Bangkok or Kerry dynasties (1782–present).[52] Thai medicine is considered Buddhist medicine due to the strong links to the faith in the Thai region. It contains an amalgamation of local as well as ancient Chinese and Indian influences due to the migrations of the people now comprising the Thai people. Thai traditional medicine generally employs a wide range of indigenous herbs in the form of tincture or tea for the cure of skin and systemic inflammatory diseases.[53] Prior to the Sukotai period, traditional medicine had been used by the Thai people to treat common diseases and some chronic diseases. Traditional medicine was outlawed in the early 1900s, as it was deemed to be "quackery." Concomitantly, the increase in the number of modern medical doctors led to an increase in the use of modern medicines and an increase in demand for imported modern medicine and pharmaceutical industry raw materials. This, unfortunately, accounts for a considerable proportion of Thailand's trade deficit. The Seventh National Economic and Social Plan (1992–1996) promoted the development of traditional wisdom in health care, including Thai traditional medicine, herbal medicine, and traditional massage. The Thai nation created the National Institute of Thai Traditional Medicine in 1993 under the supervision of the Ministry of Public Health.[54]

From the second century BC to the tenth century AD, Vietnam was ruled by China.[55] Vietnamese traditional medicine (VTM) is thus also greatly influenced by traditional Chinese medicine, and many herbs from Vietnam have also been introduced into China, such as betel nut, kudzu root, lotus seed, and so on, and some processing methods have also been introduced into China. The existing VTM was organized and developed in the 14th century after Vietnam's departure from Chinese rule by Tuê Tinh, known as the founder of Vietnamese traditional medicine.[56] Between 1858 and 1954, Vietnam was ruled by France, and Western medicine developed rapidly, while VTM was strongly suppressed and regarded by the colonial powers as quack medicine. The Vietnamese people of that time, however, did not abandon VTM, and it thus begun to coexist with Western medicine. In 1955, the Vietnamese President Ho Chi Minh proposed combining Eastern medicine with European medicine. During the Vietnam War (1955–1975), VTM played an important role in the treatment of burns, fractures, war zone plagues, and other diseases, especially when the supply of modern medicine was very short. In this environment, there was significant need for VTM, and it was reborn. Departments specializing in the study and use of herbs, such as research institutes and hospitals, modernized VTM. In 1957, the Vietnamese Ministry of

Health established the Department of Oriental Medicine, which was renamed the Ministry of Traditional Medicine in 1993. The Ho Chi Minh Institute of Traditional Medicine was established in 1976.

In its rainforests, Indonesia has the second biggest biodiversity in the world, expressed by a high number of indigenous medicinal plants. Based on this rich source of medicinal plants, most Indonesian people, especially in rural areas, use traditional herbal medicines known as *jamu* to treat disease. *Jamu* is a word in the Javanese tribal language meaning traditional medicine from plants. Minerals, animals, and parts thereof have also been used but are not the subject of this review.[57]

The Middle East

The so-called Cradle of Civilization is near the intersection of the African, Asian, and European continents. There is a rich history of civilization in this region, particularly that of Mesopotamians, Byzantines, Persians, and Egyptians, that significantly predates the Islamic era. This intersection of cultures was enhanced by the many trade routes that moved goods and ideas between the Mediterranean nations (especially Greece and the Roman Empire) and Asia, as well as sub-Saharan Africa. Unsurprisingly, this produced a very robust collection of local medical knowledge, much of which was widely disseminated by the same forces that brought it to the Middle East.

Ancient Egypt

The ancient Egyptians had a system of medicine that was very advanced for its time and influenced later medical traditions.[58] Herbal medicine played an important role in ancient Egyptian medicine. Many herbs were soaked in wine and used directly as oral medicine. The ancient Egyptians turned many materials into medicinal materials, such as plants, animals, minerals, and even animal urine and feces.[59] Many medicinal herbs, such as opium, marijuana, myrrh, frankincense, fennel, cinnamon, thyme, and flaxseed, were recorded in recovered papyri, and garlic cloves were unearthed in the tomb of Pharaoh Tutankhamun. In 1873, George Ebers acquired a remarkable papyrus originally from Thebes and dated to 1555 BC, which contained 876 remedies and the use of 500 substances (mostly from plants),[60] with dosage forms including gargles, snuffs, poultices, infusions, pills, and ointments and vehicles using beer, milk, wine, and honey.[61]

Another notable recovered document, the *Edwin Smith Papyrus*, regarded as the oldest extant medical document, asserts that in ancient Egypt, both physicians and herbalists avoided the use of magic when treating their patients because they assumed that diseases were simply produced by natural causes.[62] The best-known Egyptian pharmaceutical record is the *Ebers Papyrus* (dating back to 1500 BC), which documented some 700 herbal medicines.

After the Arabs conquered Egypt in the seventh century AD, Arabic medicine became the dominant practice of medicine, and the art of healing made use of all the available knowledge gained by the Arabs from their trading relationships with different civilizations, such as the Persians, Chinese, and Greeks, as well as the Ancient Egyptians.

The Arabs

The majority of Arabs are currently Muslims, and Arabic culture and Islamic ideology are now closely related. As such, Arabic medicine/*materia medica*/herbal medicine (AM/AMM/AHM) may also be called Greco-Arab or Islamic medicine.[63] In the ninth century AD, the Arabs translated and adapted *De Materia Medica*, a five-volume work written by the Greek physician Pedanius Dioscorides between AD 50 and 70, which contains hundreds of herbs for the treatment of different diseases. The cultural aspect of traditional Arabic medicine developed from the ancient Arab civilization, with a "magical" religious or spiritual mode of thought that prevailed throughout that civilization. Traditional Arabic medicine owes a great deal to the influences of antecedent civilizations. The medical expertise of the ancient Egyptians (the era of the Pharaohs), Greeks, Babylonians (Mesopotamia), Persians, Romans, Byzantines, Indians, and Chinese helped create a basis for later Arab-Islamic scientific explorations and discovery.[64]

During the Golden Age of Islam (eighth to 13th century AD), the herbal drug trade promoted significant commercial and scientific exchange between China and the Muslim world (see Figure 1.6). Chinese herbal drugs were described by medieval Muslim medical scholars such as Tabari (870), Rhazes (925), Haly Abbas (982), Avicenna (1037), and Jurjani (1137). In particular, the Persian Avicenna (also known as Ibn Sina) was a brilliant contributor to the sciences of pharmacy and medicine during the Arabian era. Although he wrote in Arabic, his pharmaceutical teachings were accepted as authority in the West until the 17th century and still are dominant influences in the Orient. The term *al-sin* (the Arabic word for China) is used 46 times in Avicenna's *Canon of Medicine*, as it references herbal drugs imported from China.[65] Cinnamon (*dar sini*; "Chinese herb"), wild ginger (*asaron*), rhubarb (*rivand-e sini*), nutmeg (*basbasa*), incense tree wood (*ood*), cubeb (*kababe*), and sandalwood (*sandal*) were the most frequently mentioned Chinese herbs in Islamic medical books. There are also multiple

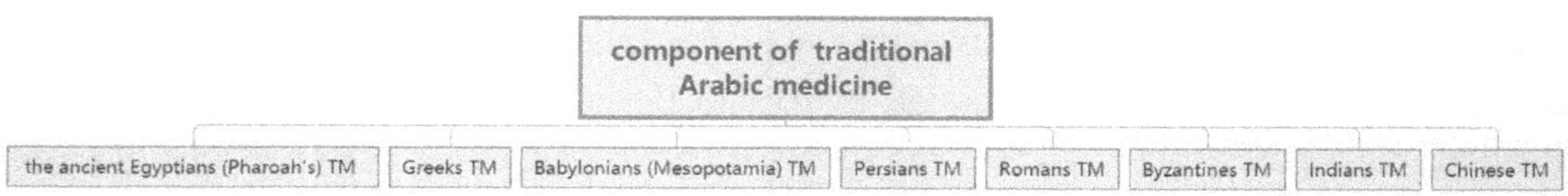

FIGURE 1.6

similarities between the clinical uses of these herbs in both medical systems. Thus, it appears that Chinese herbal drugs were a major component of the cultural exchange.

This trade route flourished in the ancient world (seventh century BC to second century AD) as a link between the Mediterranean Sea and the Eastern and Southern Asian sources of medicinal herbs and spices. It stretched from Mediterranean ports to Egypt through Northeast Africa and Arabia to India and beyond. Land routes for incense from Southern Arabia to the Mediterranean flourished from 700 through 100 BC.

Europe

Ancient Greece and Rome

The Greek philosophers systemized science and medicine while creating a lasting historical record. Theophrastus (c. 300 BC), an early Greek philosopher and natural scientist, is regarded as the "father of botany." One of his many interests was understanding and writing about the medical qualities of herbs and other plants. His observations are still mainly accurate. The most famous ancient Greek scientist/physician/philosopher, Hippocrates, practiced in the Age of Pericles and is often referred to as the "father of medicine" in recognition of his founding the Hippocratic School of Medicine, which established medicine as a discipline and ultimately a profession. Hippocrates created a variety of dosage forms, and the "pharmacy" meaning of the word *pharmakon* was first determined at that time.[66] The pharmacy gradually developed into a theoretical system, and its practitioners became the prototype of current pharmacists.[67] A Greek, Dioscorides, well-known as a historically influential physician, pharmacologist, botanist, and pharmacist, wrote the first pharmacy monograph (*De Materia Medica*) in Western history while employed by the Roman army. As noted above, *De Materia Medica* was translated throughout the civilized world of that era. One man who forged an unbreakable tie between the professions of pharmacy and medicine was Galen (AD 130–200). He practiced and taught both fields in Rome; he created many of the principles of preparing and compounding medicines used in the West until the Renaissance. "Galenical" and "Galenic preparations" are terms for pharmaceuticals, particularly botanicals, compounded by mechanical means.[68]

The European Union Countries

As noted above, the basis of Mediterranean and European medicine was laid down during Greek antiquity and during the Roman Empire by physicians and philosophers, who started building a written consensus about what was considered efficacious medical knowledge.[69] It was recorded in leechbooks "books of medical prescriptions" and apothecary texts from at least the ninth century AD (e.g., Bald's leechbook).[70] Here as well, the classic

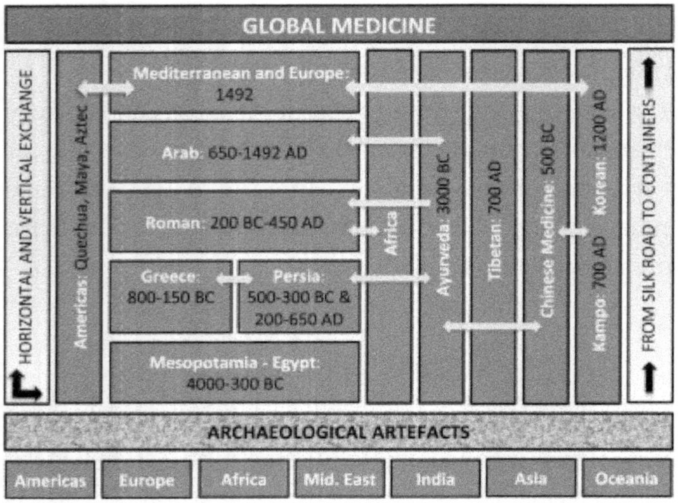

FIGURE 1.7 Mutual influence and development of major traditional medicinal systems with focus on the Mediterranean and Europe.

Mediterranean *materia medica* also influenced the structure, the literary form, and the content of the middle and northern European herbals (see Figure 1.7). During the Middle Ages, Benedictine monks were directed by monastic rule to duplicate herbal medicines and to tend medicinal herb gardens such as those of the Abbeys of Montecassino (Italy) and St. Gall (Switzerland).[71] During the Renaissance, classic Greco-Roman herbals and medical texts were critically analyzed, commented on, and translated into modern languages. This, with the burgeoning availability of the printing press, allowed dissemination of medical knowledge and herbal information to a much larger population.

The recorded use of herbs in the British Isles dates back more than 1,000 years and was initially influenced by Greek and Roman physicians and philosophers. Later, with the rich plant diversity of the British Isles and the clearly distinct nature of its climate, native herb studies also made great progress, and many notable texts on herbalism were written and published as the British Empire spread its influence through conquest, trade, and science. The 18th and 19th centuries, in particular, saw the advent of the British scientist/philosopher and an even more systemized investigation and analysis of the natural world. The ensuing Industrial Revolution, however, sidelined natural remedies in favor of pharmaceuticals, and due to restrictions on education considered to be less rigorous and other legislation, the British herbal medicine industry was out of favor by the early 20th century. As elsewhere in the West, the important role of herbal medicine in the medical system was revitalized in the late 20th century, and relevant supporting policies have emerged.[72]

Russia

Herbal medicines have been known to be used by the Russian population for centuries. In the tenth century AD, when herbs and their medical literature were first proposed, copies of some Greek texts were introduced through Eastern Orthodox Christian monasteries into Russia and eventually translated into Russian. In 1005–1010, monks from Mount Atos in

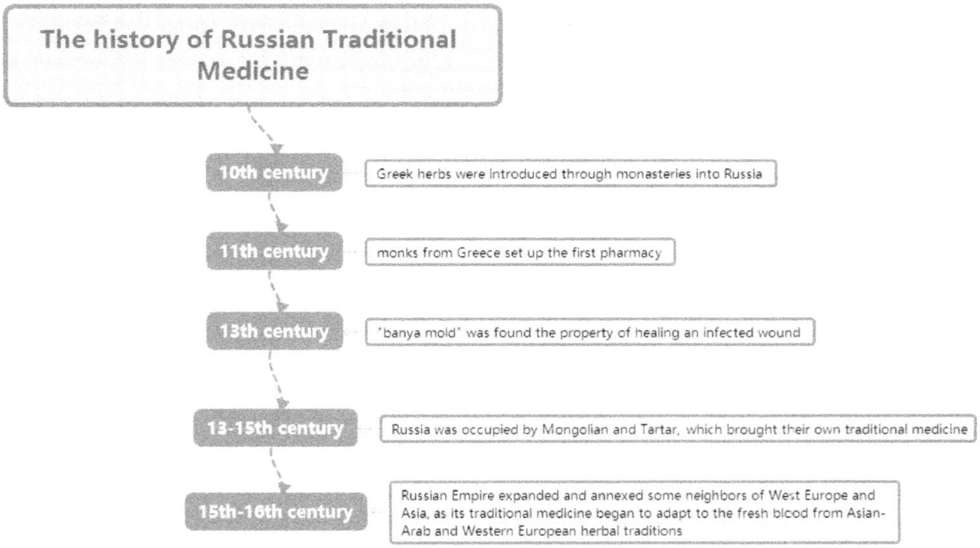

FIGURE 1.8

Greece set up their first pharmacy in Kiev-Pechora Lavra, which was likely to have strengthened Greece's influence on Russian medicine.[73] The 13th-century herbalists in the Russian city of Novgorod discovered the beneficial antimicrobial properties of mold species and successfully treated infected wounds 600 years before the introduction of antibiotics to medicine.[74] From the 15th to the 16th centuries, the Russian Empire expanded, and among its neighbors, Russia incorporated parts of Western Europe and Asia into its territory. At the same time, herbalists began to accumulate and adapt the Asian-Arab and Western European herbal traditions (see Figure 1.8) into their environment. In 1778, the Russian Academy of Sciences published the *Pharmacopoeia Rossica* in St. Petersburg. *The Pharmacopoeia* includes 770 monographs, including 316 on herbal preparations and 29 on the preparation of drugs from animal sources and complex mixtures.[76]

The Americas

North America

Herbal and plant-based medicines have been used for millennia to treat disease and augment health. Wherever humans existed, they experimented with their environment and discovered empirically both good and bad outcomes. While perhaps not as well-known as other herbal lore and traditions, such as those of China and India, the native peoples of North America had a rich indigenous health tradition. Native American traditional healing is recognized by the US National Institutes of Health/National Center for Complementary and Alternative Medicine as a "medical system," including holistic treatments for acute and chronic conditions and health and wellbeing. While there are tribal differences, there are shared beliefs often based in spiritual approaches. Positive behaviors are taught through stories that encourage observing the laws of nature.[75]

Native diets and the use of native plants for healing purposes have been used to promote health by living in harmony with the earth. Thus, before European colonization, the original people had learned the medicinal value of plants such as sage, saw palmetto, Echinacea, St. John's Wort, cohosh, dandelion, and other plants found on the continent.[76][77][78][79][80] Because of their reliance on oral tradition, these and other traditions were accurately passed on verbally from one generation to the next, and only during the last half-century or so were they committed to written records. Unfortunately, many tribes are fully integrating into the mainstream US culture and adopting the corresponding lifestyle. The abandonment of traditional practices is apparent by comparing the health of young Native Americans to their elders who rely on the medicine of their tradition.

For the rest of North Americans, they bring their cultural awareness of traditional medicine as they immigrate. As these new cultures have been incorporated into the United States, traditional herbal medicine has become far more diverse. Also, in the past few decades, the desire for a "chemical-free" life has produced a large herbal products industry manifested in nationwide chains of health food stores and nutrition centers. Thus, herbal and traditional medicine has been globalized and commoditized for the consumer.

The West Indies and Caribbean

The diversity of plants in the Caribbean Basin is unique. The geographical complexity of this region coupled with a largely tragic social history over the last five centuries have contributed to its biological diversity, which encompasses a complex mix of native and exotic species. At the onset of European contact in the 15th century, the ecosystems, resources, native tribes, and their culture components were largely doomed: the land was deforested to build large-scale plantations for sugarcane, banana, tobacco, and coffee. The native plants and animals were largely eliminated as many exotic species were introduced. Similarly, the indigenous peoples were almost totally eliminated and replaced by slaves from Africa and Asia.[81]

As the surviving indigenous populations were forced to adapt to their new culture and ecosystem, their traditional medicinal knowledge was similarly forced to adapt, and their Native pharmacopeias were radically diversified. The influences of the African slave population and their knowledge of natural medicine were particularly important in this transformation, not in small part due to the harsh conditions of their lives.[82]

South America and the Amazon Basin

After a long history of gradual screening of medicinal plants, the native people in the Amazon basin had accumulated valuable knowledge about the ingredients used in herbal medicine. Like the indigenous peoples of North America, the tribes in South America, particularly those isolated in the Amazon rainforest, did not have a written language, and their collective knowledge was passed on orally. A number of notable treatments—specifically *Petiveria alliacea L.*, a kind of plant commonly grown in the tropical regions of the Americas—were used for the treatment of various central nervous system disorders, such as anxiety, pain, memory deficits, and seizures in traditional medicine, as well as for anesthetic and sedative properties (see Table 1.1). Furthermore, the use of this species for religious ceremonies has been reported since the era of slavery in the Americas.[83][84] Also, the Ticuna, an indigenous people of the Amazon, used the roots of *P. alliacea* along with other plants to prepare curare, applied as poison to their arrows. This poison induced neuromuscular blockade, lethargy, and death by asphyxia.[85][86]

Interestingly, only in the past few years, a tribe in the Amazon, the Matsés peoples of Brazil and Peru, are creating an encyclopedia of their traditional medicine. The *Matsés Traditional Medicine Encyclopedia*, compiled by their shamans with assistance from Acaté, details every plant used in their medicine in their own language. Their use of native language is to ensure

TABLE 1.1 Indications and Forms of Traditional Use of *Petiveria alliacea L.*

No.	Indication	Forms of use
1	Buccal anti-inflammatory and analgesic	Tea of roots and leaves: 10 g in 1 L of water, four times a day.
2	Cancer	Decoction of leaves: 40 g in 1 L of water, three times a day. Plant juice (juice): 25–30 fresh leaves (green), filtered with 1 L of cold water, pure. This filtered juice should be consumed three times a day (morning, afternoon, and night).
3	Cystitis	Decoction of leaves or roots: 30 g/L.
4	Headache	Compress of macerated leaves.
5	Rheumatic pains, neuralgia, polyneuritis (beriberi), paralysis	Tincture to friction: 350 g from roots in 40% alcohol.
6	Stimulant, diaphoretic, and diuretic	Decoction from leaves or roots: 30 g in 1 L of water to be taken in tablespoons during the day.
7	Paralysis	Baths: 500 g of roots in each bath.

Source: Adapted from Gomes, P. B., 2006. Avaliação dos efeitos centrais e antinociceptivos das frações isoladas das raízes de Petiveria alliacea L. (Tipi) em camundongos (Master's Dissertation). Universidade Federal do Ceará, Fortaleza.

that their medicinal knowledge remains their intellectual property. The encyclopedia is for training young shamans in their traditional medicine before it is lost.[87]

Africa

Traditional (sub-Saharan) African medicine (TAM) also has a very long history and is an important part of the African cultural treasure.[88] Many African countries and/or tribes have their own traditional medicine. TAM refers to the use of remedies based on plants, animals, or minerals to diagnose, treat, or cure conditions, relying on knowledge handed down from generation to generation. TAM also combines religious concepts with relevant etiology, classification, and knowledge of human anatomy and physiology in the hands of folk doctors and has a set of processing and use techniques for some medicinal materials. These medical treatments, though perhaps inexplicable, are based on fundamental principles of African sociocultural and religious principles, which continue through oral transmission or are used in combination with herbal remedies. There is, unfortunately, very little historical record of TAM prior to the colonial era. And much like in other countries subject to European colonization, native remedies and practices were discouraged or outlawed.[89]

There is, however, now a growing interest in African plants with health potential. A 2013 review highlighted ten medicinal plants (*Acacia senegal*, *Aloe ferox*, *Artemisia herba-alba*, *Aspalathus linearis*, *Centella asiatica*, *Catharanthus roseus*, *Cyclopia genistoides*, *Harpagophytum procumbens*, *Momordica charantia*, and *Pelargonium sidoides*) to be of special interest for more detailed reviews. This selection is based on the criteria that these medicinal plants form part of the African herbal pharmacopeia with commercial importance or from which modern phytopharmaceuticals have been derived. [90]

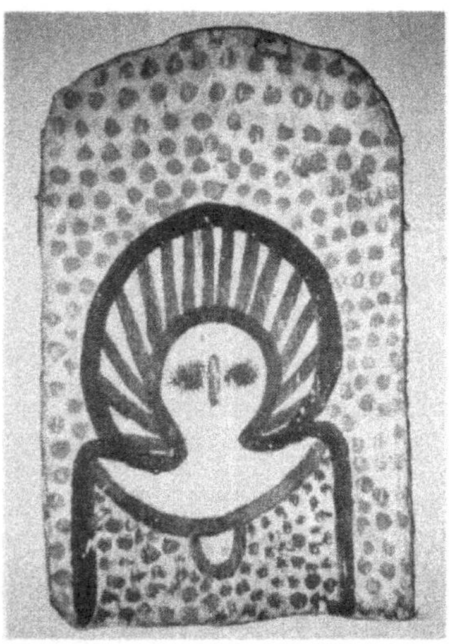

FIGURE 1.9 Rock painting of ancestral spirit.

Oceania and Australia

The Australian aborigine is one of the oldest surviving cultures in the world. The indigenous inhabitants of the Australian continent had a long tradition of using plants as therapeutic agents in the treatment of health issues and cultural ceremonies.[91] They believed that disease resulted from sorcery or disruption of the spirit[92] (see Figure 1.9). Despite their apparent preoccupation with magic, they also made extensive use of herbal remedies and had a wide knowledge of medicinal plants. The colonization of Australia and the ensuing systematic Westernization caused much of their pharmacopoeia to be lost. But even into the 1960s, knowledge of more than 124 different plant species believed to have therapeutic qualities was retained by the Australian natives.[93] Of interest is that many of the traditional medicines used by the aborigines were used topically for local or systemic effects, and relatively few were orally ingested, while some were smoked as part of their traditional use.[94] They used herbal medicine that is now found to possess antimicrobial,[95] anti-inflammatory,[96] and analgesic properties[97] to treat diseases. Most obvious are the tea tree (*Melaleuca alternifolia*) and eucalyptus tree (*Eucalyptus sp.*), used for inflammation and respiratory diseases.[98]

Historical Overview of Traditional Medicine

Many medicinal herbs have been known to have various uses throughout human history and in all regions of the globe. Herbal medicines are used for the treatment of mild and chronic diseases and as adjunct therapy, to improve well-being and delay aging, or as healthy (functional) foods.[99] In addition to their therapeutic applications, herbs were and continue to be used as spices, preservatives, perfumes, and incense.[100]

Traditional medicine has a long history worldwide, especially in Asia. China and India are the origins of most documented traditional medicine, although the ancient civilizations of the Middle East have distinctive claims as well. As the trade deepened, medicine and herbs were brought to neighboring countries and combined with local treatments, gradually evolving into different traditional medicines. Even today, most Asian countries still use traditional herbs. The Greeks and Romans began the development of modern Western medicine, starting with the accumulated knowledge of herbal medicine obtained from the East. In Western countries, in the Dark Ages up until the Renaissance, natural medicines evolved from witchcraft or philosophy, which was enriched but also limited by alchemy and chemistry. In the modern age, as the actions and interactions of drugs on the molecular scale have become more understood, the roles of herbal medicine and traditional medicine in maintaining human health have become increasingly appreciated.

In modern society, traditional medicine still plays an important role in drug therapy. The discipline is continually being enhanced, improved, and modernized in clinical applications and by new technology. We are looking forward to a day in which traditional medicine is accepted all over the world and used to complement modern Western medicine.

References

1. Berin Shah, *Textbook of Pharmacognosy and Phytochemistry* (New Delhi: Elsevier, 2009).
2. Marcy J. Alunas and A. Douglas Kinghorn, "Drug Discovery from Medicinal Plants," *Life Sciences* 78, no. 5 (2005): 431–41.

3. Ranjit Roy Chaudhary and Uton Muchtar Rafei, *Traditional Medicine in Asia* (New Delhi: World Health Organization, 2001).
4. Paul M. Dewick, *Medicinal Natural Products: A Biosyntyhetic Approach* (Chichester, UK: John Wiley & Sons, 2002).
5. Ameenah Gurib-Fakim, "Medicinal Plants: Traditions of Yesterday and Drugs of Tomorrow," *Molecular Aspects of Medicine* 27, no. 1 (2006): 1–93.
6. J. Lietava, "Medicinal Plants in a Middle Paleolithic Grave Shanidar IV?" *Journal of Ethnopharmacology* 35, no. 3 (1992): 263–66.
7. Chaudhary and Rafei, "Traditional Medicine in Asia," World Health Organization (May 1, 2002).
8. Anna De Pasquale, "Pharmacognosy: The Oldest Modern Science," *Journal of Ethnopharmacology* 11, no. 1 (1984): 1–16.
9. Mohan Bikram Gewali, *Aspects of Traditional Medicines in Nepal* (Toyama, Japan: Institute of Natural Medicines, University of Toyama, 2008).
10. Gurib-Fakim, "Medicinal Plants," 1–93.
11. Vincenzina Krymow, *Healing Plants of the Bible: History Lore and Meditations* (Cincinnati, OH, US: Novalis, 2002).
12. Enrique García Jordá, "Sacred Herbs," *Clinical and Translational Oncology* 10, no. 11 (2008): 685–87.
13. F. Stickel and D. Schuppan, "Herbal Medicine in the Treatment of Liver Diseases," *Digestive and Liver Disease* 39, no 4 (2007): 293–304.
14. Luo Xiwen, *Introductory Study of Huangdi Neijing* (Beijing: China Press of Traditional Chinese Medicine, 2009).
15. Judy Xu and Yue Yang, "Traditional Chinese Medicine in the Chinese Health Care System," *Health Policy* 90, no. 2–3 (2009): 133–39.
16. Aiping Lu et al., "Theory of Traditional Chinese Medicine and Therapeutic Method of Diseases," *World Journal of Gastroenterology* 10, no. 13 (2004): 1854–56.
17. D. Kuang, "Agricultural Advance by Yandi Sennongshi and Hunan Ancient Rice Culture," *Agricultural Archeology* 1, no. 1 (2000): 129–41.
18. Si-Yuan Pan et al., "Historical Perspective of Traditional Indigenous Medical Practices: The Current Renaissance and Conservation of Herbal Resources," *Evidence-Based Complementary and Alternative Medicine* 2014 (2014): Article ID 525340.
19. Ke He, "Traditional Chinese and Thai Medicine in a Comparative Perspective," *Complementary Therapies in Medicine* 23, no. 6 (2015): 821–26.
20. Lida Teng et al., "Herbal Medicines: Challenges in the Modern World. Part 3. China and Japan," *Expert Review of Clinical Pharmacology* 9, no. 9 (2016): 1225–33.
21. Andrea T. Borchers et al., "Shosaiko-to and Other Kampo (Japanese Herbal) Medicines: A Review of Their Immunomodulatory Activities," *Journal of Ethnopharmacology* 73, no. 1–2 (2000): 1–13.

22. Shigenobu Kanba et al., "Use of Herbal Medicine for Treating Psychiatric Disorders in Japan," *Psychiatry and Clinical Neurosciences* 52, supp. (1998): S331–33.
23. T. Hakamatsuka, "Revision of Kampo Extra Formulae That Recorded in Japanese Pharmacopoeia and Standard Approval for OTC Kampo Products (in Japanese)", *Farumashia* 47 (2011): 413–17.
24. Kaichi Matsushita, "A History of Traditional Japanese Medicine (Kampo, Acupuncture and Moxibustion) in Chiba Prefecture," *Zen Nihon Shinkyu Gakkai Zasshi* 54, no. 4 (2004): 568–80.
25. Wu Boping, "Current Status and Regulations of Korean Herbs and Their Preparations," *Chinese Journal of Information on Traditional Chinese Medicine* 2 (1994): 12–15.
26. Wung-Seok Cha et al., "Historical Difference Between Traditional Korean Medicine and Traditional Chinese Medicine," *Neurological Research* 29, no. S1 (2007): S5–9.
27. K. L. Lee, "The Publication of Hyangyakjipseongbang and the Chosŏnization of the Chinese Medicine," *Uisahak* 20, no. 2 (2011): 225–62.
28. Chan Li, *Yixuerumen* (Tianjin: Tianjin Science and Technology Press, 2000).
29. Lee Je-ma, *Longevity and Life Preservation in Oriental Medicine* (Seoul: Kyung Hee University Press, 1996).
30. Han Chae et al., "An Alternative Way to Individualized Medicine: Psychological and Physical Traits of *Sasang* Typology," *Journal of Alternative and Complementary Medicine* 9, no. 4 (2003): 519–28.
31. Jae-Young Um et al., "Angiotensin Converting Enzyme Gene Polymorphism and Traditional Sasang Classification in Koreans with Cerebral Infarction," *Hereditas* 138, no. 3 (2003): 166–71.
32. Hyun-Ja Jeong et al., "Yangkyuk-Sanhwa-Tang Induces Changes in Serum Cytokines and Improves Outcome in Focal Stroke Patients," *Vascular Pharmacology* 39, no. 1–2 (2002): 63–68.
33. H. Y. Shin et al., "Regulatory Effect of Cytokine Production in Patients with Cerebral Infarction by Yulda-Hanso-Tang," *Immunopharmacology and Immunotoxicology* 22 (2000): 183–93.
34. Chandrashekaran Girish and Suresh Chandra Pradhan, "Indian Herbal Medicines in the Treatment of Liver Diseases: Problems and Promises," *Fundamental and Clinical Pharmacology* 26, no. 2 (2012): 180–89.
35. Yogini Jaiswal, Zhitao Liang, and Zhongzhen Zhao, "Botanical Drugs in Ayurveda and Traditional Chinese Medicine," *Journal of Ethnopharmacology* 194 (2016): 245–59.
36. Nithya J. Gogtay et al., "The Use and Safety of Non-Allopathic Indian Medicines," *Drug Safety* 25, no. 14 (2002): 1005–1019.
37. Pulok K. Mukherjee et al., "Development of Ayurveda - Tradition to Trend," *Journal of Ethnopharmacology* 197 (2017): 10–24.
38. Si-Yuan Pan et al., "Historical Perspective of Traditional Indigenous Medical Practices: The Current Renaissance and Conservation of Herbal Resources," *Evidence-Based Complementary and Alternative Medicine*, 2014, 525340. https://doi.org/10.1155/2014/525340.
39. "Rigveda," http://www.indianetzone.com/2/rig_veda.htm.

40. Charaka Samhita, *Agnivesha*, revised by Charaka and Dridhbala with Ayurveda Deepika commentary, by Chakrapanidatta, edited by Vd. Jadavaji Trikamaji Acharya (Varanasi: Chaukhambha Surabharati Publications, 2013).
41. R. K. Singh and M. K. Vyas, "Surgical Procedures in Sushruta Samhita," *International Journal of Research in Ayurveda & Pharmacy* 3, no. 5 (2012): 1444–50.
42. P. V. Prasad, "Atharvaveda and Its Materia Medica," *Bulletin of the Indian Institute of History of Medicine (Hyderabad)* 30, no. 2 (2000): 83–92.
43. S. Dev, "Ayurveda and Modern Drug Development," *Proceedings of the Indian National Science Academy A: Physical Sciences* 54 (1988): 12–42.
44. P. V. V. Prasad and A. Narayana, "Biography of Narahari—the Author of Raja-Nighantu," *Bulletin of the Indian Institute of History of Medicine (Hyderabad)* 37, no. 1 (2007): 1–8.
45. Yin-Yin Siew et al., "Ethnobotanical Survey of Usage of Fresh Medicinal Plants in Singapore," *Journal of Ethnopharmacology* 155, no. 3 (2014): 1450–66.
46. Suresh Kumar B. R. et al., "A Cross-Sectional Study on Knowledge and Attitude Toward Traditional Chinese Medicine (TCM) Among Adults in Selected Regions of Malaysia," *Journal of Complementary and Integrative Medicine* 12, no. 4 (2015): 317–23.
47. World Health Organization (WHO), *Legal Status of Traditional Medicine and Complementary/Alternative Medicine: A Worldwide Review* (Geneva: WHO, 2001), 160–63.
48. Theresa Hesketh and Wie Xing Zhu, "Health in China: Traditional Chinese Medicine: One Country, Two Systems," *BMJ* 315 (1997): 115–17.
49. World Health Organization, *Legal Status of Traditional Medicine and Complementary/Alternative Medicine.*
50. N. K. Ho, "Understanding Traditional Chinese Medicine—A Doctor's Viewpoint," *Singapore Medical Journal* 42, no. 10 (2001): 487–92.
51. Chee Hong Loh, "Use of Traditional Chinese Medicine in Singapore Children: Perceptions of Parents and Pediatricians," *Singapore Medical Journal* 50, no. 12 (2009): 1162–68.
52. Xu Dongying, "A Review of Traditional Medicine in Thailand," *School of Traditional Chinese Medicine* 9 (2003): 1597.
53. Visa Thongrakard et al., "Protection from UVB Toxicity in Human Keratinocytes by Thailand Native Herbs Extracts," *Photochemistry and Photobiology* 90, no. 1 (2014): 214–24.
54. Viggo Brun, "Traditional Thai Medicine," in *Medicine Across Cultures: History and Practice of Medicine in Non-Western Cultures*, ed. Helaine Selin and Hugh Shapiro (Dordrecht, Netherlands: Springer, 2003), 129.
55. Herman J. Woerdenbag et al., "Vietnamese Traditional Medicine from a Pharmacist's Perspective." *Expert Review of Clinical Pharmacology* 5, no. 4 (2012): 459–77.
56. T. N. Dung and Gerard Bodeker, "Tue Tinh: Founder of Vietnamese Traditional Medicine," *Journal of Alternative and Complementary Medicine* 7, no. 5 (2001): 401–403.

57. Elfahmi Yaman, Herman J. Woerdenbag, and Oliver Kayser, "Jamu: Indonesian Traditional Herbal Medicine Towards Rational Phytopharmacological Use," *Journal of Herbal Medicine* 4, no. 2 (2014): 51–73.
58. Shereen K. Ali et al., "In-Vitro Evaluation of Selected Egyptian Traditional Herbal Medicines for Treatment of Alzheimer Disease," *BMC Complementary and Alternative Medicine* 13, no. 1 (2013): 121.
59. N. H. Aboelsoud, "Herbal Culture in Ancient Egyptian Medicine," *Asia-Pacific Traditional Medicine* 12, no. 20 (2016): 1–2.
60. Richard Sullivan, "A Brief Journey into Medical Care and Disease in Ancient Egypt," *Journal of the Royal Society of Medicine* 88, no. 3 (1995): 141–45.
61. Bashar Saad, H. Azaizeh, and Omar Said, "Tradition and Perspectives of Arab Herbal Medicine: A Review," *Evidence-Based Complementary and Alternative Medicine* 2, no. 4 (2005): 475–79.
62. Enrique García Jordá, "Sacred Herbs," *Clinical and Translational Oncology* 10, no. 11 (2008): 685–87.
63. Si-Yuan Pan et al., "Historical Perspective of Traditional Indigenous Medical Practices: The Current Renaissance and Conservation of Herbal Resources," Evidence-Based Complementary and Alternative Medicine, 2014.
64. Oumeish Youssef Oumeish, "Traditional Arabic Medicine in Dermatology," *Clinics in Dermatology* 17, no. 1 (1999): 13–20.
65. Mojtaba Heyadri et al., "The Use of Chinese Herbal Drugs in Islamic Medicine," *Journal of Integrative Medicine* 13, no. 6 (2015): 363–37.
66. Kanwen Ma, "Overview of Ancient Greek Medicine," *Chinese Journal of Medical History* 10, no. 1 (1980): 27.
67. Guang Xu, "A Preliminary Study on the History of Ancient Greek Medicine," *Chinese Pharmaceutical Journal* 24, no. 8 (1989): 493.
68. Zhiqi Song, "Ancient Rome's Pharmacy and Its Contribution," *Chinese Journal of Medical History* 20, no. 2 (1990): 104.
69. Marco Leonti and Robert Verpoorte, "Traditional Mediterranean and European Herbal Medicines," *Journal of Ethnopharmacology* 199 (2017): 161–67.
70. Richard Scott Nokes, "The Several Compilers of Bald's *Leechbook*," *Anglo-Saxon England* 33 (2004): 51–76.
71. A. Tschirch, *Handbuch der Pharmakognosie* (Leipzig, Germany: Chr. Herm. Tauchnitz, 1910).
72. Liying Zhang and Nianqing Ding, "The History of Herbal Usage in UK and Its Implication to the Internalization of Chinese Herbal Medicine," *Chinese Journal of Management in Chinese Medicine* 26, no. 14 (2018): 1–4.
73. A. N. Shikov et al., "Medicinal Plants of the Russian Pharmacopoeia; Their History and Applications," *Journal of Ethnopharmacology* 154, no. 3 (2014): 481–536.

74. V. A. Solovieva, *Traditional Methods of Health Promotion* [Narodnye metody ukreplenija zdorovja] (St. Petersburg: Izdatel'skiy dom "Neva," 2005).
75. Mary Koithan and Cynthia Farrell, "Indigenous Native American Healing Traditions," *The Journal for Nurse Practitioners* 6, no. 6 (2010): 477–78.
76. James D. Adams and Cecilia Garcia, "Women's Health Among the Chumash," *Evidence-Based Complementary and Alternative Medicine* 3, no. 1 (2006): 125–31.
77. James D. Adams and Cecilia Garcia, "The Advantages of Traditional Chumash Healing," *Evidence-Based Complementary and Alternative Medicine* 2, no. 1 (2005): 19–23.
78. John K. Borchardt, "Native American Drug Therapy: United States and Canada," *Drug News and Perspectives* 16, no. 3 (2003): 187–91.
79. Andrea T. Borchers et al., "Inflammation and Native American Medicine: The Role of Botanicals," *American Journal of Clinical Nutrition* 72, no. 2 (2000): 339–47.
80. Yafan Yang Y and Shuangshuang Li, "Dandelion Extracts Protect Human Skin Fibroblasts from UVB Damage and Cellular Senescence," *Oxidative Medicine and Cellular Longevity* 2015, no 1. (2015): 1–10.
81. Wendy Torres-Avilez et al., "Medicinal Plant Knowledge in Caribbean Basin: A Comparative Study of Afrocaribbean, Amerindian and Mestizo Communities," *Journal of Ethnobiology and Ethnomedicine* 11, no. 1 (2015): 18.
82. Jerome S. Handler and JoAnn Jacoby, "Slave Medicine and Plant Use in Barbados," *Journal of the Barbados Museum and Historical Society* 41 (1993): 74–98.
83. L. C. Branch and M. F. Silva, "Folk Medicine in Alter do Chão, Pará Brasil," *Acta Amazonica* 13, no. 5–6 (1983): 737–97.
84. Thereza C. M. De Lima, Gina Struffaldi Morato, and Reinaldo Takahashi, "Evaluation of Antinociceptive Effect of *Petiveria alliacea* (Guiné) in Animals," *Memórias do Instituto Oswaldo Cruz* 86, no. S2 (1991): 153–58.
85. Eliana Rodrigues and E. A. Carlini, "Plants Used by a Quilombola Group in Brazil with Potential Central Nervous System Effects," *Phytotherapy Research* 18, no. 9 (2004): 748–53.
86. Eliana Rodrigues et al., "Preliminary Investigation of the Central Nervous System Effects of 'Tira-capeta' (Removing the Devil), a Cigarette Used by Some Quilombolas Living in Pantanal Wetlands of Brazil," *Phytotherapy Research* 22, no. 9 (2008): 1248–55.
87. Jeremy Hance, "Amazon Tribe Creates 500-Page Traditional Medicine Encyclopedia," *Mongabay*, June 24, 2015, news.mongabay.com/2015/06/amazon-tribe-creates-500-page-traditional-medicine-encyclopedia.
88. Ali Arazeem Abdullahi, "Trends and Challenges of Traditional Medicine in Africa," *African Journal of Traditional, Complementary and Alternative Medicines* 8, no. 5S (2011): 115–23.
89. Abdullahi, "Trends and Challenges of Traditional Medicine in Africa," 115–23.

90. Fawzi M. Mahomoodally, "Traditional Medicines in Africa: An Appraisal of Ten Potent African Medicinal Plants," *Evidence-Based Complementary and Alternative Medicine* 2013, no. 2 (2013): 617459.
91. Aaron C. Tan et al., "Towards the Discovery of Novel Phytochemicals for Disease Prevention from Native Australian Plants: An Ethnobotanical Approach," *Asia Pacific Journal of Clinical Nutrition* 19, no. 3 (2010): 330–34.
92. Kenneth Maddock, *The Australian Aborigines: A Portrait of Their Society* (London: Penguin Press, 1972).
93. R. Byard, "Traditional Medicine of Aboriginal Australia," *CMAJ* 139, no. 8 (1988): 792–94.
94. Joseph Tucci and Sabine Wilkens, "A Brief Review of the Application and Pharmacology of Ethnomedicines of Indigenous Australians," *Australian Journal of Rural Health* 24, no. 3 (2015): doi:10.1111/ajr.12256.
95. Enzo A. Palombo and Susan J. Semple, "Antibacterial Activity of Traditional Australian Medicinal Plants," *Journal of Ethnopharmacology* 77, no. 2–3 (2001): 151–57.
96. Rachel Li et al., "A Cross-Cultural Study: Anti-Inflammatory Activity of Australian and Chinese Plants," *Journal of Ethnopharmacology* 85, no. 1 (2003): 25–32.
97. R. N. Westhorpe and Christine Ball, "Pituri and Other Aboriginal Medicines for Pain Relief," *Anaesthesia and Intensive Care* 39, no. 1 (2011): 3.
98. Nicholas J. Sadgrove and Graham Lloyd Jones, "A Possible Role of Partially Pyrolysed Essential Oils in Australian Aboriginal Traditional Ceremonial and Medicinal Smoking Applications of Eremophila longifolia (R. Br.) F. Muell (Scrophulariaceae)," *Journal of Ethnopharmacology* 147, no. 3 (2013): 638–44.
99. Teng et al., "Herbal Medicines."
100. Robert A. Halberstein, "Medicinal Plants: Historical and Cross-Cultural Usage Patterns," *Annals of Epidemiology* 15, no. 9 (2005): 686–99.

Credits

Fig 1.7: Marco Leonti and Robert Verpoorte, Global Medicine, from "Traditional Mediterranean and European Herbal Medicines," Journal of Ethnopharmacology, vol. 199, no. 6. Copyright © 2017 by Elsevier.

Fig. 1.9: Roger Byard, Rock Painting of Ancestral Spirit, from "Traditional Medicine of Aboriginal Australia," CMAJ, vol. 139, no. 8, pp. 793, 1988.

Chapter 2

Global Use of Herbal Medicine

Current Status

Hui Ouyang, Qiaozhen Lu, and Bethany A. Reinecke

OVER THE PAST TWO DECADES, HERBAL medicine (HM) has become extremely popular worldwide. The number of people using HM is growing.[1][2][3] HM is a type of complementary and alternative medicine (CAM).[4] Most HMs are utilized in conjunction with conventional therapy rather than as a replacement.[5] CAMs containing medicinal plants are used to treat nonserious, minor medical conditions, to maintain good health, and to prevent illnesses.[6][7] According to a 2018 survey, about 5 percent of patients were reported to be using natural medicine.[8]

While the use of HM is common to all cultures, HM use in the last decade has shown regionally specific tendencies both between and within countries. China and Japan have significant integration of HM within their accepted medicinal practices.[9] Other nations and regions, including Australia, New Zealand, Russia, Canada, the United States, and the European Union, utilize HM in varying degrees to prevent disease development, improve health and well-being, or, rarely, as a replacement for ineffective conventional medicine.[10][11][12]

The Use of Herbal Medicine in Different World Regions

Asia

China

Since 1949, the Chinese government has emphasized the importance of incorporating traditional Chinese medicine (TCM) into the nation's health care programs alongside conventional medicine.[13] Nowadays, Chinese herbs have become an indivisible part of the Chinese culture under the efforts of thousands of traditional Chinese medical doctors. Regarded as part of a natural and healthy lifestyle, these herbs have been used for several purposes, not just for remedies:[14]

1. Herbs for medical use. In China, doctors often use both TCM and Western medicine in conjunction to treat patients.
2. Herbs in cosmetics and hygiene products. Many research institutions and Chinese factories utilize herbs to make therapeutic cosmetics and medicated cleanliness items (e.g., shampoo, toothpaste, and underwear).
3. Herbs in food. The use of herbs in food is not a new concept in Chinese culture. Chinese people frequently cook with herbs like *Codonopsis pilosula*, pepper, and so on. In addition, with the advancement of food processing technology, they have also been developed into commercialized food products for daily consumption. For example, they make a number of health teas and wines with hawthorn, yam, honeysuckle, Hippophaë, *Prunella vulgaris*, and red dates, among others.[15][16]

There are 12,694 kinds of traditional Chinese medicine in China, including 11,020 species of medicinal plants. Additionally, there are over 1,590 known species of medicinal products derived from animals and 84 species of medicinal minerals. The exportation of Chinese herbs to other countries and regions such as Japan, Taiwan, South Korea, India, Hong Kong, Germany, Holland, other European Union nations, and the United States is constantly increasing.[17][18] The most frequently exported herbs are ginseng (*Panax ginseng*), dang Shen (*Codonopsis pilosula*), Medlar (*Mespilus germanica*), and Sheng Di huang (*Rehmannia glutinosa*) (see Figure 2.1).

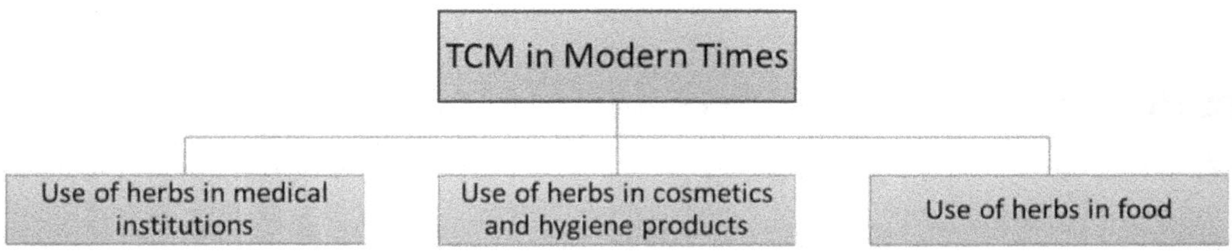

FIGURE 2.1 Common uses for traditional Chinese medicine (TCM) in modern times.

Source: Lida Teng et al., "Herbal Medicines: Challenges in the Modern World. Part 3. China and Japan," Expert Review of Clinical Pharmacology *9, no. 9 (2016): 1225–33.*

India

In modern Ayurvedic medicine, herbs are primarily utilized to treat different infirmities such as diabetes, diarrhea, fever, food poisoning, heartburn, intestinal parasites, sickness, and vomiting.[19][20][21][22][23][24] Nearly 25 percent of medications in present-day inventories are isolated from plants, while numerous others are engineered analogues of prototypical compounds separated from plants.[25]

Indian medicine has not only been used in India but has also been exported for use in other countries.[26][27]

Japan

There are two noteworthy kinds of HM available in Japan: crude drugs (*shoyaku*) and natural herbal preparations. Crude drugs originate from plant or animal parts and are utilized in making decoctions and homegrown preparations. The herbal preparations are usually prepared in a dry extract powder form and sold as over the counter (OTC) preparations. OTC drugs just require the direction of a pharmacist, while prescription medicines are prescribed by statutorily registered Western therapeutic specialists.[28]

In Japan, herbs are not only used in medical areas but are also made into dietary supplements and health foods. This means that the herbs must contain ingredients not merely listed on the "List of Raw Materials Exclusively Used as Pharmaceuticals."[29]

According to the national consumer survey, 54 percent of Japanese consumers have utilized prescription Kampo drugs.[30] Another national medical doctors survey observed that Kampo drugs are most usually prescribed for ailments such as muscle spasm (44.1%), acute upper respiratory tract aggravation (40.1%), constipation (38.5%), general discomfort and PMS (35.5%), and ileus (19.4%).[31]

Korea

There are about 4,500 types of medicinal plants in Korea, including 3,400 species, 762 varieties, and 287 subtypes. Of these, more than 2,000 are grown wild or artificially.

Traditional Korean medicine (TKM) is widely used in Korea. More than 20 percent of the Korean population uses TKM for health care purposes.[32] In addition, it was reported that about 30–40 percent of the Korean population had utilized complementary and alternative medicine (including TKM) within a five-year time frame.[33] The market for functional foods has had prosperous development within recent decades.[34] The most popular kind of herb in Korea is ginseng. For example, *Panax ginseng* can be used to treat *geonmang* (forgetfulness, amnesia, or poor memory).[35]

Singapore

In Singapore, many people choose to use locally developed medicinal herbs for health maintenance and therapeutic use, despite access to modern health care. Most people use herbs to treat ailments associated with the respiratory system, such as the common cold and flu. However, these conditions are for the most part self-limiting and do not require a lot of therapeutic intervention. In addition to treating minor illnesses, medicinal plants have also been utilized for the treatment of major illnesses such as neoplasm.[36]

Malaysia

In Malaysia, people spend more money on traditional and complementary medicine than on Western medicine.

Thailand

In Thailand, traditional medicinal plants are commonly utilized to treat basic ailments. However, there is concern that these traditions will be lost among the younger generations because of their changing lifestyle and lack of medicinal plant knowledge.[37]

Limited data has revealed that *L. ramiflora*, also known as *Chionanthus ramiflorus*, has been ethnopharmacologically used in a few countries, such as Papua New Guinea and Thailand, for treatment of malnutrition (bark and leaf), uterus infection (root), and cancer (stem).[38]

Vietnam

Today, Vietnamese traditional medicine (VTM) is well integrated into the lives of Vietnamese people, with both VTM and Western medicine playing a vital role in the health system. VTM is often used to treat common ailments such as fever, cough, indigestion, diarrhea, and adjuvant treatment for chronic diseases such as hepatitis and diabetes. Older people with chronic diseases use VTM more often. Others frequently use VTM to restore physical fitness postsurgery or postpregnancy. VTM is also regularly used as supplementary therapy to Western medicine. Some herbs can be used to make tea. These teas have antioxidant, anti-inflammatory, and antivirus effects, which can enhance the body's immunity. Herbal medicines are also available for health care, with more than 2,000 of the 10,000 drugs on the market made from herbs.

Indonesia

In Indonesia, a large national household survey showed that a large population still uses traditional medicine for self-medication.[39] In Indonesia, medicinal plants spanning 344 species, 217 genera, and 90 families are traded in the Kabanjahe market.[40]

Middle East

The Middle East also has a long history of herb usage. The first use of herbs goes back 60,000 years.[41]

Just as in the medieval era, several Islamic nations such as Iran, Turkey, and the UAE play an important role in the import of Chinese herbs to European nations.[42] Herbs that are utilized as spices are among the most regularly imported homegrown materials from China to these nations. These herbs include cinnamon, capsicum, nutmeg, ginger, and aniseed.[43][44][45] Herbs referred to in Islamic medicinal treatises as imported from China include *Asarum*, *Myristica fragrans*, *Cinnamomum cassia*, *Croton tiglium*, *Terminalia chebula*, *Cinnamomum camphora*, *Piper cubeba*, *Aquilaria sinensis*, *Santalum album*, and *Alpinia officinarum*.

Europe

United Kingdom

Britain is a paradise for Chinese medicine. The British House of Lords Science and Technology Committee gave a report that included complementary and alternative medicine. The report considered acupuncture, Western herbs, homeopathic therapy, and whole bone therapy as the first category. The Ministry of Health classified Chinese, Indian, and Western herbs together under the common name of herbal medicine. The UK herbal market is the third-largest herbal market in the EU, with a value at £10,000 of £100 million. The common herbal medicines in the UK include ginseng, garlic, food additives, and homeopathic drugs. People in the UK use herbal medicines as laxatives, treatments for colds and coughs, stomach medicines, and sedatives. As of June 2015, there were more than 3,000 Chinese medicine clinics and pharmacies in the UK, including towns and cities across the three Isles of England. In the London area alone, there were more than four million visits to the over 400 clinics and pharmacies, offering a conservative estimate of £58 million a year.[46]

A widely used natural herbal medicine, *Ginkgo biloba* (Gb) is commonly utilized to prevent and treat Alzheimer's disease (AD).[47]

Resveratrol (3,5,4′-trihydroxystilbene), a member of the polyphenolic compounds family, mostly seen in grapes, is very valuable in averting neurodegeneration in Alzheimer's disease due to its potent antioxidant activity.[48][49][50]

Green tea contains an amino acid compound called L-theanine ($C_7H_{14}N_2O_3$), which can enhance cognitive functions as well as facilitate relaxation and quality rest and improve emotional states.[51][52]

In recent years, the potential positive cognitive effects of flavanols, which are separated from *Theobroma cacao*, have been evidenced. It is thought that these flavanols directly act on the neurons and improve blood flow to the brain.[53][54]

Crocin ($C_{44}H_{64}O_{24}$), a primary ingredient in saffron, is known for its antidepressant and anti-inflammatory activities, which can essentially improve learning and memory.[55]

Below are a few botanicals and phytochemicals with well-known actions on the central nervous system (CNS) and clinically pertinent effects in modulating cognitive decline (see Table 2.1).

In addition, the application of traditional medicines in the treatment of hepatitis receives higher value in the UK (see Table 2.2). In traditional medication, the use of *Andrographis paniculate* (Burm.f.) Nees (Acanthaceae) in the cure of hepatitis is well established because of its main component, a diterpenoid lactone called andrographolide.[56]

Artemisia gmelinii Weber ex Stechm. (Asteraceae) is a perennial subshrubby plant that can be used as a remedy for chronic and acute hepatitis due to the potent hepatoprotective activity of its airy and dried flowering parts.[57][58] The existence of some key components responsible for hepatic protection,[59] such as esculetin, isofraxidin, chlorosacrorati,[60] 2,5-dihydroxycinnamic acid, O-hydroxycinnamic acid,[61] and scopoletin, show the protective activity

TABLE 2.1 Botanicals and Phytochemicals with Known Activity on the Central Nervous System in Modulating Cognitive Decline in Humans

Botanicals	Active Compounds	Beneficial Proprieties Involved in Cognitive Decline Modulating
Ginkgo biloba (EGb761)	Flavonol glycosides, proanthocyanidins, terpenoids	Neuroprotective and antiapoptotic properties
Vitis vinifera	Trans-resveratrol	Antioxidant activity and anti-inflammatory effects
Cammelia sinesis	Epigallocatechin-3-gallate, L-theanine	Antioxidant activity, anti-inflammatory activity, blood brain barrier crossing ability
Theobroma cacao	Cocoa flavanols	Antioxidant activity and neuroprotective propriety
Bacopa monnieri	Bacosides A and B, alkaloids, saponins	Anti-inflammatory, antioxidant, metal chelation, amyloid and cholinergic effects
Crocus sativus	Crocin	Antidepressant and anti-inflammatory effects, improves learning and memory
Curcuma longa	Curcumin	Antioxidant, anti-inflammatory and amyloid disaggregating activities

Source: Arrigo Francesco Giuseppe Cicero, Federica Fogacci, and Maciej Banach, "Botanicals and Phytochemicals Active on Cognitive Decline: The Clinical Evidence," Pharmacological Research *130 (2018): 204–12.*

TABLE 2.2 Herbal Formulations Commercially Used for Liver Complications

Sr #	Marketed Herbal Formulation	Plant Used in Formulation
1	Hefiaye	*Achillea millefoiliven L.*
2	Livex	*Aconitum heterophyllum Wall. ex. Royle*
3	Livin	*Acorus calamus L.*
4	Livol	*Justicia adhatoda L.*
5	Livodin	*Aloe vera (L.) Bum.f.*
6	Livomap	*Artemisia absinthium L.*
7	Jaundex syrup	*Calotropis gigantea (L.) Dryand.*
8	Amlycure	*Cassytha filiformis L.*
9	Livatona	*Glycyrrhiza glabra L.*
10	Hepatomed	*Cichorium intybus L., Eclipta prostrata (L.) L., and Solanum nigrum L.*
11	Hepa-10	*Andrographis paniculate (Burm.f.) Nees*
12	Triguliv	*Boerhavia diffusa L.*
13	Adliv	*Senna alexandrina Mill.*
14	Livarin	*Cassia fistula L.*
15	Acilvan	*Senna occidentalis (L.) Link*
16	Hepex	*Phyllanthus amarus Schumach. & Thonn.*
17	Livomycin	*Zingiber officinalis Roscoe*
18	Legalon	*Silybum marianum (L.) Gaertn.*
19	Vimlin	*Picrorhiza Kurroa Royle ex benth.*
20	Ginseng	*Ginkgo biloba L.*

Source: Bushra Sultana et al., "Escalation of Liver Malfunctioning: A Step Toward Herbal Awareness," Journal of Ethnopharmacology *216 (2018): 104–19.*

against hepatitis. In the herbal market, various commercial items produced from plants of this family, such as livomap from *A. gmelinii*, are prescribed to patients with liver issues.

Cynara cardunculus L. (Asteraceae), a perennial thistle that is well-known under the name artichoke, is commonly used in Southern Europe as a vegetable and herbal tea component. However, younger leaves and delicate artichokes are more popular for consumption. The plant is able to strengthen the functions of the liver and gall bladder due to its nutritional factors that aid in digestion.[62] The ingredients in artichoke are apigenin glycosides, naringenin, and luteolin-7-glucoside. Among them, naringenin possesses the most remarkable antihepatotoxic effects.[63]

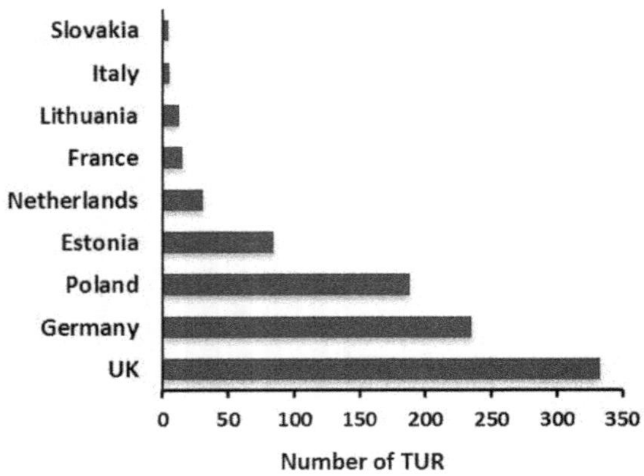

FIGURE 2.2 Number of granted traditional use registration (TUR) for traditional herbal medicinal products (THMP) in the EU since implementation of directive 2004/24/EC until December 31, 2014.

Source: Helen M. Sammons et al., "Herbal Medicines: Challenges in the Modern World. Part 2. European Union and Russia," Expert Review of Clinical Pharmacology *9, no. 8 (2016): 1117–27.*

Germany

Germany is the highest consumer of herbal medicine in Western Europe (see Figure 2.2), with more than 58 percent of Germans taking Chinese herbal medicine. Chinese herbs can be bought in any medicine store in Germany. The annual sales of *Ginkgo biloba* in Germany have exceeded $100 million. Antiasthmatic drugs made from licorice, pangolin, and Anemarrhena and youth vitality tablets made from garlic and rutin have reached annual sales of $100 million in EU countries. Since 1980, Germany has carried out more than 300 clinical studies with standardized botanicals containing garlic, ginkgo, valerian, Echinacea, kava, mistletoe, milk thistle, St. John's wort, and many others.

Valerian, a common European herbal medicine, accepted in the 17th century due to its slight sedative and tranquilizing effects, frequently appears in herbal prescriptions for sleep disorders. Essential oil components such as monoterpenes and sesquiterpenes provide its sedative properties with the clear mechanism of inhibition of the catabolism of gamma-amino butyric acid (GABA).[64]

German chamomile belongs to the daisy plant family, whose dried leaves have been used for enhancing sleep for centuries. The relaxing activity of the plant is supposedly due to chamomile's essential oil, and the mild sedative activity is due to the flavonoid apigenin, a ligand that binds to benzodiazepine receptors.[65]

The German Commission E monographs illustrate that lavender oil possesses the ability to relieve and prevent insomnia. The active compounds isolated from lavender oil have also been reported.[66]

France

Among all the western European countries giving importance to traditional Chinese medicine, France has the longest history. France believes that Chinese herbal medicine and the acupuncture-based treatment of diseases of traditional Chinese medicine are soft medicine.

St. John's wort is applied to relieve mild to minimal depression due to its antidepressant effect,[67] which can be explained by its flavonoid and phloroglucinol compounds.[68]

Corn Silk (*Stigma maydis*) is reported to have effects against ailments such as urinary tract infections (UTI), kidney stones, edema, prostate disorders, and other infections, along with enuresis and obesity.[69][70][71][72][73][74] Corn silk possesses a number of phenolic compounds, especially flavonoids,[75] and contains vitamins, proteins, carbohydrates, potassium, calcium, magnesium and sodium salts, volatile oils, and steroids such as stigmasterol, sitosterol, and alkaloids and saponins.[76] The rich flavonoid content accounts for its pharmacological effects.[77]

Russia

As indicated by the Market Analysis Report from the Canadian Markets Bureau on Health and Wellness Trends in Russia, the turnover of dietary supplements in Russia is nearly $1.2 billion, while the turnover of other various herbal items is evaluated to be $493 million.[78] The income from HM is not an independent revenue category but plays an important role in the pharmaceutical market as a whole, with volumes ranging from $1.2 billion to $1.5 billion.[79] It's reported that 14 percent of Russians frequently use herbal treatment, while 44 percent occasionally use it.[80]

Duckweed, a traditional Russian folk medicine used to treat vitiligo, is rich in iodine, bromide, and protein, which explain its potent anti-inflammatory, cholagogic, and slight analgesic effects.[81]

The number of complex glucosides, phytoncides, enzymes, vitamins (especially vitamin C), and the elements of magnesium and calcium in the leaves of Candelabra Aloe (*Aloe arborensis*) make it a potent antibacterial.

Onions have been utilized for the treatment of carbuncles and furuncles since ancient times. Aside from being 86-percent water, onions possess numerous phytoncides; vitamins B1, B2, B6, C, and E; biotin; carotene; folic acid; and microelements, thus accounting for their potent anti-inflammatory and antimicrobial properties.

The juice of viburnum berries, a rich, sugary fruit, contains vitamins K and C, saponins, pectins, and tannins, and is an effective anti-inflammatory and wound-healing drug. However, it is not safe at excess doses and may cause nausea and vomiting.

Marigolds (*Calendula officinalis*) are widely considered anti-inflammatory agents. Phytoncides, flavonoids, traces of alkaloids, proteins, glycoside, calendoside, triterpenoids (arnidol and faradiol), organic acids (hydroxysuccinic, pentadecanoic, and salicylic acids), essential oil, and ascorbic acid are the major active components in its flowery part.[82]

North America

America

More and more Americans, including the public and those in the medical profession, have begun to acknowledge the undeniable utility of TCM. Some of the most widely used traditional herbal medicines are listed here (see Table 2.3). There are more than 12,000 stores and health care providers in the United States that offer traditional Chinese medicine, with the turnover being an estimated $2 billion. The United States is one of the largest markets for Chinese natural medicine. In the United States, herbs are categorized as dietary supplements (see Table 2.4). This means the Federal Trade Commission (FTC) is responsible for herbal medicines rather than the US Food and Drug Administration (FDA).[83] Herbal supplements are under the control of some unique regulations due to their special status. In general, the United States approaches regulations from the standpoint that dietary supplements are safe until proven otherwise. The FDA and FTC supervise the manufacture, labeling, and marketing of dietary supplements that have reached the US market.[84]

TABLE 2.3 Herbs and Their Effects

Common Name	Uses
St John's Wort (*Hypericum perforatum*)	Treats mild to moderate depression, anxiety, nervous unrest, and dyspeptic complaints
Licorice (*Glycyrrhiza glabra*)	Demulcent. Expectorant. Treats stomach, mouth, and genital ulcers. Treats hypoglycemia and Addison's disease. Purifies the liver and blood. Has antiviral properties. May inhibit cancer, depression, and enzymes that cause tooth decay.
Ginkgo (*Ginkgo biloba*)	Improves blood flow to the brain. Reduces cellular lesions. Reduces edema in the retina. Antioxidant. Treats dementia. Inhibits platelet-activating factors.
Garlic (*Allium sutivum*)	Antibacterial. Lowers blood lipids. Inhibits platelet clumping. Enhances fibrolytic activity. Increases liver's ability to detoxify chemicals.
Ginseng (*Panax*)	Prevents the depletion of stress-fighting hormones. Enhances memory.
Kava Kava (*Piper methysticum*)	Controls nervous anxiety. Sedative. Muscle relaxant. Sleep-enhancing agent. Wound-healing agent.
Ephedra (*Ephedra sinica*)	Amphetamine-like actions.

Source: Cindy Brumley, "Herbs and the Perioperative Patient," AORN Journal *72, no. 5 (2000): 785–94.*

TABLE 2.4 Reported Trends in the Use of HM and Other Dietary Supplements

2001	2002	2007		2012	
Adults	**Adults**	**Adults**	**Children**	**Adults**	**Children**
Echinacea	Echinacea	Omega 3/ Essential Fatty Acid	Echinacea	Omega 3/ Essential Fatty Acid	Omega 3/ Essential Fatty Acid
Garlic	Ginseng	Glucosamine/ Chondroitin	Omega 3/ Essential Fatty Acid	Glucosamine/ Chondroitin	Melatonin
Ginkgo biloba	Ginkgo biloba	Echinacea	Combination Herb Pill	Pre-/Probiotics	Pre-/Probiotics
Saw palmetto	Garlic	Combination Herb Pill	Flaxseed Oil/ Pill	Melatonin	Echinacea
Ginseng	Glucosamine/ Chondroitin	Ginseng	Pre-/Probiotics	Coenzyme Q10	Glucosamine
Grape seed extract	St. John's Wort	Garlic Supplements	Goldenseal	Echinacea	Chondroitin
Green tea	Peppermint	Ginkgo biloba	Melatonin	Cranberry	Combination Herb Pill
St. John's Wort	Omega 3/ Essential Fatty Acid	Coenzyme Q10	Garlic	Garlic	Cranberry
Bilberry	Ginger	Saw Palmetto	Fiber/Psyllium	Ginseng	Garlic
Aloe	Soy	Cranberry	Cranberry	Ginkgo biloba	Ginseng

Source: Kathleen Job et al., "Herbal Medicines: Challenges in the Modern World. Part 4. Canada and United States," Expert Review of Clinical Pharmacology *9, no. 12 (2016): 1–13.*

Licorice (*Glycyrrhiza glabra* L.) is used to treat stomach, mouth, and genital ulcers. It also can treat hypoglycemia and Addison's disease.

Kava Kava (*Piper methysticum*) is used to control nervous anxiety. It is made into sedatives and muscle relaxants.

Hawthorn (*Crataegus*) is used for hypotensive effects and to dilate coronary arteries by potentially acting as a beta-blocker.[85]

Echinacea is a common herb that is used by patients suffering from cancer who are eager for "immune enhancing" effects.

Canada

Canada's characterization of Chinese herbal medicine products is consistent with that of EU countries, in that these products are included in the scope of "drugs" as "supplementary drugs" or "transmissible drugs." Natural health products are strictly regulated in Canada under a federal body (the Natural and Nonprescription Health Product Directorate), which is controlled with the minimum criteria for its manufacture and circulation.[84]

American ginseng (*Panax quinquefolius* L.), an herb mainly found in Northern America and Canada, is used as an antifatigue and an immunostimulant. It is reported that this herb has potent estrogenic,[86] antimutagenic,[87][88][89] and hypoglycemic[90][91][92] effects. Its memory-enhancing and learning-accelerating effects also have attracted wild attention. These effects may due to its principal ingredient, ginsenoside.[93]

Echinacea species possess a number of volatile terpenes, like polyacetylenes, germacrene D, highly unsaturated fatty acids, phenolic compounds, high molecular weight polysaccharides, and glycoproteins.[94] Today, it is primarily included in several supplements prescribed to treat immune system and respiratory disorders.[95]

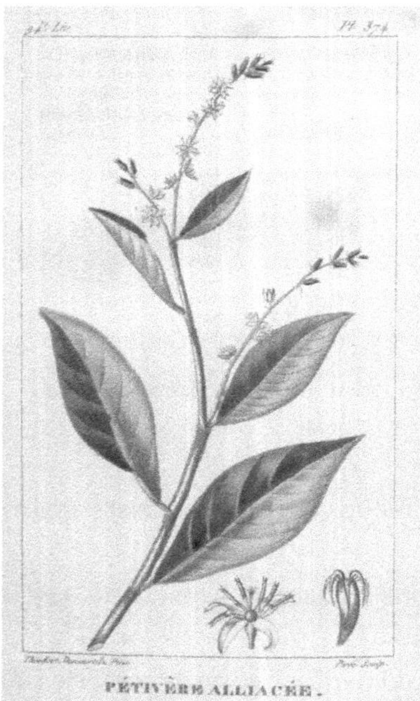

FIGURE 2.3 Principal anatomic structures of *Petiveria alliacea* L.

Source: Diandra Araújo Luz et al., "Ethnobotany, Phytochemistry and Neuropharmacological Effects of Petiveria alliacea L. (Phytolaccaceae): A Review," Journal of Ethnopharmacology *185 (2016): 182–201.*

Mexico

The Chinese herbal medicine market in Mexico is also expanding. In recent years, Gaofule, ginkgo extract powder, Baoqingchun oral liquid, Royal jelly series beauty products, and pollen series such as pollen Tianqi oral liquid and other Chinese herbal products have increased in popularity in Mexico.

Pharmacological research has found that *Petiveria alliacea* L. (see Figure 2.3) possesses antispasmodic, diuretic, analgesic, emmenagogic, anti-inflammatory, antimicrobial, anthelminthic, antileukemic, antirheumatic, and depurative properties.[96] Sulphur compounds, lipids, flavonoids, and triterpenes,[97] along with others isolated from the herb, may account for its multiple effects. It is used for the treatment of snakebites, pimples, emmenagogue, and skin diseases clinically.[98]

Oceania

Australia

Chinese herbal medicine has gradually become an important part of the Australian medicine market.[100] Australians typically utilize herbal medicines to maintain general health; however, they have also been employed to treat specific ailments both alone and in combination with conventional therapeutics.[101] A population study conducted in 2008 identified the 24 most commonly used HMs among the Australian community (see Table 2.5).[99][100][101]

TABLE 2.5 Most Commonly Used Herbal Medicines in Australia

1. Aloe vera	9. Ginseng	17. Milk thistle
2. Garlic	10. Ginkgo biloba	18. Dong quai
3. Green tea	11. Evening primrose	19. Black cohosh
4. Chamomile	12. Dandelion	20. Bilberry
5. Echinacea	13. Valerian	21. Senna
6. Ginger	14. Licorice	22. Hawthorn
7. Cranberry	15. St. John's wort	23. Saw palmetto
8. Peppermint	16. Slippery elm	24. Chasteberry (vitex)

Sources: Alastair H. MacLennan, Stephen P. Myers, and Anne W. Taylor, "The Continuing Use of Complementary and Alternative Medicine in South Australia: Costs and Beliefs in 2004," The Medical Journal of Australia *184, no. 1 (2006): 27–31; Tony Zhang et al., "A Population Survey on the Use of 24 Common Medicinal Herbs in Australia," Pharmacoepidemiology* and Drug Safety *17, no. 10 (2008): 1006–13; Y. Chen et al., "Review on the Development of Traditional Chinese Medicine in Australia: Review, Present Situation and Prospect,"* Chinese Journal of Integrated Traditional and Western Medicine *(2017): 607–11.*

Eryngium foetidum L. (see Figure 2.4), a traditional ethnomedicinal herb to treat earache, stomachache, fevers, burns, fits, hypertension, constipation, asthma, infertility complications, worms, snakebites, diarrhea, and malaria, is widely used by Aboriginal Australians.

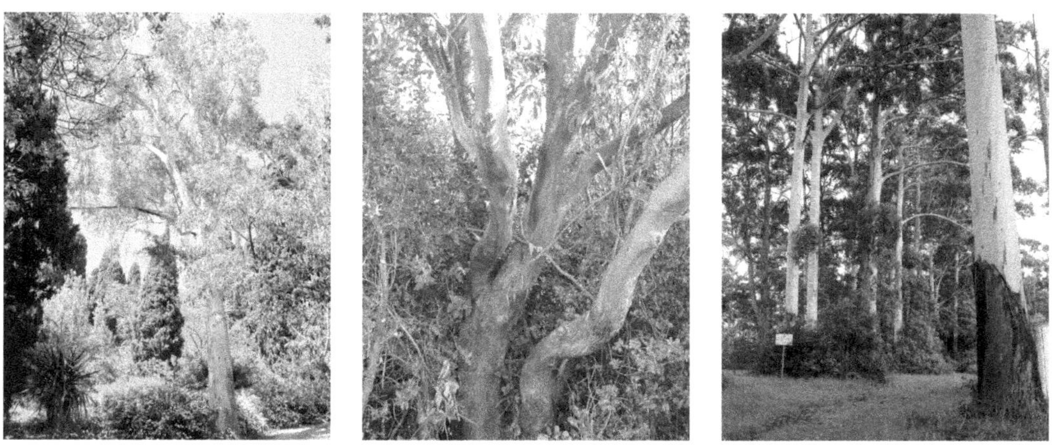

FIGURE 2.4 Selected common Eucalyptus species. (*Continued*)

Source: Q. V. Vuong, A. C. Chalmers, D. J. Bhuyan, M. C. Bowyer, & C. J. Scarlett, Botanical, phytochemical, and anticancer properties of the Eucalyptus species, Chemistry & Biodiversity *12, no. 6 (2015): 907–24.*

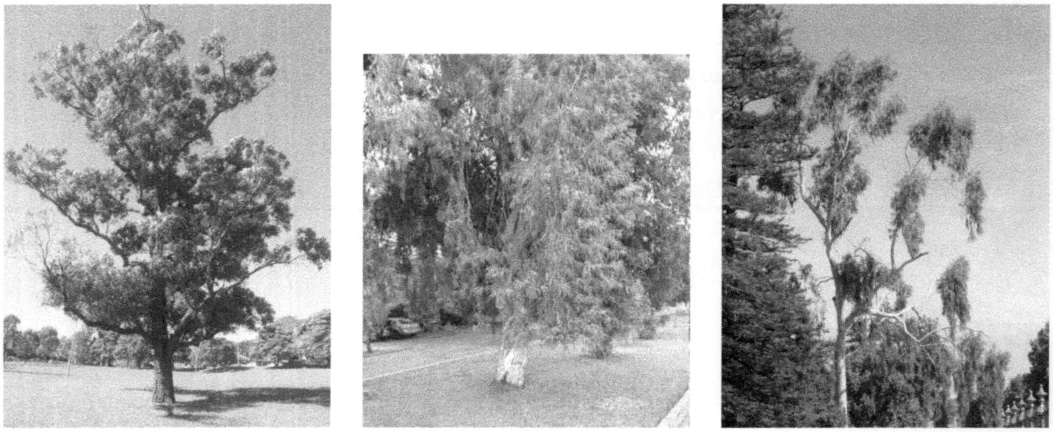

FIGURE 2.4 *(Continued)*.

Pharmacological research has found that the herb's components are tannins, flavonoids, a saponin, and various triterpenoids, while no alkaloids have been reported yet.[102]

Africa

In Africa, herbal medicine utilization is an optional or complementary type of treatment.[103] Local people use plant materials to make teas, like Honeybush (*Cyclopia intermedia* Vent, family Fabaceae), Rooibos tea (*Aspalathus linearis* [Brum.f] Dahlg., family Fabaceae), black tea (*Camellia sinensis* [L.] Kuntze, Fabaceae), and bush tea (*Athrixia phylicoides* DC, family Asteraceae). In Egypt, traditional herbal medicines have been described for use in various memory- and age-related diseases, such as Alzheimer's disease.[104]

The Expectation of Traditional Medicine

It's true that modern medicine currently dominates human health care. However, it cannot be denied that traditional medicine will certainly continue to be considered another vital source. Their "drug-like" properties guide us to explore their utility and bioactivity, as well as inspire the reinvestigation of previously used plants for therapeutic purposes. Although the fast development of modern medicine indeed limits the expansion of traditional medicine, we are still looking forward to the day that traditional medicine comes to life.

References

1. T. Smith et al., "Herbal Dietary Supplement Sales in US Increase 6.8% in 2014," *HerbalGram*, American Botanical Council (2015): 52–59. Article highlights continuous increase in US consumers' spending on HM.
2. World Health Organization. *WHO Traditional Medicine Strategy: 2014–2023* (Geneva: WHO, 2013). Available at http://apps.who.int/iris/bitstream/10665/92455/1/9789241506090_eng.pdf.
3. DSM Group, *Pharmaceutical Market in Russia* (Moscow: DSM Group, 2014). Available at http://www.dsm.ru/docs/analytics/spravka_may_2014.pdf (in Russian).
4. M. Nilsson, G. Trehn, and K. Asplund, "Use of Complementary and Alternative Medicine Remedies in Sweden. A Population-Based Longitudinal Study Within the Northern Sweden MONICA Project," *Journal of Internal Medicine* 250, no. 3 (2001): 225–33.
5. David M. Eisenberg et al., "Unconventional Medicine in the United States—Prevalence, Costs, and Patterns of Use," *New England Journal of Medicine* 328, no. 4 (1993): 246–52.
6. Eisenberg et al., "Unconventional Medicine in the United States."
7. Mary Ann Burg, Robert L. Hatch, and A. H. Neims, "Lifetime Use of Alternative Therapy: A Study of Florida Residents," *Southern Medical Journal* 91, no. 12 (1998): 1126–31.
8. Huiling Zhao, Yun Wu, and Xinyan Liu, "Development and Prospect of Traditional Chinese Medicine Culture in the United States," *World Chinese Medicine* 12 (2017): 436–39.
9. Lida Teng et al., "Herbal Medicines: Challenges in the Modern World. Part 3. China and Japan," *Expert Review of Clinical Pharmacology* 9, no. 9 (2016): 1225–33.
10. Kathleen Job et al., "Herbal Medicines: Challenges in the Modern World. Part 4. Canada and United States," *Expert Review of Clinical Pharmacology* 9, no. 12 (2016): 1–13.
11. Joanne Barnes et al., "Herbal Medicines: Challenges in the Modern World. Part 1. Australia and New Zealand," *Expert Review of Clinical Pharmacology* 9, no. 7 (2016): 905–15.
12. Helen M. Sammons et al., "Herbal Medicines: Challenges in the Modern World. Part 2. European Union and Russia," *Expert Review of Clinical Pharmacology* 9, no. 8 (2016): 1117–27.
13. Kelvin Chan, "Chinese Medicinal Materials and Their Interface with Western Medical Concepts," *Journal of Ethnopharmacology* 96, no. 1–2 (2005): 1–18.
14. Teng et al., "Herbal Medicines."
15. X. Liu and T.-F. Lin, "Application Progress on the Development of Functional Beverages with Medicinal Edible Chinese Herbs," *Journal of Anhui Agricultural Sciences* 43, no. 10 (2015): 81–86.
16. Y. Lin, J. K. Lin, and L. Wu, "Research Progress in Health Instant Tea in China (in Chinese)," *Journal of Guizhou Tea* 40, no. 2 (2012): 3–6.
17. Helmut Kaiser Consultancy, "Traditional Chinese Medicine," 2019. Available at http://www.hkc22.com/ChineseMedicine.

18. "2014 General Situation of Import and Export of Traditional Chinese Medicine Products," *Sina Finance*, April 24, 2015. Available at http://finance.sina.com.cn/money/future/20150424/095722036680.shtml
19. K. M. Nadkarni, *Indian Materia Medica*, 3rd ed. (Bombay: Popular Prakashan Publications, 1976).
20. Elizabeth M. Williamson, ed., *Major Herbs of Ayurveda* (London: Churchill-Livingstone, 2002).
21. Sushil Kumar Middha et al., "In Silico-Based Combinatorial Pharmacophore Modeling and Docking Studies of GSK-3β and GK Inhibitors of Hippophae," *Journal of Biosciences* 38, no. 4 (2013): 805–14.
22. Sushil Kumar Middha et al., "In Silico Exploration of Cyclooxygenase Inhibitory Activity of Natural Compounds Found in *Myrica nagi* Using LC–MS," *Symbiosis* 70 (2016): 169–78.
23. Usha Talambedu et al., "Rosmarinic Acid, a New Polyphenol from *Baccaurea ramiflora* Lour. Leaf: A Probable Compound for its Anti-Inflammatory Activity," *Antioxidants* 3, no. 4 (2014): 830–42.
24. Usha Talambedu et al., "Identification of Bioactive Glucose-Lowering Compounds of Methanolic Extract of *Hodgsonia heteroclita* Fruit Pulp," *Frontiers in Bioscience* 23, no. 3 (2018): 875–88.
25. K. G. Ramawat, "Secondary Metabolites in Nature," in *Biotechnology: Secondary Metabolites*, edited by K. G. Ramawat and J. M. Merillon (Enfield, CT: Science Publishers, 2007), 21.
26. Bhushan Patwardhan and Raghunath Anant Mashelkar, "Traditional Medicine-Inspired Approaches to Drug Discovery: Can Ayurveda Show the Way Forward?" *Drug Discovery Today* 14, no. 15–16 (2009): 804–11.
27. V. P. Kamboj, "Herbal Medicine," *Current Science* 78, no. 1(2000): 35–39.
28. Teng et al., "Herbal Medicines."
29. "List of Raw Materials Exclusively Used as Pharmaceuticals," 2019. Available at https://images-na.ssl-images-amazon.com/images/G/09/Restricted-Products/EN_iyakuhinlist_20190304FIX.pdf.
30. I. Arai and K. Sugiyama, "National Survey on the Views of Kampo Formulae for Prescription Use," *Journal of the Japan Society for Oriental Medicine* 59 (2008): 262.
31. Japan Kampo Medicines Manufacturers Association (JKMA). Available at http://www.nikkan-kyo.org/index.html
32. Changgi D. Hong, "Complementary and Alternative Medicine in Korea: Current Status and Future Prospects," *The Journal of Alternative and Complementary Medicine* 7, no. S1 (2001): S33–S40.
33. Victor Kuete et al., "Cytotoxicity and Pharmacogenomics of Medicinal Plants from Traditional Korean Medicine," *Evidence-Based Complementary and Alternative Medicine* 2013 (2013): 341724.
34. Hyunjin Park and Hyun-Sook Kim, "Korean Traditional Natural Herbs and Plants as Immune Enhancing, Antidiabetic, Chemopreventive, and Antioxidative Agents: A Narrative Review and Perspective," *Journal of Medicinal Food* 17, no. 1 (2014): 21–27.

35. Hemant Kumar et al., "Traditional Korean East Asian Medicines and Herbal Formulations for Cognitive Impairment," *Molecules* 18, no. 12 (2013): 14670–93.
36. Yin-Yin Siew et al., "Ethnobotanical Survey of Usage of Fresh Medicinal Plants in Singapore," *Journal of Ethnopharmacology* 155, no. 3 (2014): 1450–66.
37. Angkhana Inta, Paritat Trisonthi, and Chusie Trisonthi, "Analysis of Traditional Knowledge in Medicinal Plants Used by Yuan in Thailand," *Journal of Ethnopharmacology* 149, no. 1 (2013): 344–51.
38. Nguyen Thuy Duong et al., "Xanthine Oxidase Inhibitors from *Archidendron clypearia* (Jack.) I.C. Nielsen: Results from Systematic Screening of Vietnamese Medicinal Plants," *Asian Pacific Journal of Tropical Medicine* 10, no. 6 (2017): 549–56.
39. Supa Pengpid and Karl Peltzer, "Utilization of Traditional and Complementary Medicine in Indonesia: Results of a National Survey in 2014–15," *Complementary Therapies in Clinical Practice* 33 (2018): 156–63.
40. Marina Silalahi et al., The Local Knowledge of Medicinal Plants Trader and Diversity of Medicinal Plants in the Kabanjahe Traditional Market, North Sumatra, Indonesia," *Journal of Ethnopharmacology* 175 (2015): 432–43.
41. Solecki R. Shanidar IV, "A Neanderthal Flower Burial in Northern Iraq," *Science* 190 (1975): 880–81.
42. Saad Bashar, Azaizeh Hassan, Said Omar, "Tradition and Perspectives of Arab Herbal Medicine: A Review," *Evidence-Based Complementary and Alternative Medicine* 2, no. 4, (2005): 475–79. doi:10.1093/ecam/neh133.
43. Aus AID, *Trade Information Brief: Spices*.
44. N. Ashayeri et al., "The More Prevalent Medicinal Herbs which Have Been Purchased from Herbal Medicine Stores in Tehran, 2008," *Journal of Islamic and Iranian Traditional Medicine* 3, no. 4 (2013): 477–82.
45. Mojtaba Heydari et al., "The Use of Chinese Herbal Drugs in Islamic Medicine," *Journal of Integrative Medicine* 13, no. 6 (2015): 363–67.
46. Ru Su, Yan Chen, and Peng Sun, "Traditional Medicines Legislation Status of 7 European Participating Countries TC 249," *Chinese Journal of Traditional Chinese Medicine* 21 (2014): 1–4.
47. Arrigo Francesco Giuseppe Cicero, Federica Fogacci, and Maciej Banach, "Botanicals and Phytochemicals Active on Cognitive Decline: The Clinical Evidence," *Pharmacological Research* 130 (2018): 204–12.
48. Jiangli Shi et al., "The Comparative Analysis of the Potential Relationship Between Resveratrol and Stilbene Synthase Gene Family in the Development Stages of Grapes (Vitis quinquangularis and Vitis vinifera)," *Plant Physiology and Biochemistry* 74 (2014): 24–32.
49. Amirhossein Sahebkar et al., "Lack of Efficacy of Resveratrol on C-Reactive Protein and Selected Cardiovascular Risk Factors—Results from a Systematic Review and Meta-Analysis

of Randomized Controlled Trials," *International Journal of Cardiology* 189 (2015): 47–55. doi: 10.1016/j.ijcard.2015.04.008.

50. Jiyoung Kim, Hyong Joo Lee, and Ki Won Lee, "Naturally Occurring Phytochemicals for the Prevention of Alzheimer's Disease," *Journal of Neurochemistry* 112 (2010): 1415–30.
51. Sebastian Aguiar and Thomas Borowski, "Neuropharmacological Review of the Nootropic Herb *Bacopa monnieri*," *Rejuvenation Research* 16, no. 4 (2013): 313–26. doi: 10.1089/rej.2013.1431
52. Duygu Türközü and Nevin Şanlier, "Unique Aminoacid of Tea, and Its Metabolism, Health Effects, Safety," *Critical Reviews in Food Science and Nutrition* 57, no. 8 (2017): 1681–87. doi: 10.1080/10408398.2015.1016141
53. Davide Grassi, Claudio Ferri, and Giovambattista Desideri, "Brain Protection and Cognitive Function: Cocoa Flavonoids as Nutraceuticals," *Current Pharmaceutical Design* 22, no. 2 (2016): 145–51.
54. Astrid Nehlig, "The Neuroprotective Effects of Cocoa Flavanol and Its Influence on Cognitive Performance," *British Journal of Clinical Pharmacology* 75, no. 3 (2013): 716–27. doi: 10.1111/j.1365-2125.2012.04378.x.
55. Mathias Schmidt, Georges Betti, and Andreas Hensel, "Saffron in Phytotherapy: Pharmacology and Clinical Uses," *Wiener Medizinische Wochenschrift* 157, no. 13–14 (2007): 315–19.
56. Bushra Sultana et al., "Escalation of Liver Malfunctioning: A Step Toward Herbal Awareness," *Journal of Ethnopharmacology* 216 (2018): 104–19.
57. C. Y. Li et al., eds., *Northeast Herbaceous Flora*, vol. 9 (Shenyang, China: Shenyang Institute of Applied Economy, The Chinese Academy of Sciences, 2004).
58. G. C. Piao and Y. C. Quan, "Protective Effects of Extracts of *Artemisia sacrorum* Ledeb. on Acute Hepatic Injury" *Li Shizhen Medicine and Materia Medica Research* 18 (2007): 1646–47.
59. F. Y. Fan et al., "Research Advances on Chemical Constituents and Pharmacological Activities of *Artemisia sacrorum* Ledeb," *Li Shizhen Medicine and Materia Medica Research* 18 (2007): 1779–80.
60. D. Z. Zhang, "Studies on New Susquiterpenes in *Artemisia sacrorum* Ledeb," *Guangdong. Trace Elements. Science* 13 (2006): 59–63.
61. D. Z. Zhang, "Studies on Cinnamic Acids in *Artemisia sacrorum* Ledeb," *Journal of Jiangxi University of Traditional Chinese Medicine* 14 (2002): l5.
62. Qing Shen, Zhiyuan Dai, and Yanbin Lu, "Rapid Determination of Caffeoylquinic Acid Derivatives in *Cynara scolymus* L. by Ultra-Fast Liquid Chromatography/Tandem Mass Spectrometry Based on a Fused Core C18 Column," Journal of Separation Science 33, no. 20 (2010): 3152–58.
63. Florinda Fratianni et al., "Polyphenolic Composition in Different Parts of Some Cultivars of Globe Artichoke (*Cynara cardunculus* L. var. scolymus (L.) Fiori)," *Food Chemistry* 104, no. 3 (2007): 1282–86.
64. Peter John Houghton, "The Scientific Basis for the Reputed Activity of Valerian," *Journal of Pharmacy and Pharmacology* 51, no. 5 (1999): 505–512.

65. Jorge H. Medina et al., "Neuroactive Flavonoids: New Ligands for the Benzodiazepine Receptors," *Phytomedicine* 5 (1998): 235–43.
66. Keith I. Block, Charlotte Gyllenhaal, and Mark N. Mead, "Safety and Efficacy of Herbal Sedatives in Cancer Care," *Integrative Cancer Therapies* 3, no. 2 (2004): 128–48.
67. A. Bouron and Eric Lorrain, "Cellular and Molecular Effects of the Antidepressant Hyperforin on Brain Cells: Review of the Literature," *Encephale* 40, (2014): 108–113.
68. Daniel Jean, M. Pouligon, and A. C. Henriot, "Pharmacological Activity of Three Commercial *Hypericum perforatum* Preparations in Mice," *Phytotherapy Research* 20, no. 8 (2006): 653–54.
69. Qing-Lan Hu et al., "Purification and Anti-Fatigue Activity of Flavonoids from Corn Silk," *International Journal of Physical Sciences* 5, no. 4 (2010): 321–26.
70. J. W. Bastien, "Pharmacopeia of Qollahuaya Andeans," *Journal of Ethnopharmacology* 8 (1982): 97–111.
71. Armando Cáceres, Lydia M. Girón, and Ana M. Martinez, "Diuretic Activity of Plants Used for the Treatment of Urinary Ailments in Guatemala," *Journal of Ethnopharmacology* 19, no. 3 (1987): 233–45.
72. D. D. Dat et al., "Studies on the Individual and Combined Diuretics Effects of Four Vietnamese Traditional Herbal Remedies (*Zea mays*, *Imperatacylindrica*, *Plantago major* and *Orthosiphonstamineus*)," *Journal of Ethnopharmacology* 36, no. 3 (1992): 225–31.
73. F. Grases et al., "The Influence of *Zea mays* on Urinary Risk Factors for Kidney Stones in Rats," *Phytotherapy Research* 7, no. 2 (1993): 146–49.
74. Erdem Yesilada et al., "Traditional Medicine in Turkey. V. Folk Medicine in the Inner Taurus Mountains," *Journal of Ethnopharmacology* 46, no. 3 (1995): 133–52.
75. Jun Liu et al., "Supercritical Fluid Extraction of Flavonoids from *Maydis stigma* and Its Nitrite-Scavenging Ability," *Food Bioproducts Processing* 89, no. 4 (2011): 333–39.
76. Mohammad Ali Ebrahimzadeh, Fereshteh Pourmorad, and Samira Hafezi, "Antioxidant Activities of Iranian Corn Silk," *Turkish Journal of Biology* 32, no. 1 (2008): 43–49.
77. Khairunnisa Hasanudin, Puziah Hashim, and Shuhaimi Mustafa, "Corn Silk (Stigma maydis) in Healthcare: A Phytochemical and Pharmacological Review," *Molecules* 17, no. 8 (2012): 9697–715.
78. Editorial comments, "The Development Status and Prospect of Traditional Chinese Medicine in Russia," *World Journal of Integrated Traditional and Western Medicine* 6, no. 5 (2011): 445.
79. Sammons, "Herbal Medicines: Challenges in the Modern World. Part 2. European Union and Russia."
80. Our Journal, "History and Application of Medicinal Plants in the Russian Pharmacopoeia," *Asia-Pacific Traditional Medicine* 13, no. 3 (2017): 1–3.
81. V. I. Ivanov, "Remedies in Traditional Medicine" (Military Publishing House of the Ministry of Defense of the Russian Federation, 1992), 227–29.

82. Olga Y. Olisova et al., "Russian Traditional Medicine in Dermatology," *Clinics in Dermatology* 36, no. 3 (2018): 325–37.
83. Job, "Herbal Medicines."
84. Job, "Herbal Medicines."
85. Cindy Brumley, "Herbs and the Perioperative Patient," *AORN Journal* 72, no. 5 (2000): 785–94.
86. Rosemary B. Duda, "pS2 Expression Induced by American Ginseng in MCF-7 Breast Cancer Cells," *Annals of Surgical Oncology* 3 (1996): 515–20.
87. Duda, "pS2 Expression Induced by American Ginseng in MCF-7 Breast Cancer Cells."
88. Yasuo Fujimoto et al., "Cytotoxic Acetylenes from *Panax quinquefolium*," *Chemical and Pharmaceutical Bulletin* 39, no. 2 (1991): 521–23.
89. Yuan S. Chang et al., "Evaluation of the Mutagenic Potential of American Ginseng (*Panax quinquefolius*)," *Planta Medica* 4 (1986): 338–39.
90. Vladimir Vuksan et al., "American Ginseng (*Panax quinquefolius* L.) Attenuates Postprandial Glycemia in a Time-Dependent but Not Dose-Dependent Manner in Healthy Individuals," *American Journal of Clinical Nutrition* 73, no. 4 (2001): 753–58.
91. Vladimir Vuksan et al., "American Ginseng (Panax quinquefolius L.) Reduces Postprandial Glycemia in Nondiabetic Subjects and Subjects with Type 2 Diabetes Mellitus," *Archives of Internal Medicine* 160, no. 7 (2001): 1009–13.
92. Yoshitero Oshima, Kuniko Sato, and Hiroshi Hikino, "Isolation and Hypoglycemic Activity of Quinquefolans A, B, and C, Glycans of *Panax quinquefolium* Roots," *Journal of Natural Products* 50, no. 2 (1987): 188–90.
93. Valerie A. Assinewe et al., "Phytochemistry of Wild Populations of *Panax quinquefolius* L. (North American ginseng)," *Journal of Agricultural and Food Chemistry* 51, no. 16 (2003): 4549–53.
94. I. Mistrikova and S. Vaverkova, "Echinacea—Chemical Composition, Immunostimulatory Activities and Uses," *Thaiszia Journal of Botany* 16 (2006): 11–26.
95. Javad Sharifi-Rad et al., "Echinacea Plants as Antioxidant and Antibacterial Agents: From Traditional Medicine to Biotechnological Applications," *Phytotherapy Research* 32, no. 9 (2018): 1653–63.
96. M. R. Duarte and J. F. Lopes, "Leaf and Stem Morphoanatomy of *Petiveria alliacea*," *Fitoterapia* 76, no. 7–8 (2005): 599–607.
97. Paulo José Coelho Benevides et al., "Antifungal Polysulphides from *Petiveria alliacea* L.," *Phytochemistry* 57, no. 5 (2001): 743–47.
98. Diandra Araújo Luz et al., "Ethnobotany, Phytochemistry and Neuropharmacological Effects of *Petiveria alliacea* L. (Phytolaccaceae): A Review," *Journal of Ethnopharmacology* 185 (2016): 182–201.
99. Alastair H. MacLennan, Stephen P. Myers, and Anne W. Taylor, "The Continuing Use of Complementary and Alternative Medicine in South Australia: Costs and Beliefs in 2004," *The Medical Journal of Australia* 184, no. 1 (2006): 27–31.

100. Tony Zhang et al., "A Population Survey on the Use of 24 Common Medicinal Herbs in Australia," *Pharmacoepidemiology and Drug Safety* 17, no. 10 (2008): 1006–13.
101. Y. Chen et al., "Review on the Development of Traditional Chinese Medicine in Australia: Review, Present Situation and Prospect," *Chinese Journal of Integrated Traditional and Western Medicine* (2017): 607–11.
102. J. H. A. Paul, C. E. Seaforth, T. Tikasingh, "*Eryngium foetidum* L.: A Review," *Fitoterapia* 82, no. 3 (2011): 302–308.
103. Werner Cordier and Vanessa Steenkamp, "Drug Interactions in African Herbal Remedies," *Drug Metabolism and Drug Interactions* 26, no. 2 (2011): 53–63.
104. Shereen K. Ali et al., "In-Vitro Evaluation of Selected Egyptian Traditional Herbal Medicines for Treatment of Alzheimer Disease," *BMC Complementary and Alternative Medicine* 13, no. 1 (2013): 121.

Credits

Fig. 2.1: Lida Teng, et al., "TCM in Modern Time," Herbal Medicines: Challenges in the Modern World. Part 3. China and Japan., Expert Review of Clinical Pharmacology, vol. 9, no. 9. Copyright © 2016 by Taylor & Francis.
Fig. 2.2: Helen M. Sammons, et al., "Number of granted Traditional Use Registration (TUR) for Traditional Herbal Medicinal Products (THMP) in EU since the implementation of Directive 2004/24/EC until December 31, 2014," Herbal Medicines: Challenges in the Modern World. Part 3. China and Japan., Expert Review of Clinical Pharmacology, vol. 9, no. 8. Copyright © 2016 by Taylor & Francis.
Fig 2.3: Source: https://commons.wikimedia.org/wiki/File:Flore_m%C3%A9dicale_des_Antilles,_ou,_Trait%C3%A9_des_plantes_usuelles_(Pl._374)_(7795752696).jpg.
Fig 2.4a: Source: https://commons.wikimedia.org/wiki/File:Eucalyptus_camaldulensis_(villa_Hanbury,_Italy).jpg.
Fig 2.4b: Copyright © 2006 by Auckland Museum, (CC BY 4.0) at https://commons.wikimedia.org/wiki/File:Eucalyptus_saligna_J.Sm._(AM_AK298016-1).jpg.
Fig 2.4c: Copyright © 2010 by Tatiana Gerus, (CC BY 2.0) at https://commons.wikimedia.org/wiki/File:Eucalyptus_grandis_2.jpg.
Fig 2.4d: Copyright © 2012 by Casliber, (CC BY-SA 3.0) at https://commons.wikimedia.org/wiki/File:Eucalyptus_robusta_robson2.jpg.
Fig 2.4e: Source: https://commons.wikimedia.org/wiki/File:E._Globulus.png.
Fig 2.4f: Copyright © 2005 by Manuel Anastácio, (CC BY 2.0) at https://commons.wikimedia.org/wiki/File:EUCALYPTUS_CITRIODORA.jpg.

Part II

Herbal Medications

Chapter 3

Dietary Supplements

Scope, Regulation, and Evidence

Lisa B. Phipps

What Is a Dietary Supplement?

Before we can understand how dietary supplements are regulated, we must first understand the scope of products this category contains. As defined in the Dietary Supplement Health and Education Act of 1994 (DSHEA),[1] a dietary supplement is a product (other than tobacco) that

- is intended to supplement the diet;
- contains one or more of the following dietary ingredients: vitamins, minerals, herbs or other botanicals, amino acids, or other dietary substances for use by man to supplement the diet, or their constituents, metabolites, extracts, or a combination thereof;
- is intended to be taken by mouth as a pill, capsule, tablet, or liquid; and
- is labeled on the front panel as being a dietary supplement.

In taking a closer look at this definition, we find that dietary supplements encompass a broad scope of potential substances and products, including the following categories.

Vitamins

Vitamins are organic compounds that are required by plants and animals in small amounts for healthy functioning. While they do not directly provide energy to the body or serve as building blocks for other compounds (e.g., amino acids), they support biochemical processes in the organism that do so, often serving as coenzymes or precursors thereof. The 13 vitamins essential for humans are A, B1 (thiamine), B2 (riboflavin), B3 (niacin), B5 (pantothenic acid), B6 (pyridoxine), B7 (biotin), B9 (folic acid), B12 (cyanocobalamin), C, D, E, and K.

Minerals

Minerals are inorganic compounds or elements that support enzymatic processes in the body, as well as having some direct actions. Functions involving minerals include acid-base balance, constriction and relaxation of blood vessels, nerve cell firing, and bone formation, among others. Minerals such as iron and zinc are needed in much smaller quantities than minerals such as calcium, sodium, and potassium and are thus termed "trace minerals."

The Food and Nutrition Board of the National Academies of Science, Engineering, and Medicine, together with input from the Department of Agriculture, put out the Dietary Reference Intake (DRI) values for vitamins and minerals. DRI values include Recommended Daily Allowances (RDAs) and/or Adequate Intakes (AIs), depending on the quantity and quality of evidence available for a given nutrient. In addition to how much we should be taking in, Tolerable Upper Intake Levels (ULs) are determined. The UL is the greatest amount of a nutrient that someone in the general population can consume with a very low likelihood of posing a risk to their health. It is important to note that these levels may be different for special populations such as children, pregnant women, and those with altered kidney or liver function. With the advent of things like hypervitamin therapy and people consuming acutely high doses of vitamins, minerals, and other substances to try to stave off colds and flu, for example, gathering data on tolerable upper levels is of increasing importance. Fat soluble vitamins and some minerals can cause various problems when taken in very large amounts, especially for long periods of time. DRIs and ULs for selected vitamins and minerals are shown in Table 3.1. The information shown was adapted from several tables and encompasses both males and females in age groups from nine to less than 70 years of age and does not include recommendations in pregnancy and lactation.[2][3][4][5] The most complete and up to date information about DRIs and ULs for vitamins and minerals can generally be found online from various sources, such as the Food and Drug Administration (FDA), National Institutes of Health Office of Dietary Supplements (NIH ODS), and the Health and Medicine Division of the National Academies of Science, Engineering, and Medicine (NASEM).

TABLE 3.1 Dietary Reference Intake and Tolerable Upper Intake Level for Selected Vitamins and Minerals[2][3][4][5]

Nutrient	DRI (Either an RDA or an AI)	UL
Vitamin A	700–900 micrograms/day	2,800–3,000 micrograms/day
Vitamin D	15–20 micrograms/day (600–800 IU/day)	100 micrograms/day (4,000 IU/day)
Iron	8–18 mg/day	45 mg/day
Sodium	1.2–1.5 g/day	2.3 g/day

Tolerable Upper Intake Levels for some substances, such as vitamin K, thiamin, riboflavin, pantothenic acid, biotin, and cyanocobalamin, are unavailable because of a lack of sufficient data.[4][5]

Herbs or Other Botanicals

Extracts and/or parts of plants, fungi, and algae are often marketed as dietary supplements. Their use is often rooted in herbalist traditions from medicine systems like Ayurveda and traditional Chinese medicine. It is not uncommon for people to believe that herbal products are completely safe because they are "natural"; however, it is important to remember that compounds in botanical products may have effects, adverse effects, and interactions with medications or disease states. One of the most well-characterized examples of this is the induction of the enzyme cytochrome P450 3A4 by St. John's wort.[6][7][8] Induction of an enzyme can result in other medications using the same pathway to be metabolized or broken down more quickly than usual, making them less effective. Care should be taken when recommending or using any herbal product, particularly when other medications and disease states are at play.

Amino Acids

Amino acids are the building blocks of protein and can be found separately or in combination with other amino acids or proteins. They are most often used by those seeking to either gain muscle (bodybuilders and other athletes) or maintain muscle while losing weight and may be used as part of a high protein and/or low carbohydrate diet. Sources of amino acid and protein supplements may include whey, soy, casein, hemp, pea, and rice, among others. While proteins and amino acids are often discussed together and may both be present in dietary supplements, it should be noted that manufacturers may not claim protein on their product labels if their supplement contains only amino acids.[9]

Other Substances

Other substances that may be classified as dietary supplements include fatty acids, probiotics, and substances from animal sources. Omega-3 and Omega-6 fatty acids may come from seed, nut, fish, and algae extracts. A few other supplements that may come from both animal and nonanimal sources are listed in Table 3.2.[10][11] This is an important consideration for those with allergies or other dietary restrictions, such as vegetarians or those who do not consume pork products, for example.

Often termed "good bacteria," probiotic products contain bacteria and yeast of various species and concentrations. Some of these are classified as dietary supplements, and some

TABLE 3.2 Commonly Used Supplements Often Derived from Animal Sources

Supplement	Animal Sources	Nonanimal Sources
Glucosamine	Shellfish	Corn fermentation, *Aspergillus niger*
Chondroitin	Shark, pig, cattle	Fermentation processes (Mythocondro and Phytodroiton)*
Collagen	Cattle, pig, poultry, fish	None; vegetarian options are marketed as "collagen builders" or "collagen boosters" and may contain silica (for topical use) or a combination of plant-derived amino acids
Hyaluronic acid	Rooster combs	Various bacteria species

***Note: These two products, released in 2013 and 2016, respectively, do not have exactly the same structure as chondroitin, so they are not actually plant sources of the identical compound.**

are regulated as medical foods. Medical foods are regulated and labeled differently from dietary supplements and are intended to be used under the supervision of a physician.

Box 3.1

Dietary supplements may contain the following:

- Vitamins
- Minerals
- Herbs/Botanicals
- Amino Acids/Proteins
- Other Substances (Probiotics, Fatty Acids, etc.)

Dietary supplements are intended only to add to the diet and augment nutritional benefits from the food supply; however, their use for increasing wellness and health has blurred the lines between being food and being used for therapeutic purposes. In the next section, we will explore the history and legislation surrounding these special products.

Do We Regulate Dietary Supplements?

A common myth about dietary supplements is that they are not regulated or that the manufacturing and marketing of them has no oversight whatsoever. Conventional foods, dietary supplements, and medications are all regulated by the FDA, but they have different guidelines and legislation governing them. Oftentimes, the classification of a product as a food, dietary supplement, or medication is largely based on its intended use. Some pieces of legislation address more than one of these categories, and others are specific to one type of product. Some provide definitions to help clarify when something should be classified as a food, a dietary supplement, a medication, or a medical device. Let's dive into some of the history and legislation most relevant to how dietary supplements came to be regulated as they are today.

Early 1900s

In 1906 and 1907, significant advances in regulation and consumer protection efforts were made with the Pure Food and Drug Act, the creation of the Board of Food and Drug Inspection, and the creation of the Food, Drug, and Insecticide Administration (FDIA), which would later be renamed the FDA.[12] This is where a drug was defined as a substance used to cure, mitigate, or prevent a disease. Foods were not required at this time to have nutrition labels but were required to declare if they contained one or more of 11 specific substances that were considered to be dangerous; among them were alcohol, morphine, opium, cocaine, and cannabis.

1938–1941

The more comprehensive Federal Food, Drug, and Cosmetic Act of 1938, which was spurred on by more than 100 deaths related to a new sulfanilamide preparation containing diethylene glycol, gave the FDA the authority to oversee the safety of food, drugs, cosmetics, and medical devices used in the United States.[13] Prohibited acts were spelled out, and misbranded and adulterated drugs, cosmetics, and medical devices were defined. One aspect of this law that holds interesting for the history of dietary supplements was a redefining of a drug to be an "article (other than food) intended to affect the structure or any function of the body of man or other animals."[14] Additionally, a food was considered misbranded if it "purports to be or is represented for special dietary uses." Given the scientific knowledge and technology of the time, it was acknowledged that certain populations and disease states had different dietary requirements, though they were not well characterized. As vitamins were also being discovered and isolated at this time and marketed for health benefits, one can see how the matter of dietary supplements became complicated. At that point, and still to some effect today, the intention of the words played an important part in whether a substance was classified as a food, a drug, or a dietary supplement.

In 1940 and 1941, two FDA rules came into effect that dealt primarily with special dietary requirements, such as preventing deficiency of nutrients. These rules established minimum daily requirements of certain vitamins and minerals and required that the supplements be labeled with the relative amounts of the nutrients they contained. These and other dietary supplements were required to include on their labels the quantity of each substance present, directions for use, and a statement that the need for supplementing the substances had not been established.[15][16]

1990s–2006: NLEA, DSHEA, and MedWatch

Next, the Nutrition Labeling and Education Act of 1990 (NLEA) gave the FDA the authority to require that most foods and dietary supplements contain nutrient labeling.[17] It established requirements for nutrient claims, such as stating that something is "high in" or "a good source of" a particular nutrient. Any health claims made by foods or dietary supplements were subject to FDA regulations. We will further explore details of current label requirements for dietary supplements in another section of this chapter.

Perhaps the single most important piece of legislation surrounding the regulation of dietary supplements came about in October 1994, with the signing into law of the Dietary Supplement Health and Education Act (DSHEA).[18] The DSHEA provided us with a legal definition of a dietary supplement and showed the broad scope of substances classified as dietary supplements, as was discussed in the first section of this chapter. Additionally, it established the Office of Dietary Supplements within the National Institutes of Health, whose mission is to support, coordinate, and evaluate research on dietary supplements, disseminate research results, and educate the public on issues related to dietary supplements.[19] The DSHEA requires that manufacturers meet standards of good manufacturing practices (GMPs) equivalent to those for foods, and this rule was finalized for dietary supplements in 2007. GMPs are a system of checks and balances for manufacturers to ensure proper quality control and consistency in all aspects of dietary supplement manufacture, including raw materials, personnel, facilities management, and content and purity testing of products; this is discussed in more detail in another chapter. Finally, the DSHEA created the Commission on Dietary Supplement Labels, which put forth a report establishing label requirements for supplement facts panels and nutrient content, as well as defining claims that can and cannot be made by dietary supplement manufacturers.[20] These label requirements will be discussed in more detail later in this chapter.

Box 3.2 Important Point

The DSHEA is the most important piece of legislation surrounding the regulation of dietary supplements in the United States.

One of the major differences between regulations for dietary supplements and regulations for medications is the burden of the manufacturer in proving safety and efficacy, which is required for FDA-approved medications before they reach the market but not for dietary supplements. In 1993, a voluntary adverse event reporting system called MedWatch was rolled out to allow health care providers and manufacturers the ability to report adverse events to the FDA. The FDA could then keep track of these occurrences and determine if there was cause for reevaluation of the safety of a product on the market based on frequency and causal relationship investigations. MedWatch collects data for all FDA-regulated products, including medications, medical foods, devices, cosmetics, and infant formulas, as well as dietary supplements. In 2006, the Dietary Supplement and Nonprescription Drug Consumer Protection Act required reporting of serious adverse events associated with dietary supplements and over-the-counter medications through the MedWatch system.[21] Serious adverse events are those that result in death, inpatient hospitalization, a life-threatening experience, persistent or significant disability or incapacity, a congenital anomaly or birth defect, or require medical or surgical intervention. Informing consumers and their health care providers with point-of-sale information in the form of bottle labeling requirements is an important step in helping to prevent these adverse events from occurring.

What Do Labeling Requirements Entail?

As previously stated, the NLEA and DSHEA provided the FDA with the authority to set forth labeling requirements and definitions guiding those requirements. In May 2016, updated requirements for the Supplement Facts panel (the nutrition label for dietary supplements) were put into effect. These recommendations were based on the latest scientific information about the link between diet and chronic disease states, common nutrient deficiencies, and ease of information available to the consumer.[22] The Supplement Facts panel is just one of the required items on a label. Manufacturers have until January 1, 2020 or 2021, depending on their average annual sales, to comply with new labeling requirements. As of the writing of this chapter, a label on a dietary supplement must contain the following:

1. The name of the supplement.
2. A statement indicating that it is a dietary supplement.
3. The net quantity of the contents.
4. The updated Supplement Facts panel, which includes the following:
    a. Serving size and servings per container (note: serving size may be in capsules, tablets, etc., depending on the formulation of the product).
    b. Calories per serving.
    c. Total fat, saturated fat, and trans-fat content and Percent of Daily Value (%DV).

d. Cholesterol content and %DV.
e. Sodium content and %DV.
f. Carbohydrate content and %DV:
    i. Fiber content and %DV.
    ii. Total sugars and %DV.
    iii. Added sugars and %DV.
g. Protein content and %DV.
h. List of nutrients (currently required nutrients include Vitamin D, calcium, iron, and potassium) with content and %DV.
i. Explanation of %DV: The Percent of Daily Value (%DV) tells you how much a nutrient in a serving of food contributes to a daily diet; usually, 2,000 calories a day is used for general nutrition advice.

5. The complete ingredient list by their common names, in descending order by weight.
6. The name and address of the manufacturer, packer, or distributor.
7. The part of the plant used if it is an herb or botanical product. If the supplement contains a proprietary blend, the net weight of the blend must be included in addition to the list of ingredients in descending order by weight.
8. Safety information and directions for use.
9. Disclaimer statements, such as the following:
    a. This statement has not been evaluated by the FDA.
    b. This product is not intended to diagnose, treat, cure, mitigate, or prevent any disease.

As previously stated, GMPs have been put into place in order to help ensure quality and purity of products. While manufacturers are required to do some internal quality assurance and quality control, some manufacturers put their products through outside quality testing. This can offer an additional seal of approval that a product contains what the label claims to, in the correct amounts, and does not contain contaminants or other impurities. Four of the most commonly used organizations offering outside testing for dietary supplements are the US Pharmacopeia, NSF International, ConsumerLab.com, and Informed Choice. These organizations offer testing for raw ingredients, finished products, and/or site inspections. It is important to know what these seals of approval tell us and what they do not. They may tell us that the manufacturer's facilities, procedures, raw materials, and/or finished products meet certain standards; however,

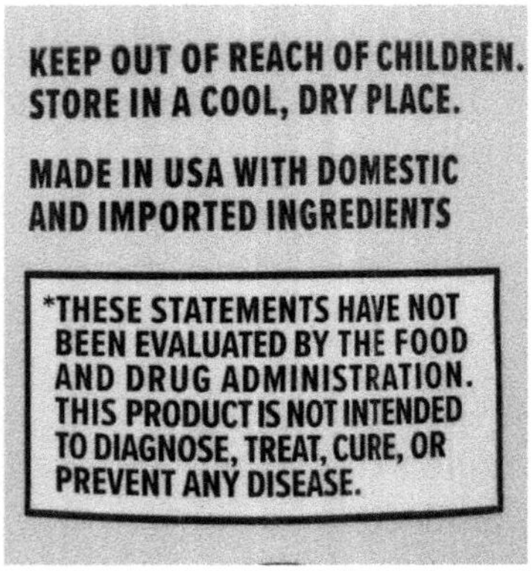

FIGURE 3.1

they do not provide us with any information about efficacy or effectiveness of the product. Figures 3.2 and 3.3 show examples of stamps from NSF and Informed Choice. As you can see in the figures, the manufacturer indicates for what aspect they used the third-party testing. The manufacturer who used Informed Choice for the determination that their product is "clean, tested, and trusted for sport," which implies that it does not contain any of the currently banned substances for competing athletes, also had an NSF gluten-free stamp on the same product.

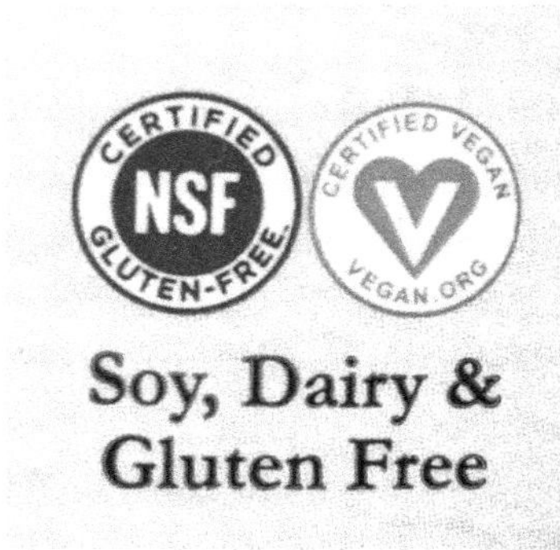

FIGURE 3.2

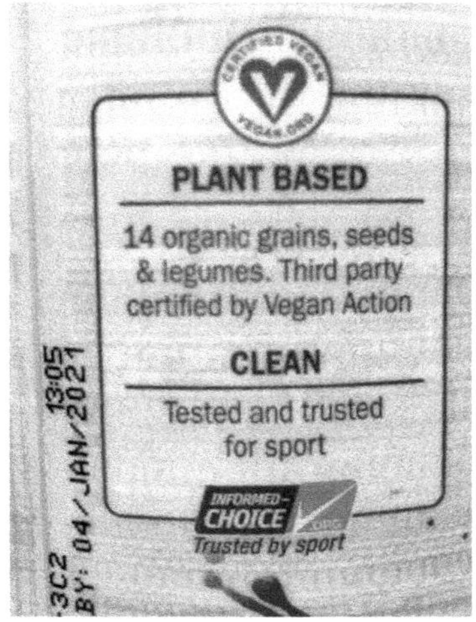

FIGURE 3.3

What Can Manufacturers Say About Their Products?

While dietary supplement manufacturers must have a disclaimer that their product is not intended to diagnose, treat, mitigate, cure, or prevent a disease, there are three types of claims that can be made: nutrient content claims, structure/function claims, and health claims.[23]

Nutrient content claims characterize how much of a nutrient a product contains in relative terms. A product may want to claim it is a "good" source of a nutrient or is "high" or "low" in a particular nutrient. The FDA provides requirements a manufacturer must meet in order to make these claims. For example, a product containing 10–19 percent of the %DV of a nutrient may say that it is a "good source" of that nutrient; if it were to contain 20 percent or more of the %DV, the product could claim it is "high in" that nutrient.[24]

A structure/function claim describes how a nutrient affects a particular organ or system but cannot make any mention of a specific disease. For example, a general claim stating that a product "supports bone and joint health" would be a structure/function claim; however, statements that mention decreasing the risk of osteoporosis or even "supporting those with osteoarthritis" would not be categorized as structure/function claims. Note that the claims in Figure 3.4, from a supplement label, do not specifically

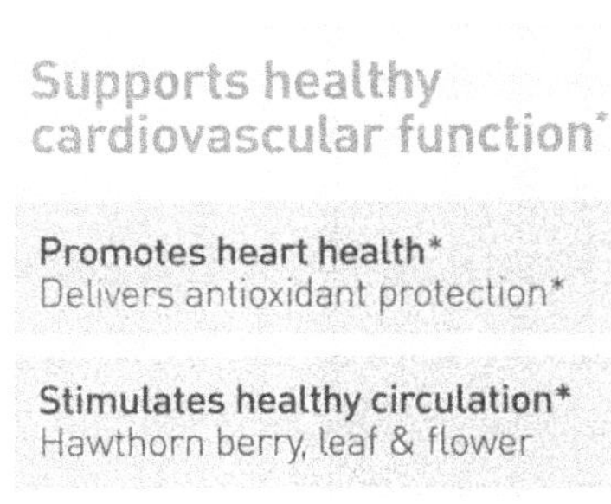

FIGURE 3.4

mention cardiovascular disease, hypertension, heart failure, or other cardiovascular conditions and thus are classified as structure/function claims.

Health claims, which require prior FDA approval for use, make statements about the relationship between a substance and its possible effect in reducing the risk of a specific disease state. Sticking with our bone and joint health theme, an example of a health claim might be "calcium may reduce the risk of osteoporosis."

Who Keeps Track of the Claims Made for These Products?

Two agencies are responsible for oversight of the Dietary Supplement Industry. While we have primarily covered legislation related to the authority of the FDA, the Federal Trade Commission (FTC) also has a role in consumer protection with regard to dietary supplements. The FDA handles the regulation of the manufacturing side of the dietary supplement industry, while the FTC is more marketing-centered. The two basic principles behind the FTC truth-in-advertising law are that 1) advertising must be truthful and not misleading and 2) before disseminating an ad, advertisers must have adequate substantiation for all objective product claims.[25] Both the FTC and the FDA monitor claims made by dietary supplement manufacturers; the difference lies in where the claims occur. The FDA oversees claims made on bottle labels, whereas the FTC would pay attention to claims made in advertising materials on an advertisement appearing in social media, for instance. Advertising claims may be direct or implied in nature. Even the name of a supplement can have implications; for example, a supplement called Cardiocure may imply that it cures a cardiovascular condition. Omission of important information is also considered to be deceptive and therefore misleading. A dietary supplement claiming to be useful in relieving a symptom associated with a specific condition may imply to consumers that it is useful for relieving that symptom generally, regardless of the underlying cause of it. If a known drug interaction can occur, a warning should be present in any advertisements. Even differences in font sizes for claims and disclaimers are evaluated closely. Consumers who have a question or concern about any claim made about a dietary supplement can contact either agency, as the two work closely together to investigate any questionable practices. Table 3.3 summarizes the responsibilities of the two agencies.

How Are New Dietary Ingredients Handled?

Any dietary ingredient that was not marketed as a dietary supplement in the United States prior to the DSEHA in 1994 is considered a new dietary ingredient (NDI).[26] Manufacturers are responsible for determining whether or not their anticipated new product will contain any new dietary ingredients, and the FDA puts out guidance for manufacturers in helping

TABLE 3.3 Responsibilities of Agency Oversight

Agency:	Federal Trade Commission (FTC)	Food and Drug Administration (FDA)
Responsibilities:	Focus = Marketing-centered Investigate questionable trade practices Challenge or stop unsubstantiated advertising Investigate complaints about false advertising	Focus = Manufacturing-centered Maintain a registry of dietary supplement manufacturers Stop distribution of toxic or unsanitary products Take action if risk of injury occurs or illness occurs (e.g., adverse reactions) Stop manufacturing and marketing if safety information is not received within specified time Ensure that manufacturers comply with good manufacturing practices (GMPs) Inspect manufacturing, storage, and distribution facilities

them determine whether or not they need to go through the NDI process.[27] If it is determined that an NDI is present, the manufacturer must notify the FDA a minimum of 75 days before market and provide sufficient evidence of the safety of the NDI. Information included in the safety profile should include the name and address of the manufacturer or distributor, the name of the NDI, and a description of the dietary supplement containing it. Botanical ingredients must be identified with their genus and species, along with the citation for the scientist who named it. Evidence for safety can include documentation of historical use or current studies demonstrating that the NDI will be reasonably expected to be safe when used per the directions suggested in the label. Ninety days after a manufacturer files a safety profile for an NDI, the evidence submitted supporting its safety will be made public. This excludes, of course, any trade secrets and/or proprietary information.

What About the Evidence for Dietary Supplements?

As we just discussed for NDIs, safety information will become more and more available. The many supplement ingredients grandfathered in that have been on the market since before the DSHEA are being monitored by MedWatch and other regulations looking for adverse events and contaminated products. Efficacy and effectiveness of ingredients contained in dietary supplements, however, are a different story altogether. First, let's briefly tease out the terms *efficacy* and *effectiveness*. *Efficacy* is most often used to refer to how a substance works in clinical trials, where many variables are controlled and patient populations may or may not be very representative of the population at large. We do this in clinical trials to increase the chances that any effect we see is because of the intervention (medication, etc.) that we are testing. *Effectiveness*, on the other hand, tends to be used in describing how well a substance works in "the real world," where there are many other issues, such as lifestyle changes, comorbid disease states, drug interactions, patient adherence, and other circumstances or variables that we may not have controlled for during clinical trials. Effectiveness is generally determined postmarketing and can take a long time to characterize. Aside from those differences, there are many factors that influence the quantity and quality of the evidence available for dietary supplements. Randomized controlled trials (RCTs), currently considered the gold standard for efficacy of new medications, are very expensive, so if it is not required, a manufacturer would not likely spend the money for an unbiased objective trial to be conducted. Additionally, the differences in regulation of dietary supplements mean that not all dietary supplements are created equally; in other words, one manufacturer's version of St. John's wort might not be anything like another. One may use the entire dried plant, and another may process the plant in order to obtain a standardized extract. Trials using the two different products may give very different results. This would mean that even if RCTs were conducted by researchers, their results would have to be product-specific and could not be generalized to all products containing the ingredient.

The National Center for Complementary and Integrative Health (NCCIH) has a growing body of knowledge about integrative health practices, including dietary supplements. Their website has a section called "Herbs at a Glance," which provides monographs that include what we currently know about selected dietary supplements. Natural Standard, a database that may be available to students and faculty in academic centers at no cost, is another source of information that can provide some insight about the use of dietary supplements and the levels of evidence we currently have. Access to Natural Standard is also available to individuals at a cost for subscription. PubMed is a search engine that accesses biomedical science articles. Many articles there are available for free as well, and others may be available for purchase, depending on an organization's subscriptions. Much of the information we have about how well dietary supplements work is currently based on case reports, testimonials, and very small pilot studies. As we learn more about the active compounds in herbal and botanical products and are able to isolate them with consistency, perhaps better data are on the way in the future.

References

1. "Dietary Supplement Health and Education Act of 1994," Pub. L. 103-417, 108 Stat. 4325 (1994), https://www.govinfo.gov/content/pkg/STATUTE-108/pdf/STATUTE-108-Pg4325.pdf.

2. Institute of Medicine (US) Committee to Review Dietary Reference Intakes for Vitamin D and Calcium, "Dietary Reference Intakes (DRIs): Recommended Dietary Allowances and Adequate Intakes, Elements," in *Dietary Reference Intakes for Calcium and Vitamin D*, edited by A. Catherine Ross et al. (Washington: National Academies Press, 2011), https://www.ncbi.nlm.nih.gov/books/NBK56068/table/summarytables.t3/?report=objectonly.
3. Institute of Medicine (US) Committee to Review Dietary Reference Intakes for Vitamin D and Calcium, "Dietary Reference Intakes (DRIs): Recommended Dietary Allowances and Adequate Intakes, Vitamins," in *Dietary Reference Intakes for Calcium and Vitamin D*, edited by A. Catherine Ross et al. (Washington: National Academies Press, 2011), https://www.ncbi.nlm.nih.gov/books/NBK56068/table/summarytables.t2/?report=objectonly.
4. Institute of Medicine (US) Committee to Review Dietary Reference Intakes for Vitamin D and Calcium, "Dietary Reference Intakes (DRIs): Tolerable Upper Intake Levels, Vitamins," in *Dietary Reference Intakes for Calcium and Vitamin D*, edited by A. Catherine Ross et al. (Washington: National Academies Press, 2011), https://www.ncbi.nlm.nih.gov/books/NBK56068/table/summarytables.t7/?report=objectonly.
5. Institute of Medicine (US) Committee to Review Dietary Reference Intakes for Vitamin D and Calcium, "Dietary Reference Intakes (DRIs): Tolerable Upper Intake Levels, Elements," in *Dietary Reference Intakes for Calcium and Vitamin D*, edited by A. Catherine Ross et al. (Washington: National Academies Press, 2011), https://www.ncbi.nlm.nih.gov/books/NBK56068/table/summarytables.t8/?report=objectonly.
6. Sompon Wanwimolruk, and Virapong Prachayasittikul, "Cytochrome P450 Enzyme Mediated Herbal Drug Interactions (Part I)," *EXCLI Journal* 13 (2014): 347–91.
7. Erin N. Berry-Bibee et al., "Co-Administration of St. John's Wort and Hormonal Contraceptives: A Systematic Review," *Contraception* 94, no. 6 (2016): 668–77, https://doi.org/10.1016/j.contraception.2016.07.010.
8. Samaneh Soleymani et al., "Clinical Risks of St. John's Wort (Hypericum perforatum) Co-Administration," *Expert Opinion on Drug Metabolism and Toxicology* 13, no. 10 (2017): 1047–62, https://doi.org/10.1080/17425255.2017.1378342.
9. "Nutrition Labeling of Dietary Supplements," 21 CFR 101.36(b)(2)(i), https://www.govinfo.gov/app/details/CFR-2012-title21-vol2/CFR-2012-title21-vol2-sec101-36.
10. Glucosamine animal sources: Michael T. Murray, "Glucosamine," in *Textbook of Natural Medicine* (4th ed.), edited by Joseph E. Pizzorno, Jr., and Michael T. Murray (Edinburgh: Churchill Livingstone, 2012), 790.
11. Chondroitin plant source: Nicola Volpi et al., "Oral Bioavailability and Pharmacokinetics of Nonanimal Chondroitin Sulfate and Its Constituents in Healthy Male Volunteers," *Clinical Pharmacology in Drug Development* 2018, https://doi.org/10.1002/cpdd.587.
12. 1906 law: "Federal Food and Drugs Act," Pub. L. 59-384, 34 US Stat. 768, 1906.

13. 1938 law: "Federal Food, Drug, & Cosmetic Act," Pub. L. 75-717, 53 US Stat. 1040, 1938.
14. 1938 law specific definition of drug: "Federal Food, Drug, and Cosmetic Act," Public Law 75-717, 52 US Stat. 1040, 1938, Sec. 201(g)(3), 403(j), 502(f).
15. 1940 rule: National Archives and Records Administration, *Federal Register: 5 Fed. Reg. Sept. 5, 1940*. September 5, Thursday. [Periodical], 5 Fed. Reg. 3565-3566, 1940, https://www.loc.gov/item/fr005173/.
16. 1941 rule: National Archives and Records Administration, *Federal Register: 6 Fed. Reg. 5909*. Saturday. [Periodical], 6 Fed. Reg. 5921-5926, 1941, https://www.loc.gov/item/fr006227/.
17. "Nutrition Labeling and Education Act," Pub. L. 101-535, 104 US Stat. 2353, 1990, https://www.govinfo.gov/content/pkg/STATUTE-104/pdf/STATUTE-104-Pg2353.pdf.
18. "Dietary Supplement Health and Education Act of 1994."
19. National Institutes of Health, Office of Dietary Supplements, "Mission, Origin, and Mandate," n.d., https://ods.od.nih.gov/About/MissionOriginMandate.aspx.
20. Commission on Dietary Supplement Labels, "Report of the Commission on Dietary Supplement Labels," (Washington, DC: US Government Printing Office, 1997), Stock no. 017-001-00531-2.
21. "Dietary Supplement and Nonprescription Drug Consumer Protection Act," Pub. L. 109-462, 120 US Stat. 3469, 2006, https://www.congress.gov/109/plaws/publ462/PLAW-109publ462.pdf.
22. US Food and Drug Administration, "New and Improved Supplement Facts Label: Key Changes," 2018, https://www.fda.gov/downloads/food/labelingnutrition/ucm511646.pdf.
23. US Food and Drug Administration, "Label Claims for Dietary Foods and Supplements," 2018, https://www.fda.gov/food/labelingnutrition/ucm111447.htm.
24. US Food and Drug Administration, "Claims," in *Dietary Supplement Labeling Guide*, 2005, https://www.fda.gov/Food/GuidanceRegulation/GuidanceDocumentsRegulatoryInformation/DietarySupplements/ucm070613.htm.
25. Federal Trade Commission, "Dietary Supplements: An Advertising Guide for Industry," 2001, https://www.ftc.gov/tips-advice/business-center/guidance/dietary-supplements-advertising-guide-industry.
26. US Food and Drug Administration, "New Dietary Ingredients in Dietary Supplements: Background for Industry," 2011, https://www.fda.gov/food/new-dietary-ingredients-ndi-notification-process/new-dietary-ingredients-dietary-supplements-background-industry.
27. US Food and Drug Administration, "Draft Guidance for Industry: New Dietary Ingredient Notifications and Related Issues," 2016, https://www.fda.gov/downloads/Food/GuidanceRegulation/GuidanceDocumentsRegulatoryInformation/UCM515733.pdf.

Chapter 4

Background of Botanical Ingredients

Katie E. Alix

What Is a Botanical Ingredient?

A *botanical* can be described as a material originating from or relating to plants or botany. Botanicals may be derived from plants but also from algae and fungi; it may refer to the whole plant, a part of the plant, or an extract of the parts.[1] The plant (in whole or part) is valued for therapeutic or medicinal properties, flavor, and/or aroma; herbs would be considered a subset of botanicals.[2] Products containing herbal, botanical, or phytomedicinal ingredients are all classified as botanicals and are used to maintain or improve health.

Botanicals may be sold in many forms, including fresh, dried, or extracted products. Extracts may be liquids or solids; additionally, extracts can be delivered or consumed from tablets, capsules, powders, and tea bags. For example, different forms of echinacea have been used throughout generations. The echinacea plant, purple cone flower, was used by Native Americans in the Great Plains region as traditional medicine. Today, liquid extracts of the root and plant or dried whole herbs may be found in the dietary supplement aisle. Whole dried herbs may be packaged and sold as herbal teas.

Some common preparations of botanicals include teas, decoctions, tinctures, and extracts.[2] Teas are infusions of fresh or dried botanicals steeped in boiling water. A decoction is made through simmering roots, bark, or some berries in boiling water for longer periods of time. This is usually done when a more forceful treatment is necessary to extract the desired ingredients. A tincture is made by soaking the botanical in a solution of water and alcohol, usually ethanol. The solutions are sold as liquids and used for preserving or concentrating the botanical. A single chemical or group of chemicals may be isolated from botanicals by soaking them in a solution and then drying them; the dried material (extracted material) is then sold as a tablet or capsule.

The solution used to isolate the desired chemicals depends on the solubility of the chemicals to be extracted.

An *extract* is not a dried, ready-to-ship, *crude* botanical, but it is not a finished product either;[3] it is an herbal product ingredient. In some cases, the bioactive material of an herb is known, for example, anthocyanin from bilberry fruit. Anthocyanins represent a class of flavonoids and are made up of several different chemicals. Anthocyanins give some plants their dark red, purple, or blue color and have shown antioxidant properties *in vitro*. An extract of bilberry fruit would contain anthocyanins, as well as many other extracted constituents such as sugars and other plant materials. In other cases, the active ingredient is not known and an extract would be a mixture of unknown compounds.

Extracts can be standardized to specific ingredients to ensure batch-to-batch consistency.[2] This process involves quantitating and adjusting the level of specific chemicals in the extract, known as markers. The standardization process provides a level of quality control but is not required in the United States, and there is no regulatory or legal definition of standardization of botanical ingredients.

Classification of Botanical Ingredients

If the botanical is intended for ingestion and is not considered a food, the Food and Drug Administration (FDA) would classify this material as a *dietary supplement*.[4][5] The Dietary Supplement Health and Education Act (DSHEA) defines the term "dietary supplement" to mean a product (other than tobacco) intended to supplement the diet that bears or contains one or more dietary ingredients, including a vitamin; a mineral; an herb or other botanical; an amino acid; a dietary substance for use by man to supplement the diet by increasing the total dietary intake; or a concentrate, metabolite, constituent, extract, or combination of any of the aforementioned ingredients. To differentiate between foods and dietary

Box 4.1

A dietary supplement is a product (other than tobacco) that

- is intended to supplement the diet;
- contains one or more dietary ingredients (including vitamins, minerals, herbs or other botanicals, amino acids, or other substances) or their constituents;
- is intended to be taken by mouth as a pill, capsule, tablet, or liquid; and
- is labeled on the front panel as being a dietary supplement.

supplements, products intended to be dietary supplements are to be labeled on the front panel as dietary supplements.

Botanicals may also be used in personal care products and cosmetics, which are covered under the US Food, Drug, and Cosmetic Act.[6] Any botanical claiming to cure, treat, or prevent human disease is classified as a drug, and the manufacturer would be required to file a New Drug Application (NDA) providing evidence of its safety and efficacy in humans. Additional information regarding the regulatory aspects of botanicals will be covered in another chapter.

Regulatory Controls for Quality

While the FDA is responsible for the regulations of dietary supplements, the Federal Trade Commission (FTC) is responsible for advertising regulations. The product safety and proper labeling of dietary supplements, and *botanicals*, are the responsibility of the manufacturer. To meet the requirements for ensuring product quality, manufacturers provide due diligence, which includes but is not limited to following good manufacturing practices (GMP) as per part 111 of the Code of Federal Regulations (21 CFR Part 111). The GMP regulations require manufacturers to make safe, pure, and effective products. They cover the manufacture, packaging, labeling, and holding of materials. In addition, the regulations address personnel, records, facilities, equipment, and quality control.

There are three general product quality requirements that apply to a wide range of products including small drug products, large molecule drug products, and dietary supplements. These three main criteria are identity, purity, and potency. Identity ensures the identification of the active ingredient in the sample; purity assesses the presence of impurities or degradants in the sample; potency is a quantitative measurement of the major active ingredient or preservative in the sample. A sample could be the raw material or the finished product. Identity and purity are generally assessed on the raw material, while potency is generally assessed on the finished product. Potency in this context can also be considered the assay or content of the active ingredient typically found in the finished product.

There are a wide range of resources and guidance available for dietary supplements and botanicals; sources of monograph tests include the United States Pharmacopeia (USP),[7] the World Health Organization (WHO), the American Herbal Pharmacopeia (AHP), and the Association of Official Analytical Chemists (AOAC).[1] Compendial *monograph* tests are standardized methods and specification tests for generic raw materials and finished products. The International Council for Harmonization (ICH) of Technical Requirements for Pharmaceuticals for Human Use,[8] USP, and the AOAC all have published documents outlining their requirements and guidance for analytical method validations.

Safety and Risks

While botanicals are derived from plants and are *natural*, this does not mean they are *safe*.[2][4][5] Like anything else, the safety depends on many factors, including the chemical makeup, how it works in the body, how it is prepared, the form, and the dosage. For example, peppermint tea is generally considered safe to drink, but peppermint oil is much more concentrated and may be toxic. While both methods of preparation may contain some of the same chemicals, the method in which they are prepared, the form, and the dosage levels are dramatically different.

It is important to note that the FDA does not review dietary supplements for safety and effectiveness prior to commercialization; if a botanical ingredient was used as a food ingredient prior to 1994, it is considered an old dietary ingredient and does not need premarket notification. And if the ingredient was used in food prior to 1958, it is generally regarded as safe (GRAS). For personal care products, there is a Cosmetic Ingredient Review (CIR) providing self-regulation of the industry.[6] An expert independent panel provided by the CIR reviews the relevant data to decide whether these products are safe under their current conditions of use. The panel is made up of voting members (toxicologists, dermatologists, academic affiliated chemists) and nonvoting members (representatives from FDA, consumer groups, industry).

Whether labeled as GRAS or deemed safe by a CIR panel for a specific use, botanical ingredients can have many interactions with other supplements and drugs. For example, St. John's wort, which is sold as a dietary supplement for depression, can also speed the breakdown of many drugs, including warfarin, cyclosporine, digoxin, birth control pills, antidepressants, and some cancer and HIV medications.[2]

Product Quality

Identity

Identification of botanical ingredients can vary greatly depending on the state of the raw material. Dried herbs can be identified through macroscopic or microscopic techniques. Powders that would lack the plant structure may require other techniques, such as colorimetric, infrared spectroscopy, or thin-layer chromatography. A botanical identification method answers the question, "Is this the botanical it claims to be?" in a yes or no fashion. The method must be robust and specific enough to give a negative result for similar botanical ingredients.

As with any plants, the quality and therapeutic value of herbal products is dependent on several factors related to the growth and harvest of the plants themselves. Water, humidity, light exposure, temperature, and nutrient levels in the soil can impact the growth of the plant. The time of year harvested, how the plants are harvested, and how they are dried, packaged, and stored can impact the stability of the therapeutic agents. In addition, the *part of the plant* collected can change the therapeutic value of the plant. The whole plant of evening primrose was used by Native Americans to treat bruises, while the roots were used to treat hemorrhoids. The leaves were traditionally used to treat minor wounds, gastrointestinal complaints, and sore throats. In the case of the elder tree, the flower and prepared berries may relieve flu symptoms, but the leaves, stems, and raw and unripe berries contain a toxic substance that may cause nausea, vomiting, and severe diarrhea.

Identification techniques for whole plants is quite different than those used for powders, liquids, and other extracts. Macroscopic and microscopic identification testing looks at the appearance of the botanical substance in comparison to a known reference material. Visual identification can be useful for determining foreign matter and monographs may specify size, shape, color of material, and part of plant. The size, shape, and color may indicate the incorrect material or material that has been improperly prepared, such as improperly dried.

A newer technique starting to gain traction is the use of DNA for identification.[9] This technique involves using polymerase chain reaction (PCR) to amplify the DNA present in the sample. Sections of DNA, or a DNA barcode, are then compared against a database of known material. While this would be beneficial for samples in which the plant DNA is still present, particularly in crude powders, it is not as beneficial in highly processed samples, in which any DNA fragments may have been lost.

Box 4.2 Characteristics of *Cinnamomum cassia* Twig

Macroscopic

- Long, cylindrical, branched, 30–75 cm long, 0.3–1 cm in diameter
- Externally brown to reddish brown, longitudinal ridges, fine wrinkles
- Texture hard and fragile, easily broken

Microscopic

- In the transverse section, epidermis consists of one layer of cells; unicellular non-gladular hairs visible in young branches
- Cork consists of 3–5 layers of cells; innermost cells with thickened outer walls
- Oil and stone cells scattered in the cortex

Where there are no macroscopic or microscopic details to be assessed, other methods must be implemented. Historically this has been done using thin-layer chromatography (TLC). With TLC, a solution of sample is spotted onto a thin layer of adsorbent material, such as silica gel on a glass plate or plastic sheet. The adsorbent layer is known as the stationary phase. A solvent or mixture of solvents, known as the mobile phase, is then drawn up the plate through capillary action. Generally, the compounds in the sample are separated based on differences between their affinity for the stationary phase and the mobile phase; most commonly, the affinity differences are based on the polarities of the sample and mobile phase.

Advancements have been made to allow for more reproducible and quantitative results using high-performance thin-layer chromatography (HPTLC). The use of automation overcomes differences in droplet size and position and gives the analyst a higher resolution. This newer technique is quickly taking the place of traditional TLC methods within compendial monographs.

Other chemical techniques for identification include colorimetric tests and spectroscopy. Colorimetric tests involve reacting the material with a chemical, which produces a change in color. One of the USP identification tests for ginger reacts the sample with sulfuric acid and vanillin; a positive result would turn blue. There are different types of spectroscopy techniques used for identification; most common techniques would include FTIR, NIR, and Raman. Fourier transform infrared (FTIR) passes infrared radiation through a sample. The radiation that passes through, or is transmitted, results in a signal that can be detected. The Fourier transform converts the detector output to a spectrum that can be interpreted. Near-infrared (NIR) and Raman spectroscopy both obtain spectra based on molecular vibrations. NIR uses near-infrared light, while Raman uses either visible or near-infrared laser light. NIR is based on the absorption of light in the near-infrared region, while Raman relies on nonelastic scattering of photons from the laser source.

Purity

Purity testing looks at the contaminants present in the sample. This may include looking at the microbial load, pesticides, residual solvents, ash, heavy metals, and loss upon drying. Generally, monographs require the raw material to meet specific limits for the presence of *E. coli* and *Salmonella* and limit the total aerobic microbial, mold, and yeast counts. Microbes found in samples could be from the soil, harvesting method, storage method, or any processing that may have occurred.

Pesticide testing looks for *residual pesticides* that may have been used on the plant prior to harvest. These pesticide residues may be enriched or reduced on the material compared to their plant materials, depending on how the raw material was processed. The USP limit for pesticides in extracts of botanicals can be calculated using this equation:

$$if\ E \leq 10, Limit\left(\frac{mg}{kg}\right) = L \times E$$

$$if\ E > 10, Limit\left(\frac{mg}{kg}\right) = \frac{A \times M}{100 \times B}$$

where L is the limit in the original article, E is the plant extract ratio, A is the acceptable daily intake, M is body weight, and B is the daily dose of the extract.

The EPA has a tolerance level, while the FDA has an action level, for specific pesticides. In addition, the acceptable pesticides for use in products labeled as organic are different than those not labeled as organic.

Box 4.3 Aspects of Purity

- Microbial growth
- Residual pesticides
- Residual solvents
- Ash
- Heavy metals
- Loss on drying
- Related substances

If a raw material was prepared with solvents other than alcohol, water, or alcohol-water mixture, then *residual solvents* would need to be determined. Both USP and ICH have guidelines on the acceptable limits of residual solvents allowed in raw materials. Solvents are classified into three classes based on toxicity or environmental effects.[10] Class 1 solvents, human carcinogens, and environmental hazards should be avoided; examples include benzene (carcinogen), carbon tetrachloride (toxic and environmental hazard), 1,2- and 1,1-dichloroethane (toxic), and 1,1,1-trichlorethane (environmental hazard). Class 2 solvents, nongenotoxic animal carcinogens, and possible neurotoxicity or tetrogenicity should be limited; examples include acetonitrile, chloroform, cyclohexane, methanol, toluene. Class 3 solvents generally have low toxic potential; examples include acetic acid, acetone, ethanol, formic acid, and propanol.

Ashing samples involves burning the material; any water or organic matter will burn off, while inorganic matter will remain. The total ash level is the amount of material left, which is then subjected to additional tests to determine the composition. If the ash is insoluble in acid, then it is likely sand or silica.

Heavy metals are monitored and regulated by the FDA in certain foods and dietary supplements due to their potential to cause serious health problems. Typical analysis of the sample is performed for high levels of lead, mercury, arsenic, and/or cadmium. These materials could be present due to pollution or inherent from the environment. Historically, these had been tested by colorimetric techniques, which have been replaced by inductively coupled plasma-mass spectrometry (ICP-MS). In ICP-MS, a sample solution is atomized with plasma, and the metal ions are detected and quantified with a mass spectrometer.

Loss on drying determines the amount of volatile matter that is driven off, including water. Different botanical ingredients have different acceptable levels of moisture. Additional purity factors to consider would include being able to differentiate the sample from related substances. Failure with any of the purity tests may indicate the presence of adulterants or contaminants or that the material is not authentic.

Potency

To allow for an accurate statement on the content of an analyte in the finished product, the *potency* must be assessed. In general, potency determinations are done through chromatographic analysis of the finished product. Different types of detectors are available for different types of chromatography systems; the most widely used is a liquid chromatography system with a UV detector.

A sample solution is applied to a stationary phase within a column, then eluted using a solvent mixture called the mobile phase. The solvent flows through the column to a detector, where the detection of the different components can be graphed versus time spent on the column. This time on the column is called the retention time. Different stationary phases and mobile phases can change the order of elution and the resolution of components. *Resolution* (R_s) is defined with respect to chromatography as twice the difference of retention times (t) divided by the sum of the two peak widths (w).

$$R_s = \frac{2 \times (t_2 - t_1)}{(w_1 + w_2)}$$

Another important factor when considering chromatographic data would be the overall peak shape. An optimal peak would show a Gaussian distribution that was relatively narrow. The sample will broaden as it elutes from the column due to diffusion, slow equilibration between the phases, and irregular flow paths on the column.[11] The way analytical chemists examine the result of these three reasons for peak broadening is captured in the van Deemter equation:

$$H \approx A + \frac{B}{u} + C_u$$

This equation shows that the plate height (H) is a function of the flow rate (u), the flow path (A), diffusion (B), and equilibration time (C). A column is divided into discrete sections called theoretical plates; these are not actual divisions in the column but a way of thinking about the column. The plate height is based on the length of the column divided by the number of theoretical plates. While the number of theoretical plates differs for each specific compound, it is based on the retention time and width of the peak and half-height of the peak. More simply, narrow peaks, which are a result of a small plate height, are preferred to achieve optimal separations.

Fronting or tailing of the peak produce a non-Gaussian distribution. Fronting typically occurs from an overload of solute in a band—the solute is so soluble in the concentrated part of the band that very little solute trails behind the concentrated region. Decreasing the amount of sample or the strength of the solution the sample is in will decrease fronting by not overloading the column. Tailing is when the peak shape at the trailing region is elongated. This usually occurs when the solute is more strongly retained by the column. Changing the column chemistry to reduce interactions between the stationary phase and solute can help reduce trailing.

Gas chromatography systems, unlike liquid chromatography systems, do not always use a packed column but more often use an open tubular column. This column is a long, hollow capillary that has an interior thin coating of stationary phase. Peak broadening is not seen, as there aren't multiple flow paths. While an open tubular column may have more theoretical plates and therefore better resolution, it cannot handle as much solute as a packed column. An open tubular column can be 100 m, while a packed column would only be a fraction of that, 2–3 m due to the pressures required to push the gas through the column.

After separating the solute into individual compounds with a chromatographic system, there needs to be a way to detect the separated components. In gas chromatography (GC), this is usually through a flame ionization detector (FID), which measures the ions of the analyte in the gas stream. In liquid chromatography (LC), this is usually through a diode array detector, in which the sample is irradiated with light (white or UV) and the absorbance at a specific wavelength is monitored. For both GC and LC systems, mass spectrometry detectors are also used. A mass spectrometer ionizes the analyte and produces a spectrum showing the relative abundance of an analyte ion versus its mass to charge ratio.

The quantitative output from the chromatographic analysis represents the potency. The method would be optimized so that the area of the chromatographic peak is proportional to the amount of the analyte of interest. The Gaussian peak would represent 96 percent of the peak area (1/2 base × height). The amount in a sample would be quantitated based on the peak area of the sample chromatogram and the peak area of a known standard chromatogram. To show that the method is suitable for use, the method should be validated, typically by USP, AOAC, or ICH guidelines.

Method Validation

The accuracy of the analysis is determined by how close the measured value is to the true value. This should not be confused with precision, which is determined by how close multiple sample results are to each other. Other characteristics of a potency assay to be aware of include the detection and quantitation limits, the linear range of the method, and the robustness. The detection limit is the lowest amount of sample that can be reliably detected, while the quantitation limit is the lowest amount of sample that can be quantitatively determined with suitable precision and accuracy. Linearity is the method's ability to produce results directly proportional to the concentration within upper and lower concentration limits. The robustness of the method describes the bounds of what small changes in the method parameters are tolerable and still provide reliable results. Robustness is sometimes referred to as the ruggedness of the method.

Box 4.4 Components of a Method Validation

- Accuracy
- Specificity
- Repeatability
- Limits
- Linearity
- Robustness

Accuracy, Specificity, Precision, and Repeatability

The *accuracy* or trueness of the method must be determined and is reported in terms of recovery. An analyte-free material, also called a placebo, is used, and the analyte is then added at known concentrations. If no placebo is available, then standard addition may be used. Standard addition is a method in which a known concentration (usually 2–3 times higher) of the standard analyte is added to the sample. There are two ways to calculate the recovery: total recovery (spiked plus inherent) and marginal recovery (based only on the spiked amount). The AOAC[1] provides a sliding scale of what they consider acceptable accuracy recovery values at a specific concentration based on the weight to weight (w/w) concentration of the analyte in the finished product. Typically, accuracy is assessed at multiple levels. The ICH[7] recommends nine determinations at a minimum of three concentration levels (i.e., three replicates at each of the three concentrations).

A placebo can also be used to determine *specificity*. This is the ability to assess the analyte in the presence of impurities, degradation products, matrix components or other components anticipated to be present. The placebo should be run using the method to show a lack of interference for the analyte of interest. When no placebo is present, standard addition can be used to determine specificity; the slope of standard addition should be close to 1. To determine if there are any chromatographic interferences, the most useful technique is evaluating the resolution. As shown earlier, the resolution (R_s) is a function of the absolute separation distance expressed as retention times (t_1 and t_2) and the baseline widths (W_1 and W_2).[1] A resolution of 1.0 would be considered the minimum usable separation; typically a resolution of at least 1.5 is desired.

One type of *precision* is the closeness of repeated measurements, known as *repeatability* precision; this would be validated through repeating discrete sample preparations from a single bulk material. The ICH[7] indicates that six determinations should be made and that the relative standard deviation (RSD) is calculated. The AOAC[1] provides a sliding scale of what they consider acceptable RSDs based on w/w concentration of the analyte in the finished product. The repeatability precision is typically done by a single analyst.

Another precision value to examine would be the intermediate precision or the within laboratory precision. In most cases, this is validated by different analysts, on different days, using different equipment, where possible. The relative standard deviation of six replicates from both analysts is calculated. Once again, the AOAC[1] provides a sliding scale of what they consider acceptable RSDs based on w/w concentration of the analyte in the finished product.

Limits, Linearity, and Robustness

There are two limits to be concerned with in an analytical method—detection and quantitation. The *detection limit*, or limit of detection (LOD), is the lowest level of the analyte that can be detected with the method. One approach to determine LOD is looking at the signal-to-noise ratio. This is done by comparing measured signals from samples with low concentrations with those of blanks. A signal-to-noise ratio between 3:1 and 2:1 is generally considered acceptable for the detection limit.[8] The LOD can also be determined from the standard deviation of the response and slope of a calibration curve as seen in the equation below, where DL is the detection limit, σ is the standard deviation of the response, and S is the slope of the calibration curve.

$$DL = \frac{3.3\sigma}{S}$$

The *quantitation limit*, or limit of quantitation (LOQ), is the lowest level of the analyte that can be quantitated with the method. This level must be determined with acceptable precision and accuracy under the experimental conditions. One approach to determine LOQ is looking at the signal-to-noise ratio; generally, a signal-to-noise ratio of 10:1 is considered acceptable. Like the detection limit, the quantitation limit can also be determined from the standard deviation of the response and the slope of the calibration curve, as seen below, where QL is the quantitation limit.

$$QL = \frac{10\sigma}{S}$$

Linearity of the method refers to the relationship of the concentration and the assay measurement. When the concentration and the assay measurement are proportional, either as is or with a mathematical transformation (log, square root, reciprocal), the assay is found to be linear.[7] If linearity cannot be achieved, then a nonlinear model may be used, but this is not ideal. Some assays or detectors do not produce linear assay measurements, such as evaporative light scattering detectors or immunoassays.[8] The range of the linear portion should be broader than the anticipated concentration range of the analyte, typically 80–120 percent or wider of the expected concentration.

Robustness can also be considered the ruggedness of the method. It is assessed by making small, deliberate changes to different elements of the method and observing any impact on the result. Examples of typical variations regardless of method type include sample stability over time and sample preparation extraction time. For LC methods, typical variations may include variations in pH of mobile phase, variations in mobile phase composition, different column lots or suppliers, temperature, and flow rate. For GC methods, typical variations may include different column lots or suppliers, temperature, and flow rate.[8] Most robustness testing is done by changing one variable at a time. A Youden Ruggedness Trial[12] can examine the effects of less important factors simultaneously; this trial can examine up to seven factors in a single experiment that has eight determinations.

Conclusion

Determining the purity and content of a botanical is much more in-depth than it appears at first glance. As presented in this chapter, to determine what a botanical is and how much is present takes a wide range of analytical techniques. The identity, purity, and potency are very important product quality aspects that need to be considered for any ingredient, including botanicals. Considering the complexity of plants and plant material, these aspects of product quality are much more difficult with botanical ingredients than other, synthetic ingredients. The product safety and proper labeling are the responsibility of the manufacturer. However, consumers should be aware of the impact that botanicals may have on other drugs and supplements they may be taking and should consult their doctor or pharmacist for "guidance."

References

1. AOAC International, "Appendix K: Guidelines for Dietary Supplements and Botanicals," in *Official Methods of Analysis* (Rockville, MD: AOAC, 2013).
2. National Institutes of Health Office of Dietary Supplements, *Botanical Dietary Supplements* (Bethesda, MD: National Institutes of Health, 2011). https://ods.od.nih.gov/factsheets/BotanicalBackground-HealthProfessional/
3. Steven Dentali, "Botanical Basics: Botanical Extracts: Not Single Chemical Ingredients," *Nutraceuticals World*, April 1, 2013.
4. National Institutes of Health Office of Dietary Supplements, *Dietary Supplements: What You Need to Know* (Bethesda, MD: National Institutes of Health, 2011). https://ods.od.nih.gov/HealthInformation/DS_WhatYouNeedToKnow.aspx
5. U.S. Food and Drug Administration, *Food Facts Dietary Supplements* (Silver Spring, MD: U.S. Food and Drug Administration, 2017).
6. Eric Antignac et al., "Safety of Botanical Ingredients in Personal Care Products/Cosmetics," *Food and Chemical Toxicology* 49, no. 2 (2010): 324–41.
7. United States Pharmacopeia and National Formulary, "<1225> Validation of Compendial Procedures USP41-NF36," United States Pharmacopeia and National Formulary, 2017.
8. International Council for Harmonisation, "Validation of Analytical Procedures: Text and Methodology Q2(R1)," ICH Harmonised Tripartite Guideline, 1996.
9. United States Pharmacopeia and U.S. Food and Drug Administration, "DNA Standards for Botanical Identification Workshop and Botanical ID Methodology Test Course," United States Pharmacopeia, 2018.
10. United States Pharmacopeia and National Formulary, "<467> Residual Solvents," United States Pharmacopeia and National Formulary, 2018.

11. Daniel C. Harris, *Exploring Chemical Analysis*, 2nd ed. (New York: W. H. Freeman and Company, 2001).
12. William J. Youden and E. H. Steiner, "Statistical Manual of the Association of Official Analytical Chemists" (Rockville, MD: AOAC International, 1975), 50–55.

Chapter 5

Herbal Bioavailability, Pharmacokinetics, and Mechanism of Herb-Drug Interactions

Phillip M. Gerk

MANY TEXTBOOKS HAVE BEEN WRITTEN ON pharmacokinetics, ranging from introductory and practical to advanced and theoretical. This brief overview will hopefully stimulate the readers toward wanting to learn more about how these concepts apply to natural products. It is also aimed at giving an appreciation of the impact for this topic, which seems to be understudied in the clinical utilization of natural products. Although the term *pharmacokinetics* specifically refers to drugs, all of the concepts similarly apply to natural products; thus, not seeing the need for a separate term, we will use *pharmacokinetics.*

What Is "Pharmacokinetics," and Why Does It Matter for Herbal Products?

From a clinical perspective, pharmacokinetics can be described simply as the science of how the body handles xenobiotic compounds (all foreign compounds, including drugs, natural products, and environmental toxins). This knowledge can be used to predict how a given patient may handle a dose of a particular compound. It can also be used to design and adjust individual dosage regimens. It is used extensively in the development of new drugs, thus enabling safe and effective application of "useful poisons" to treat diseases. Finally, it is used to make sound drug/herbal therapy decisions.

How Do We Know What Dose to Take, and What Happens to Xenobiotics When They Get in the Body?

Many patients can all be given the same dose of some drugs, which are highly effective and have very little toxicity. But patients are not all the same, so it is no surprise when patients respond differently to the same doses of other drugs. When the response to a given dose varies considerably among different patients, then it may be necessary to dose patients differently in order to achieve the desired therapeutic effect and to avoid toxicity. This would be especially important for drugs, which show a relatively small difference between efficacious doses and toxic doses. These drugs are said to have a narrow therapeutic window. This means that there is a narrow range of concentrations in the blood (or plasma) where the likelihood of efficacy is maximized and the likelihood of toxicity is minimized.

If a drug did have a narrow therapeutic window and standardized uniform dosing was used, one would expect an appreciable incidence of both toxicity and therapeutic inefficacy. The toxicities could conceivably result in patient injury, hospitalization, and possibly even death. On the other hand, the lack of therapeutic effects could allow disease progression and increased patient suffering. Additionally, some of these events could even lead to increased cost of patient therapy. For these drugs, certain knowledge is required to individualize the patient's drug therapy. This is where clinical pharmacokinetics comes in.

Clinical pharmacokinetics involves applying knowledge of how the body handles an administered drug (drug disposition) to the care of the patient. The disposition of a drug in the body can be broken down into four parts: absorption, distribution, metabolism, and excretion. Absorption is how the unchanged drug moves from the administration site to the site of measurement, which is usually blood or plasma. Distribution describes the movement of the drug to and from the site of measurement. Metabolism is the conversion of the administered drug to a chemically different molecule (metabolite); this process is usually associated with the liver. Excretion consists of the loss of unchanged drug from the body, usually into the urine. Metabolism and excretion specify how the body gets rid of the drug (elimination). These concepts form the basic outline for understanding pharmacokinetics.

We will focus only on the simplest case (one-compartment model with first-order elimination, for future reference). Since the concentrations of most drugs are measured in plasma, we will commonly refer to plasma concentrations. The discussions on pharmacokinetics in this chapter are based on the texts by Rowland and Tozer,[1] Evans, Schentag, and Jusko,[2] and Shargel and Yu.[3] For further explanations, consult these texts or other highly regarded sources. Additionally, a glossary of commonly used pharmacokinetics terms and a list of basic pharmacokinetic equations are appended to this chapter as study aids.

How Do Xenobiotics Get in the Body in the First Place?

Unless they are given by intravascular injection, they would first need to undergo the process of absorption. Absorption is the process of a molecule moving from the administration site to the blood. For products applied to the skin, the active compounds may be absorbed transdermally, and inhaled products would be absorbed through the alveolar epithelium. Most commonly, herbal and dietary supplements are given orally, so the site of absorption is the gastrointestinal tract, and this discussion will focus on oral administration.

Oral doses in the form of tablets and capsules would first need to undergo disintegration into granules, followed by deaggregation into fine particles, all of which is leading to dissolution in gastrointestinal fluids. The solubility of natural compounds ranges from extremely high (sugars and sugar conjugates) to very low (various kinds of fats).

We stated earlier that absorption, distribution, metabolism, and excretion characterize the disposition of a drug. Let us explore each of these further, beginning with absorption. Absorption is how the unchanged drug moves from the administration site to the active site (usually the blood). When a drug is administered orally, it must go through several steps to get to the blood and circulate systemically. First, it must be released from the dosage product; then it must dissolve; then it must avoid degradation in the gut; then it must pass through the gut wall (with or without the help of certain transporters, discussed below) and enter the hepatic portal vein; then it must escape the liver before it reaches the rest of the body (hepatic first pass effect). Each of these steps can potentially reduce the actual amount reaching systemic circulation, as well as how fast it gets there. The rate and extent of absorption from the site of administration to the active site is termed bioavailability.

OK, the Compound Is in the Blood, Now What?

Next on the agenda is distribution, which is the movement of a drug to and from the site of measurement (blood or plasma). Commonly, compartment models are used to illustrate the distribution behavior of a drug. In these depictions, compartments are imagined where the drug can enter, be distributed into a certain volume, and be cleared from the compartment. For simplicity, this discussion will focus only on a one-compartment model, which is useful to understand the distribution characteristics of many drugs.

The size of the imaginary compartment is described by volume of distribution. Hypothetically, let us pretend that when a drug goes into the body, it is mostly confined to the plasma volume. Here the volume of distribution would be only three liters. In another simple case, let us assume that after administration, a drug distributes evenly throughout all body fluids. In this simple case, the volume of distribution would be equal to total body water, about 42 liters. Now, to complicate the picture, there are proteins in the plasma and/or in the tissues to which drugs may bind, depending on their physicochemical properties. The most important drug binding proteins are albumin, α1-acid glycoprotein, and lipoproteins. Consider that if a molecule of a drug is bound to one of these proteins, then it is no longer free in solution, and while bound, it cannot cross any biologic membranes. However, it is

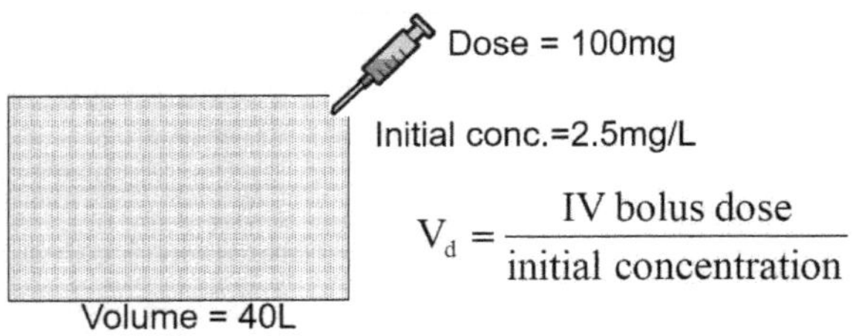

FIGURE 5.1 Volume of distribution.

necessary to think of protein binding as a reversible process, with individual drug molecules associating with and dissociating from a given protein molecule. If the binding is strong, then the "on" rate (drug associating with a protein) is much faster than the "off" rate (drug dissociating from a protein), and a large percentage of the total drug amount may be bound. If the molecule is bound strongly to a protein in the plasma, then it is not free to leave the blood vessels and enter the tissue. If the drug also has very little binding in the tissue, then this drug may have a low volume of distribution.

Consider the opposite scenario: If a drug molecule is bound strongly to a protein in the tissues, then it is not free to leave the tissue and reenter the blood circulation. If it also has very little binding to plasma proteins, then it may also have a very large volume of distribution.

Volume of distribution is a parameter for which it may be difficult to achieve a physiologic understanding in many cases. When it comes to dosing, one can think of volume of distribution as the size of a given tank. Since concentration is mass divided by volume, if the "size of the tank" (volume of distribution) is known, then one can easily determine the amount (dose, in mg) to give the patient by an intravenous bolus to reach an initial desired concentration in the plasma. This is a commonly used method for loading dose calculations.

How Does the Compound Get out of the Body?

To answer this question, let us discuss clearance. Clearance is said to have the greatest application to the patient, being crucial for maintenance dosing, predicting steady state concentrations, and understanding drug interactions. Clearance is the volume of blood (or plasma) completely cleared of a drug in a given time; think of the flow rate (e.g., liters per hour) of "dirty" blood getting "cleaned" from the drug. The body organs associated with drug clearance are the liver and the kidneys.

Systemic (total) clearance describes the sum of the elimination activity of the entire body. Usually, the liver and the kidneys are the main players in removing most drugs from the body. Therefore, systemic clearance can be broken down into its two main components: hepatic clearance and renal clearance, respectively. Some drugs are eliminated primarily by the kidneys, some primarily by the liver, and others by any proportion of both. Other organs may also be involved in eliminating some drugs, but this discussion will focus on the liver and the kidneys.

Hepatic clearance is the contribution that the liver makes to systemic clearance. The liver has a certain efficiency for removing drugs from the blood, termed hepatic extraction ratio (E). If this extraction ratio is high, the liver will remove much of the drug from the blood as it flows through. Hepatic clearance is the product of liver blood flow and hepatic extraction ratio. It can also be defined as the apparent volume of blood cleared of the drug as it passes through the liver.

In order to better understand hepatic clearance, an additional discussion on hepatic extraction ratio is necessary. For our purposes, suffice it to say that for a given drug, E depends on the liver's ability to metabolize that drug (termed *intrinsic clearance*), the fraction unbound in the blood, and the blood flow through the liver. Hepatic clearance is also dependent on these parameters. When drugs are categorized generally as low E, intermediate E, or high E, it allows us to gain a clinical understanding of the pharmacokinetics of a specific drug. For a low-E drug, hepatic clearance will depend on intrinsic clearance and the fraction unbound in blood. For a high-E drug, hepatic clearance is determined only by blood flow. The hepatic clearance of an intermediate-E drug will be dependent on all three determinants.

Another type of clearance is oral clearance. This term is useful when one desires to evaluate clearance in an oral dosing situation. Oral clearance differs from systemic clearance in that the hepatic first-pass effect contributes to the observed clearance. For a low-E drug, oral clearance would be about the same as systemic clearance, because the liver is not efficient at extracting drugs from blood coming from the intestines, so the first-pass effect would have very little impact on bioavailability. For a high-E drug, oral clearance will depend on the fraction unbound and intrinsic clearance. Since the liver is very efficient at clearing the drug, a large first-pass effect will be seen, resulting in a low bioavailability.

Next let us focus our discussion on renal clearance. Recalling the anatomy of the kidneys, the functional units (nephrons) basically perform three tasks. First is filtration of bulk fluid in the glomerulus. Glomerular filtration removes the bulk of substances from the blood, including creatinine. Therefore, creatinine clearance is considered an index of glomerular filtration rate, as well as overall kidney function in general. A patient's creatinine clearance is useful to know how well that patient's kidneys are working compared to a normal value (120 mL/min). To estimate a patient's creatinine clearance, see the appended equation sheet. Second, there is active secretion of specific substances by the renal tubules (tubular secretion), which is another mechanism for excretion of wastes. Third, there is reabsorption of some selected substances also in the renal tubules. In contrast to glomerular filtration and tubular secretion, tubular reabsorption decreases the amount of a substance excreted in urine.

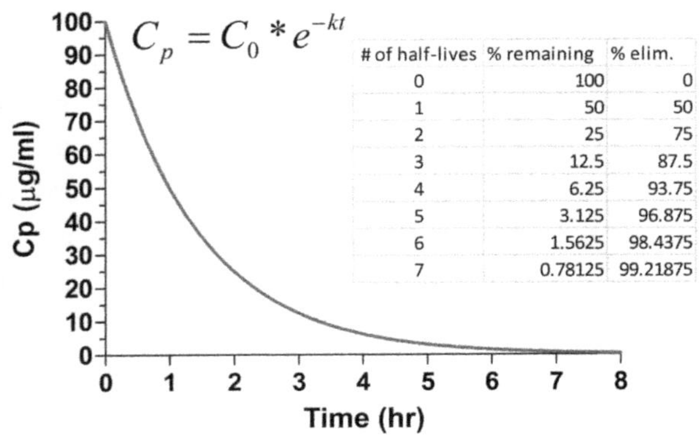

FIGURE 5.2 Monoexponential drug elimination.

When these are taken together, glomerular filtration rate (as indicated by creatinine clearance) and tubular secretion contribute positively to renal clearance, whereas tubular reabsorption contributes negatively.

How Long Do the Compounds Stay in the Body?

We have discussed clearance and volume. With these in mind, the course of plasma concentrations of a drug over time can be described by first-order elimination for many drugs. This means that the elimination rate is dependent on concentration, so that when the concentration in plasma is high, the elimination rate will also be high. As time goes on and elimination proceeds, the plasma concentration falls exponentially. In this case, we can describe the half-life of the drug, which is the time it takes for the plasma concentration to fall by a factor of one-half. When dosing is stopped, after five half-lives, a compound will be 97 percent eliminated. So, for practical purposes, we can say that the compound is "mostly gone" after five half-lives.

What Is a Dosing Regimen, and How Do We Choose One?

A dosing regimen comprises a dose to be given (e.g., 100 mg) and an interval between doses (dosing interval; e.g., every day). Clearance and half-life are important in choosing a dosage regimen. As stated earlier, half-life and the pharmacologic properties of the drug determine the dosing interval. To achieve a desired average steady-state concentration, dosing rate (dose divided by dosing interval) divided by the appropriate clearance term is a simple formula one can use in many cases.

The two most important pharmacokinetic concepts to understand are clearance and volume. With these, it is easier to understand dosing, pharmacokinetic drug interactions, and dosing regimen adjustments for different patient populations and disease states. Additionally, volume and clearance terms can be used to determine loading doses and maintenance doses, respectively.

Half-life can be used in conjunction with knowledge of a drug's pharmacologic properties to determine the appropriate dosing interval. Also, in first-order elimination, clearance is independent of concentration, so doubling the daily dosing rate will double the plasma concentration.

How Can I Use This Information?

Pharmacokinetics can be directly applied for those drugs whose dosing is extensively based on the pharmacokinetics of a drug in each patient. These concepts can be quite useful for clinicians. Many drug interactions can be evaluated, and dosage adjustments can be made for specific patient populations. Again, a detailed discussion will not be given for each of these; however, a few of these situations will be briefly reviewed.

Interactions between xenobiotics (drugs or herbal compounds) can be classified as either pharmacodynamic or pharmacokinetic. Pharmacokinetic drug interactions can then be described as altering the bioavailability, the clearance, and/or the volume of distribution of the target compound.

Other types of pharmacokinetic drug interactions are those resulting in an altered metabolism of the drugs. Generally, these interactions can be classified as those which increase the metabolic activity of the involved enzyme (enzyme induction) and those which decrease it (enzyme inhibition). Again, depending on the situation, these alterations in intrinsic clearance may or may not necessitate dosage regimen changes. To illustrate the scope of these drug interactions, a list of drugs interacting through the cytochrome P-450 complex is continually updated and available online at https://drug-interactions.medicine.iu.edu/clinical-table.aspx, courtesy of Dr. David Flockhart. One should remember that there are several other drug metabolism pathways as well. Drug interactions involving these other metabolic pathways would also work to alter hepatic clearance. Additionally, a few drug interactions may alter renal clearance, if there is appreciable tubular secretion or tubular reabsorption of the target drug. Metabolic interactions will be discussed below.

Pharmacokinetics is valuable in making dosage adjustments in special patient populations. In these special populations, their characteristics may result in altered protein binding, organ blood flow, body fluid composition, metabolic activity, gastrointestinal motility, and function of the liver and kidneys. Another example of patient populations requiring dosage adjustments due to pharmacokinetic differences from the normal adult population are seen at the age extremes. In geriatric populations, kidney and liver function are decreased, which may result in decreased renal and hepatic clearances, as well as a decreased first-pass effect. Decreases in muscle mass and increases in fat mass, as well as altered protein binding, may result in altered volumes of distribution.[2] In pediatric populations, changes in absorption may be seen due to increases in gastric pH and decreases in gastrointestinal motility. Depending on their age, increases or decreases in intrinsic clearance may be seen. Neonates may have immature kidney function, resulting in decreased renal clearance. Also, they have an increase in the weight-adjusted total body water, causing potential changes in volume of distribution.[2] In addition to physiologic differences associated with geriatrics and pediatrics, many other conditions may alter drug disposition.

How Do Natural Products Differ from Conventional Drugs in Their Pharmacokinetics?

First, it is quite rare for natural products to be given intravascularly in humans, so we can never really know several important pharmacokinetic parameters, such as systemic clearance, volume of distribution, and absolute oral bioavailability as they pertain to humans. However, even if only oral doses are given, and if plasma samples are obtained, we can determine the half-life and steady-state concentrations. Also, oral bioavailability can be compared between formulations or producers of herbal medications. Unfortunately, natural product pharmacokinetic properties are quite often not well established, and information provided to consumers is often based only on animal and in vitro studies.

Natural products include quite a diversity of chemical structures, and no attempt to be comprehensive will be made here. However, in order for any compound to be well absorbed orally, it must pass through three challenges: solubility, permeability, and presystemic metabolism. The active compound must reach the site of action in adequate concentrations to exert its effects, and in order to achieve sustained effects between dosing, it must not be eliminated too quickly.

How Do the Challenges of Solubility, Permeability, and Presystemic Metabolism Pertain to Natural Products?

As mentioned above, natural compounds include a wide range of solubility in water. For those with low solubility, doses may not dissolve adequately in gastrointestinal fluids before they are passed in the feces. For those with high solubility, dissolution is not problematic. However, once dissolved, the molecule must permeate the cell membranes of the intestinal epithelium in order to reach the blood. This presents a problem for molecules that carry a positive or negative charge, are large in structure (molecular weight >500 Daltons), or have too many hydrophilic (water-loving) functional groups (hydrogen bond donors and acceptors).[4] Many natural products fall outside of this chemical space and may thus be expected to have problematic absorption. Examples include glycosides (sugar conjugates), which have many hydroxyl (–OH) groups, such as procyanidin type-A polymer, found in cinnamon extract. On the other hand, molecules that are very lipophilic (fat-loving) are also

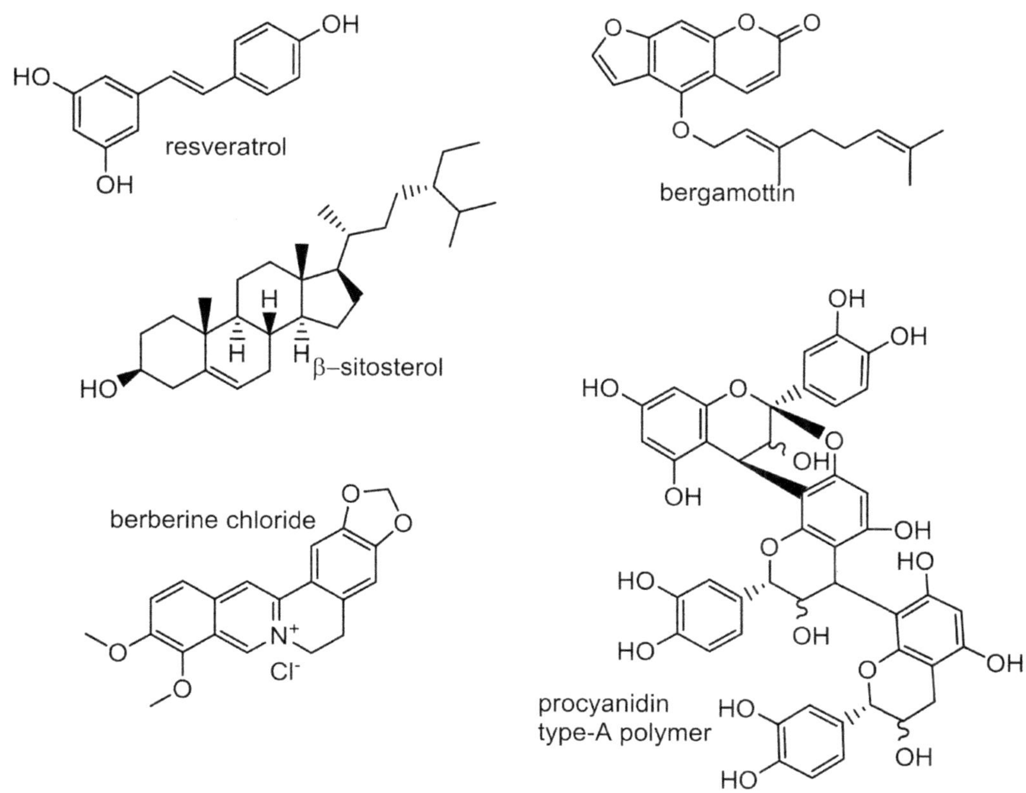

FIGURE 5.3 Chemical structures of some natural compounds.

problematic in terms of not only solubility but also membrane permeability.[4] Examples include plant sterols such as β-sitosterol.

Furthermore, there are proteins in the membranes of the cells lining the gastrointestinal tract, which may either help or hinder the absorption of certain compounds. This is illustrated in Figure 5.4 (courtesy of Absorption Systems, LLC), which represents the outer cell membrane of intestinal cells; the top of the membrane is facing the intestinal contents while the bottom is facing the inside of the intestinal cell (cytoplasm).

Once a molecule dissolves into gastrointestinal fluids and permeates the intestinal epithelium, it must still survive the exposure to xenobiotic-metabolizing enzymes in the intestinal cells and the liver. Although the specific enzymes and their expression levels differ, both the intestine and the liver express enzymes that can change the structures of various compounds in certain ways. Generally, the cytochrome P450 (CYP) family carries out oxidation reactions; the uridine diphosphate glucuronosyltransferase (UGT) family conjugates some hydrophilic groups with glucuronic acid; the sulfotransferase (SULT)

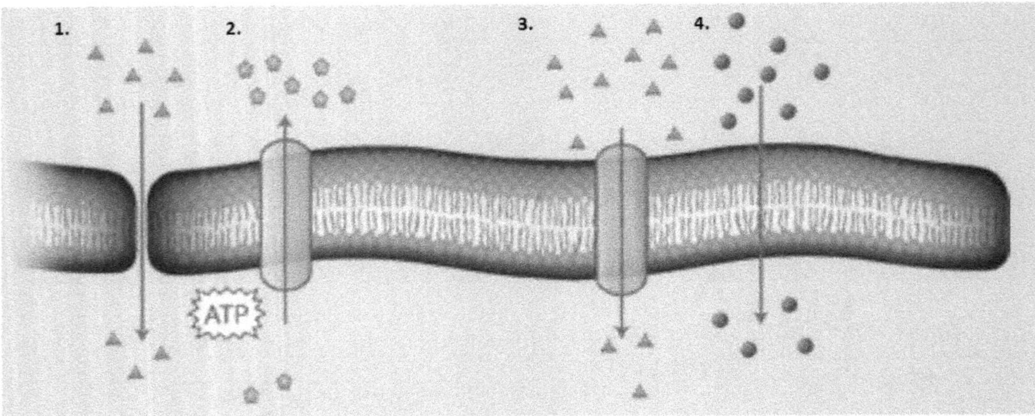

FIGURE 5.4 Membrane transport processes.
While some molecules may pass between the cells (process 1; paracellular diffusion) and other molecules may pass directly through the cell membrane (process 4; simple transcellular diffusion), some may interact with certain groups of transporters (processes 2 and 4). For example, the ATP-Binding Cassette transporters, such as P-glycoprotein, the Breast Cancer Resistance Pump, and the Multidrug Resistance-associate protein 2, may pump the compound back into the intestinal lumen (process 2).[5] Berberine is transported by P-glycoprotein, which works against its absorption.[6]

family conjugates hydroxyl groups with sulfate, as shown in the general scheme below (see Figure 5.5).

Additionally, several other enzymes, including esterases and saccharidases, can change the molecular structures. If a molecule survives metabolism in the intestine, the blood flow from the intestine will take it to the liver. Then the enzymes in the liver get a chance to metabolize the molecule. These enzymatic alterations to the molecular structures are called presystemic metabolism. In addition to metabolism in the human intestine and liver, molecules remaining in the gastrointestinal tract may be subject to metabolism by bacteria in the intestine. These gut bacteria may reduce carbon-carbon double bonds and cleave off sugar-like molecules.

An example of a natural product undergoing extensive presystemic metabolism is resveratrol. While resveratrol is hoped to have many beneficial effects, it undergoes rapid presystemic

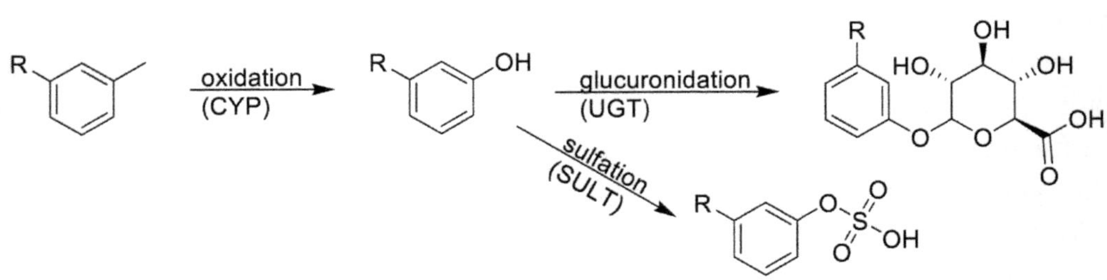

FIGURE 5.5 Examples of metabolism.

metabolism by SULT and UGT enzymes in the intestine and liver, forming multiple glucuronide and sulfate metabolites and various combinations thereof. Together, such extensive metabolism results in an absolute oral bioavailability of <1 percent.[7] Thus, many disappointments may occur when attempting to translate promising results from in vitro studies or animal experiments into human clinical benefits, unless this issue is overcome.

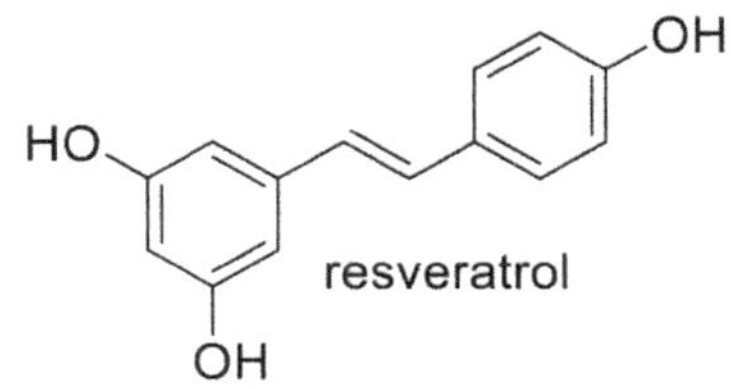

FIGURE 5.6 Structure of resveratrol.

What About Interactions Among Specific Natural Products and Medications?

Some people have mistakenly believed that because herbal substances are natural, they don't cause any problems like adverse interactions with medications. Instead, there are several well-established "herb-drug interactions" that can pose a serious health threat. For example, grapefruit juice contains components that can inhibit several CYP enzymes and cause severalfold increases in drug exposure.

To understand pharmacokinetic interactions among xenobiotics, two terms are commonly considered. One is peak concentration after the dose (C_{max}). The other term is total drug exposure, which is quantified by determining the area under the plasma concentration time curve (AUC). Following a single oral dose of any compound, the total AUC is determined by the compound's bioavailability, dose, and total clearance. So if one substance (perpetrator) causes either an increase in the bioavailability or a decrease in the clearance of another substance (victim), then the AUC of the victim substance will increase.

Back to grapefruit juice: it causes a fivefold increase in AUC of nisoldipine (antihypertensive drug), which could cause blood pressure to decrease dangerously low. It also causes a threefold increase in the AUC of cyclosporine, a drug which is an immunosuppressant used in organ transplant patients. Such an increase could cause excessive immune suppression; additionally, since cyclosporine is toxic to the kidneys, it could also result in kidney damage. Additionally, grapefruit juice nearly doubles the AUC of atorvastatin (antihyperlipidemic), and some patients have experienced serious side effects, such as muscle breakdown (rhabdomyolysis), on account of it. These adverse herb-drug interactions occur by components of grapefruit juice (such as naringin, bergamottin, and 6',7'-dihydroxybergamottin) inhibiting several CYP enzymes, including CYP3A4.[8] Thus we may expect that any compound that depends heavily on CYP3A4 for its clearance would show an increase in AUC when dosed along with grapefruit juice.

How Do Compounds Like Bergamottin Actually Inhibit Enzymes Like CYP3A4?

The nature of the interactions between enzyme inhibitors (perpetrators) and the enzymes they inhibit is worth at least a brief discussion. There are several types of enzyme inhibition interactions. The most common type is competitive inhibition, in which the inhibitor binds to the same site on the enzyme as the substrate (compound getting metabolized). The two compounds compete for binding, so that the inhibitor makes the substrate appear to bind with lower affinity, thus lowering the enzyme activity at concentrations usually seen *in vivo*. The interaction is entirely reversible, so that if the inhibitor disappears, the interaction stops. Other types of reversible inhibition mechanisms exist, and descriptions can be found elsewhere.[9] In addition, mechanism-based inhibition may occur, in which a compound gets metabolized into a reactive product, which then forms a covalent bond with the enzyme, making it inactive and thus incapable of metabolizing other substances. This is called mechanism-based or suicide inhibition and is thought to be how 6',7'-dihydroxybergamottin inhibits CYP3A4.[8] Many other compounds may inhibit enzymes in a competitive/reversible fashion, as described above.

Could Any of These Interactions Be Used in a Good Way?

Drug-drug, herb-drug, or herb-herb interactions involving enzyme inhibition could be bad or good, depending on whether the effects are desirable or undesirable. However, some interactions may be desirable. In the pharmaceutical industry, occasionally intentional drug-drug interactions are built into the product. For example, KALETRA® is a coformulation of lopinavir (as the active antiretroviral agent) with ritonavir (a strong inhibitor of CYP3A4).[10] Thus in this product, ritonavir inhibits the metabolism of lopinavir, increasing its oral bioavailability and decreasing its clearance, thus improving the patient's systemic exposure to lopinavir (increased AUC).

In the dietary supplement industry, piperine is used to inhibit metabolism of curcumin and demonstrates a 20-fold increase in AUC when the two compounds are combined.[11] Another example is silibinin (from milk thistle), which is used to treat amatoxin poisoning from poisonous mushrooms.[12] Pterostilbene inhibits the intestinal and hepatic metabolism of buprenorphine, a drug used to treat opioid use disorder.[13][14] Thus pterostilbene may also be useful for enhancing the oral bioavailability of buprenorphine.

Which Herb-Drug Interactions Should I Watch Out For?

Some herbs may interact through mechanisms similar to certain drugs, thus showing increased effects, and some of these effects are difficult to predict. Other natural

TABLE 5.1

Natural Product	Drug Affected
black pepper	nevirapine
St. John's wort	various drugs
peppermint	antacids
peppermint	felodipine, other calcium channel blockers
gingko biloba	nifedipine
berberine	cyclosporine A
grapefruit juice	various drugs

products have been demonstrated clinically to have notable effects on drugs, as listed in Table 5.1.[15]

Furthermore, a list of 18 herbal products of concern for herb-drug interactions has been published.[16] These include black cohosh, coenzyme Q10, cranberry, echinacea, evening primrose oil, valerian, St. John's wort, saw palmetto, melatonin, kava, ginseng, yohimbe, feverfew, gingko biloba, goldenseed, garlic, green tea, and ginger. It is best to check with your health care providers before using these dietary supplements with other medications.

Where Can I Go for More Information About Herb-Drug Interactions?

Although there is a tremendous amount of information available on the internet, the reliability of much of it is difficult to determine. Even if the information is reliable, its application to a particular patient situation is difficult to interpret. However, your local pharmacist is trained in understanding the mechanisms involved (as discussed above, and much more!) and can also help evaluate a certain specific situation or combination. You should also talk with your physician before making any changes to your medication regimen. Beware of information from advertisers, which have been found to contain biased interpretations of data. The United States Food and Drug Administration (FDA) also has helpful information regarding dietary supplements on their website: https://www.fda.gov/food/dietary-supplements/information-consumers-using-dietary-supplements.

References

1. Malcolm Rowland and Thomas N. Tozer, *Clinical Pharmacokinetics: Concepts and Applications*, 2nd ed. (Philadelphia: Lea & Febiger, 1989).
2. William E. Evans, Jerome J. Schentag, and William J. Jusko, *Applied Pharmacokinetics: Principles of Therapeutic Drug Monitoring*, 3rd ed. (Vancouver, WA: Applied Therapeutics, Inc., 1992).
3. Leon Shargel L. and Andrew B. C. Yu, *Applied Biopharmaceutics and Pharmacokinetics*, 7th ed. (New York: McGraw-Hill Education, 2016).
4. Christopher A. Lipinski et al., "Experimental and Computational Approaches to Estimate Solubility and Permeability in Drug Discovery and Development Settings," *Advanced Drug Delivery Reviews* 46, no. 1–3 (2001): 3–26.
5. Young Hee Choi and Ai-Ming Yu, "ABC Transporters in Multidrug Resistance and Pharmacokinetics, and Strategies for Drug Development," *Current Pharmaceutical Design* 20, no. 5 (2014): 793–807.
6. Weibin Zha et al., "Inhibition of P-Glycoprotein by HIV Protease Inhibitors Increases Intracellular Accumulation of Berberine in Murine and Human Macrophages," *PLoS One* 8, no. 1 (2013): e54349.
7. Thomas Walle, "Bioavailability of Resveratrol," *Annals of the New York Academy of Sciences* 1215, no. 1 (2011): 9–15.
8. A. M. Evans, "Influence of Dietary Components on the Gastrointestinal Metabolism and Transport of Drugs," *Therapeutic Drug Monitoring* 22, no. 1 (2000): 131–36.
9. K. Sandy Pang, A. David Rodrigues, and Raimund M. Peter, eds., *Enzyme- and Transporter-Based Drug-Drug Interactions* (New York: Springer, 2010).
10. Wolters Kluwer Health, "Lopinavir and Ritonavir," *UpToDate*, https://www.uptodate.com/contents/lopinavir-and-ritonavir-drug-information/print.
11. G. Shoba et al., "Influence of Piperine on the Pharmacokinetics of Curcumin in Animals and Human Volunteers," *Planta Medica* 64, no. 4 (1998): 353–56.
12. Ulrich Mengs, Ralf-Torsten Pohl, and Todd Mitchell, "Legalon(R) SIL: The Antidote of Choice in Patients with Acute Hepatotoxicity from Amatoxin Poisoning," *Current Pharmaceutical Biotechnology.* 13, no. 10 (2012): 1964–70.
13. Neha Maharao, Jurgen Venitz, and Phillip M. Gerk, "Use of Generally Recognized as Safe or Dietary Compounds to Inhibit Buprenorphine Metabolism: Potential to Improve Buprenorphine Oral Bioavailability," *Biopharmaceutics and Drug Disposition* 40, no. 1 (2019): 18–31.
14. Neha V. Maharao, Anand A. Joshi, and Phillip M. Gerk, "Inhibition of Glucuronidation and Oxidative Metabolism of Buprenorphine Using GRAS Compounds or Dietary Constituents/Supplements: *In Vitro* Proof of Concept," *Biopharmaceutics and Drug Dispositions* 38, no. 2 (2017): 139–54.

15. Elizabeth Williamson, Samuel Driver, and Karen Baxter, eds., *Stockley's Herbal Medicines Interactions* (Grayslake, IL: Pharmaceutical Press, 2009).
16. L. Anderson, "18 Herbal Supplements with Risky Drug Interactions," Drugs.com, July 8, 2019, https://www.drugs.com/slideshow/herb-drug-interactions-1069.

Credits

Fig 5.1b: Source: https://commons.wikimedia.org/wiki/File:Filled_Syringe_icon.svg.

Fig 5.4: Copyright © by Absorption Systems. Reprinted with permission.

Appendix 1: Basic Pharmacokinetic Equations (Adapted from Rowland and Tozer, 1989)

$$\text{volume of distribution} = \frac{\text{(IV dose)}}{\text{(initial concentration)}}$$

$$\text{volume of distribution} = \frac{\text{plasma volume + (tissue volume) * (fraction unbound in plasma)}}{\text{(fraction unbound in tissue)}}$$

systemic clearance = hepatic clearance + renal clearance

hepatic clearance = (liver blood flow) * (hepatic extraction ratio)

$$\text{hepatic clearance} = \frac{\text{(liver blood flow) * (fraction unbound in plasma) * (intrinsic clearance)}}{\text{(liver blood flow) + (fraction unbound in plasma) * (intrinsic clearance)}}$$

renal clearance = glomerular filtration + tubular secretion – tubular reabsorption

$$\text{oral clearance} = \frac{\text{systemic clearance}}{\text{bioavailability}}$$

$$\text{creatinine clearance} = \frac{\text{(140 – age) * (ideal body weight)}}{\text{72 * (serum creatinine conc.)}}$$ [Multiply by 0.85 for females]

$$\text{elimination rate constant} = \frac{\text{systemic clearance}}{\text{volume of distribution}}$$

$$\text{half-life} = \frac{0.693}{\text{(elimination rate constant)}}$$

IV loading dose = (desired concentration) * (volume of distribution)

IV maintenance dosing rate = (desired concentration) * (systemic clearance)

Part III

Natural Products

Chapter 6

Introduction to Natural Products

Yan Zhang and Yi Zheng

NATURAL PRODUCTS HAVE BEEN APPLIED FOR medicinal purposes for thousands of years, and they are still playing very important roles in our lives, especially in drug discovery and development. With the development of technologies nowadays, diverse kinds of natural products have been isolated, identified, and characterized from natural resources, such as plants, animals, microorganisms, and marine environments. For example, quinine (see Figure 6.1) was isolated from the cinchona tree and used for curing malaria and babesiosis for a long time.[1] Zetekitoxin AB (see Figure 6.1) was found in the Panamanian gold frog and used as a potent neurotoxin.[2] Penicillin and its analogues (see Figure 6.1), a group of antibiotics, were discovered by Alexander Fleming in 1928, and they are still widely used for bacterial infections today.[3] Tetrodotoxin (see Figure 6.1), a potent neurotoxin, was discovered in some ocean fishes and can act as a sodium channel blocker.[4]

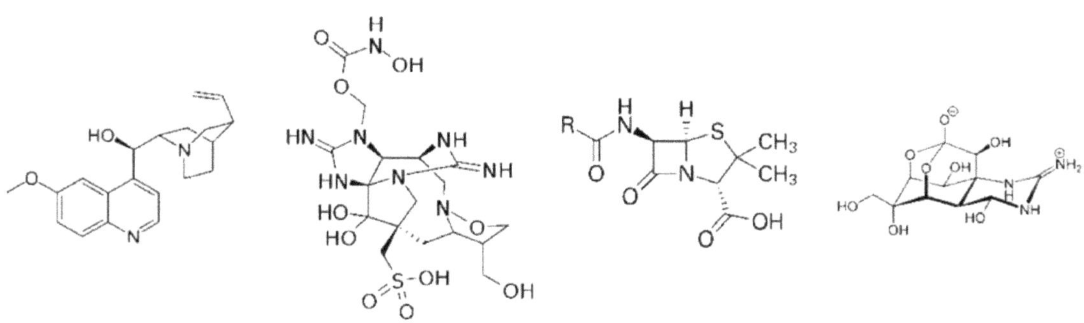

Quinine | Zetekitoxin AB | Penicillin | Tetrodotoxin

FIGURE 6.1 The structures of Quinine, Zetekitoxin AB, Penicillin, and Tetrodotoxin.

Natural products may not only be directly applied for treating diseases as drugs but also may act as a precious source for drug discovery and development.[5][6] Newman, Cragg, and Snader summarized and analyzed the number of natural products (NPs), semisynthesized natural products (SSNPs), and natural product derivatives (NPDs) from 1981 to 2002.[7] They found that natural products played an important role in drug discovery, especially in the fields of hypertension and cancer. Butler summarized and analyzed the number of NPs, SSNPs, and NPDs on the market in the United States, Europe, and Japan in 2005, 2008, and 2013.[8][9][10] Fifty-nine NP drugs, SSNP drugs, and NPD drugs were approved from 1998 to 2013. If we pay attention to small molecule drugs launched on the market from 2005 to 2013, the important role of NPs or NPDs in drug discovery will be further supported: 22 percent in 2005 (six of 25), 9 percent in 2006 (two of 21), 24 percent in 2007 (five of 21), 14 percent in 2008 (three of 19), 17 percent in 2009 (five of 24), 32 percent in 2010 (six of 19), 14 percent in 2011 (three of 21), 21 percent in 2012 (six of 28), and 8 percent in 2013 (two of 25).[8][9][10][11][12][13][14]

With an in-depth study of natural products by adopting modern analytical technology development, we may understand the critical structural features of natural products and how these structural features may provide us valuable information in designing and synthesizing novel chemical entities.[15] First, the typical structures of natural products are of architectural complexity and have many stereogenic centers, such as vancomycin (see Figure 6.2). It is to be noted that these complex structures always include special functional groups, such as calicheamicin. The structure of calicheamicin contains highly active function groups, enediynes and trisulphide.[16] Both of these are redox-active groups and can induce the generation of radical intermediates to damage DNA. The dithian-1,3-oxide group in leinamycin (see Figure 6.2) reacts with DNA by formatting episulphonium intermediate.[17] Both expoxomicin and fumagillin inhibit the activity of proteases by forming a covalent trap with their epoxide groups. These examples reveal that the special structural features of natural products play an import role in their activation mechanism. Second, compared with synthesized compounds, most natural products are composed of carbon, hydrogen, oxygen, and nitrogen, with less heteroatom. The structures of natural products have significantly conformational preferences, such as ring systems, and special crosslinks. For example, telomestatin (see Figure 6.2) has a macrocyclizations ring system. Staurosporine has a special fused-ring system. These conformational preferences demonstrate the low entropy status of natural products, which will allow natural products to bind with their targets more efficiently. That is why many natural products have a potency range of 10-7 to 10-9 M. Third, many molecular masses of natural products are more than 500 Daltons and present high solubility in water. Based on Lipinski's Rule of Five, oral administration may not be a good option for most natural products.

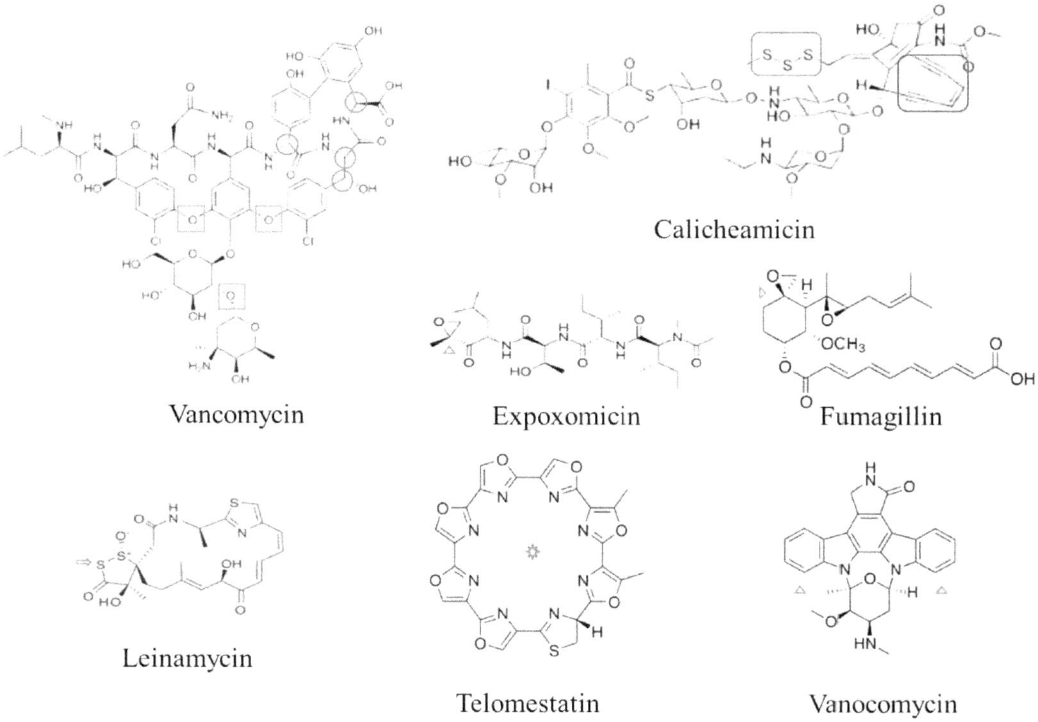

FIGURE 6.2 The structures of Vancomycin, Leinamycin, Calicheamicin, Expoxomicin, Fumagillin, Telomestatin, and Vanocomycin.

Though natural products are a valuable resource for drug discovery, there are still multiple challenges that need to be addressed. One of them is how to supply the useful natural products in a cost- and time-feasible way. To tackle this problem, diverse methods are developed in chemistry, biochemistry, molecular biology, and genetics. Taking paclitaxel as an example, paclitaxel (see Figure 6.3) is a very famous natural product used for treating a number of cancers, such as ovarian cancer, breast cancer, lung cancer, and so on.[18] It was first isolated from Pacific yew in 1971 and displayed impressive pharmacological effect.

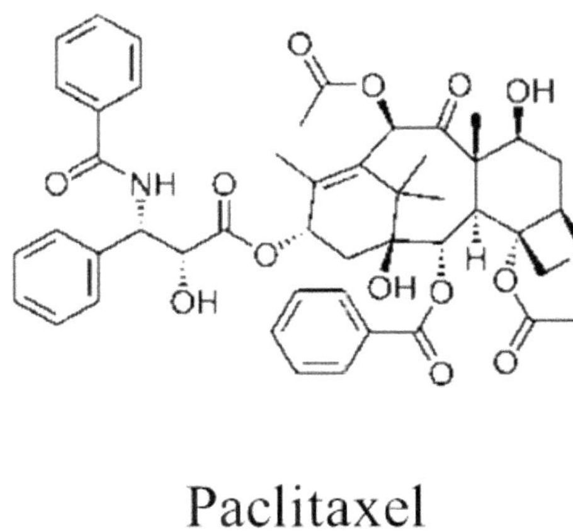

FIGURE 6.3 The structure of Paclitaxel.

However, the yield of pure paclitaxel is very low (10 g from 1,200 kg of bark).[19] Keeping this in mind, different methods are used for preparing pure paclitaxel, such as total synthesis,[20][21] semisynthesis,[19] and biosynthesis;[22][23] cell culture is also used to manufacture it now. Although we have made great progress in synthesis chemistry, finding an effective route to mass supply a natural product is still a challenge to the medicinal chemistry program.

References

1. G. Dennis Shanks, "Historical Review: Problematic Malaria Prophylaxis with Quinine," *American Journal of Tropical Medicine and Hygiene* 95, no. 2 (2016): 269–72.
2. Shenping Liu et al., "Structure of Human Methionine Aminopeptidase-2 Complexed with Fumagillin," *Science* 282, no. 5392 (1998): 1324–27.
3. Nelson Kardos and Arnold L. Demain, "Penicillin: The Medicine with the Greatest Impact on Therapeutic Outcomes," *Applied Microbiology and Biotechnology* 92, no. 4 (2011): 677–87.
4. Max Niko Lorentz et al., "Tetrodotoxin," *Current Biology* 26, no. 19 (2016): R870–72.
5. Frank E. Koehn and Guy Thomas Carter, "The Evolving Role of Natural Products in Drug Discovery," *Nature Reviews Drug Discovery* 4, no. 3 (2005): 206–220.
6. David J. Newman and Gordon M. Cragg, "Natural Products as Sources of New Drugs over the 30 Years from 1981 to 2010," *Journal of Natural Products* 75, no. 3 (2012): 311–35.
7. David J. Newman, Gordon M. Cragg, and Kenneth M. Snader, "Natural Products as Sources of New Drugs over the Period 1981–2002," *Journal of Natural Products* 66, no. 7 (2003): 1022–37.
8. Mark S. Butler, "Natural Products to Drugs: Natural Product Derived Compounds in Clinical Trials," *Natural Product Reports* 22, no. 2 (2005): 162–95.
9. Mark S. Butler, "Natural Products to Drugs: Natural Product Derived Compounds in Clinical Trials," *Natural Product Reports* 25, no. 3 (2008): 475–516.
10. Mark S. Butler, "Natural Products to Drugs: Natural Product Derived Compounds in Clinical Trials," *Natural Product Reports* 31, no. 11 (2014): 1612–61.
11. A. I. Graul and J. R. Prous, "The Year's New Drugs," *Drug News and Perspectives* 19, no. 1 (2006): 33–53.
12. A. I. Graul et al., "The Year's New Drugs and Biologics—2006," *Drug News and Perspectives* 20, no. 1 (2007): 17–44.
13. Shridhar Hegde and Michelle Schmidt, "To Market, to Market," in *Annual Reports in Medicinal Chemistry.* 42, edited by John E. Macor (Amsterdam: Academic Press, 2007), 505–54.
14. A. I. Graul et al., "The Year's New Drugs and Biologics—2007," *Drug News and Perspectives* 21, no. 1 (2008): 7–35.
15. Jon Clardy and Christopher Walsh, "Lessons from Natural Molecules," *Nature*, 432, no. 7019 (2004): 829–37.

16. May D. Lee et al., "Calicheamicins, a Novel Family of Antitumor Antibiotics," *Journal of the American Chemical Society* 109 (1987): 3464–66.
17. Masataka Konishi et al., "Crystal and Molecular Structure of Dynemicin A: A Novel 1,5-diyn-3-ene Antitumor Antibiotic," *Journal of the American Chemical Society* 112, no. 9 (1990): 3715–16.
18. Beth A. Weaver, "How Taxol/Paclitaxel Kills Cancer Cells," *Molecular Biology of the Cell* 25, no. 18 (2014): 2677–81.
19. Jordan Goodman and Vivien Walsh, *The Story of Taxol: Nature and Politics in the Pursuit of an Anti-Cancer Drug* (Cambridge, UK: Cambridge University Press, 2001).
20. Robert A. Holton et al., "First Total Synthesis of Taxol. 1," *Journal of the American Chemical Soc*iety 116, no. 4 (1994): 1597–98.
21. Robert A. Holton et al., "First Total Synthesis of Taxol. 2. Completion of the C and D Rings," *Journal of the American Chemical Society* 116, no. 4 (1994): 1599–1600.
22. Brett A. Boghigian et al., "Simultaneous Production and Partitioning of Heterologous Polyketide and Isoprenoid Natural Products in an *Escherichia coli* Two-Phase Bioprocess," *Journal of Industrial Microbiology and Biotechnology* 38, no. 11 (2011): 1809–20.
23. Benedikt Engels, Pia Dahm, and Stefan Jennewein, "Metabolic Engineering of Taxadiene Biosynthesis in Yeast as a First Step Towards Taxol (Paclitaxel) Production. *Metabolic Engineering* 10, no. 3–4 (2008): 201–206.

Chapter 7

Natural Products for Pain Management

Shijun Zhang, Hallie M. Blevins, Jakob C. Green, and Liu He

Opiates

History

Opium poppy belongs to the *Papaver somniferum* species and is cultivated worldwide. The history of the opium poppy plant dates back to the ancient time of Mesopotamia, around 4000 BC.[1] Opium poppy seeds are edible and are widely used for baking. Poppy plants provide white, pink, red, and purple flowers; therefore they are also known as the common garden poppy. Opium poppy is well known to produce raw opium, dried latex from the unripe *P. somniferum* seedpods, and for its powerful analgesic effects (see Figure 7.1).[1]

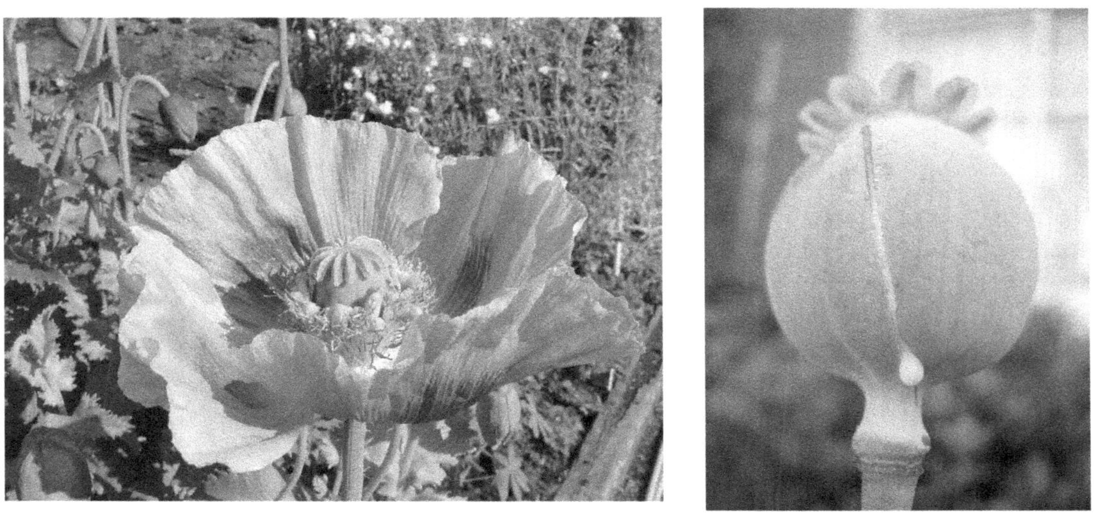

FIGURE 7.1 Images of opium poppy and seedpod with latex.

The writing of Theophrastus around 200 BC described the tonic use of opium.[2] In the early 17th century, many viewed opium as an effective medicine to treat pain, without realizing its abuse liability. Therefore, raw opium was freely available from pharmacy stores around Europe during that period of time.[1] In the United States of America, products of opium also gained popularity around the same time due to its strong analgesic effects.[3]

Chemical Composition of Opium

The opium from *P. somniferum* contains various alkaloids, and the four principle ingredients are morphine, codeine, thebaine, and papaverine (see Figure 7.2). Structurally, among these four principle ingredients, morphine, codeine, and thebaine share a morphinan core scaffold, while papaverine is an isoquinoline-based compound. Pharmacologically, morphine and codeine have analgesic effects, while papaverine shows vasodilating effects. Thebaine does not have any analgesic effects and is mainly used as a starting material to produce morphine analogs.

Morphine was first isolated from opium in 1805 by a German pharmacist, Friedrich Wilhelm Sertürner. In view of its dream-inducing properties, the compound was named *morphine* after Morpheus, the Greek god of dreams. The chemical structure of morphine was elucidated in 1925, and the total synthesis of morphine was achieved in 1952.[4][5]

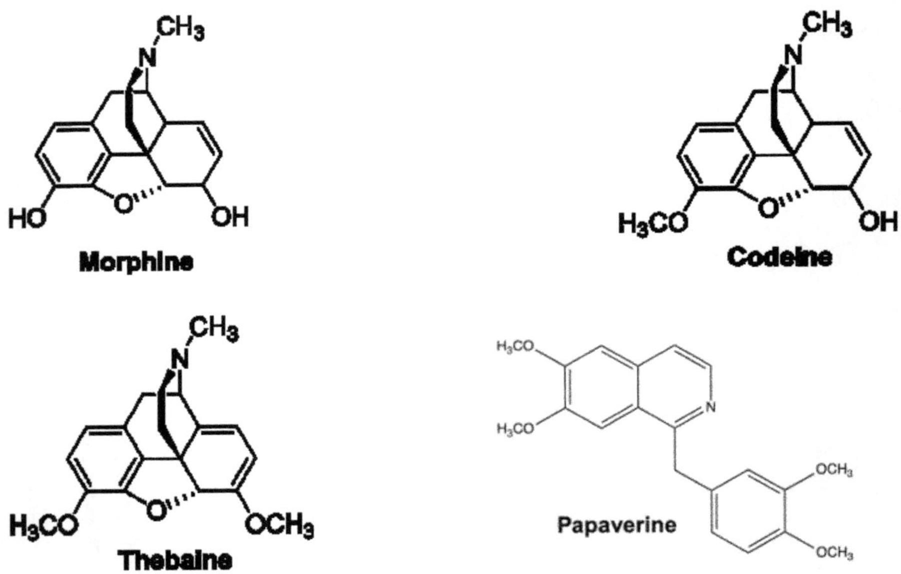

FIGURE 7.2 Major chemical constituents isolated from opium.

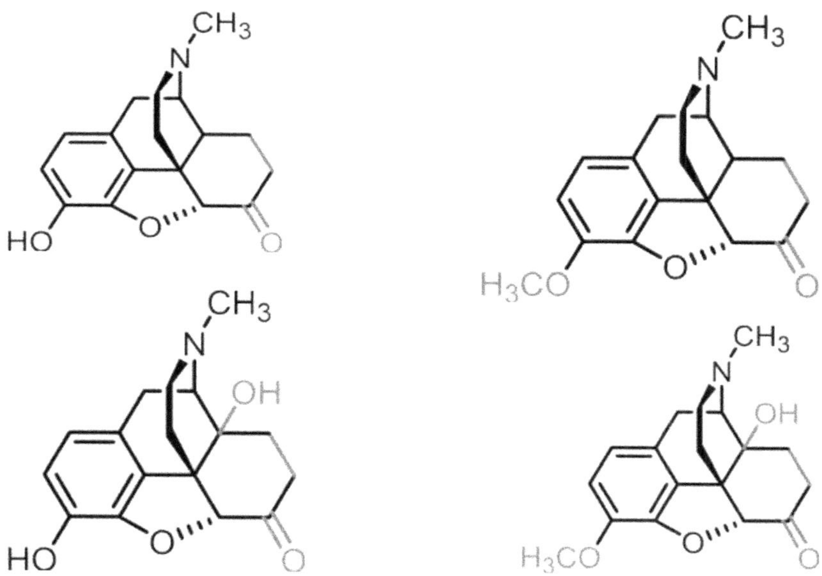

FIGURE 7.3 Chemical structures of synthetic morphine analogs.

Codeine was first isolated from opium in 1832 by French pharmacist Pierre Jean Robiquet. The total synthesis of codeine was achieved in 1973.[1]

Due to the abuse liability of morphine, extensive studies have been conducted to develop newer analogs without abuse and dependence side effects. A series of synthetic analogs (opioids) have been successfully developed (see Figure 7.3), but most of them still have abuse liability.[6][7][8][9][10][11][12]

There has also been a nomenclature change for opioids. Historically, opioids have been termed narcotics, and this is mainly because the addictive side effects of opioids can cause sleep. Since the isolation and identification of morphine, the terminology of opiates was extensively used to refer to any structurally morphine-like compounds until the 1980s.[6] With the identification of endogenous opioid receptor peptides in the 1970s, the term opioid was introduced to indicate any compounds that can produce morphine-like pharmacological actions, and these actions can be antagonized by naloxone.[6]

Mechanism of Action

The biological targets through which morphine and opioid analogs exert analgesic effects are opioid receptors.[13][14] Three classes of opioid receptors have been cloned and established, namely μ-receptor (MOR), κ-receptor (KOR), and δ-receptor (DOR).[15][16] Most of the analgesic effects are produced through interactions with the MOR.[17]

Capsaicin

History

Capsaicin (8-methyl-N-vanillyl-6-nomenamide) is one of the active chemical components found in chili peppers, which belong to the genus *Capsicum* (see Figure 7.4). Several structurally similar compounds, capsaicinoids, have also been isolated from the chili pepper plant, though not as much as capsaicin. Members of the genus *Capsicum* have long been used in culinary and medicinal applications. In many areas of the world, the spice and heat add a painfully pleasant flavor. Capsaicin is a vanilloid analog and comprises 69–80 percent of the total capsaicinoids isolated from chili peppers, though the concentration may vary depending on the species of pepper studied. Dihydrocapsaicin, the saturated analog of capsaicin, comprises 22 percent of the total capsaicinoids isolated.[18] Capsaicin is mostly enriched in the pepper placental tissue that surrounds the seeds.[19] This is probably related to its biological functions in seed germination.[20] The compound was first isolated in 1816, and total synthesis was achieved in 1930.[21]

Dosage and Uses

Capsaicin is currently available as an 8-percent transdermal patch for the treatment of neuropathic pain associated with postherpetic neuralgia. It is also available as an over-the-counter (OTC) product in various concentrations as a cream (0.025%, 0.075%, or 0.75%) for minor pain relief. Capsaicin is also under clinical trials for rheumatoid arthritis, spinal cord injury–related neuropathic pain management, preventive agent for prostate cancer, and cyclical vomiting.

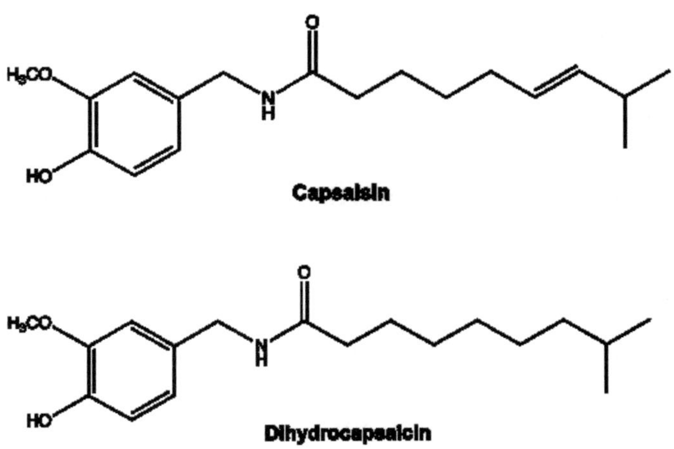

FIGURE 7.4 Structures of capsaicin and dihydrocapsaicin.

Mechanisms of Action

Capsaicin works by activating transient receptor potential cation channel subfamily V member 1 (TRPV1) to induce pain. TRPV1 is a six transmembrane helix membrane spanning channel and is a nonselective cation channel with homology to the voltage-gated potassium channels. It allows permeability to Na^+, K^+, Cs^+, Rb^+, Li^+, and several divalent cations such as Ca^{2+} and Mg^{2+}.[22] TRPV1 is activated by heat at 42°C and sensitized to activation by acidity, depending on the concentration.[23] Low pH concentrations (<6.2) result in the activation of the channel and at the same time will desensitize the conductance of TRPV1.[24][25][26][27] Once activated, ions are allowed to flow through the channel, promoting depolarization and propagation of the stimulus. Because of the role of TRPV1 in the transmission of signals of heat, TRPV1 plays important roles in inflammation and pain. Capsaicin is a selective TRPV1 agonist with high binding affinity.[28] Repeated exposure of TRPV1 to capsaicin gradually leads to desensitization of this receptor, then inhibition of the receptor function. Studies also suggested other analgesic mechanisms for capsaicin, such as inhibition of Piezo protein, degeneration of sensory fibers, and depletion of substance P centrally.[29][30][31][32]

References

1. Paul L. Schiff, "Opium and Its Alkaloids," *American Journal of Pharmaceutical Education* 66, no. 2 (2002): 186–94.
2. John Scarborough, "Theophrastus on Herbals and Herbal Remedies," *Journal of the History of Biology* 11, no. 2 (1978): 353–85.
3. Gillian R. Hamilton and Thomas F. Baskett, "In the Arms of Morpheus: The Development of Morphine for Postoperative Pain Relief. *Canadian Journal of Anesthesia* 47, no. 4 (2000): 367–74.
4. B. N. Dhawan et al., "International Union of Pharmacology XII. Classification of Opioid Receptors," *Pharmacological Reviews* 48, no. 4 (1996): 567–92.
5. Sándor Benyhe, "Morphine: New Aspects in the Study of an Ancient Compound," *Life Sciences* 55, no. 13 (1994): 969–79.
6. Mariana Spetea et al., "The μ Opioid Receptor and Ligands Acting at the μ Opioid Receptor as Therapeutics and Potential Therapeutics," *Current Pharmaceutical Design* 19, no. 42 (2013): 7415–34.
7. Mariana Spetea et al., "Effect of a 6-Cyano Substituent in 14-Oxygenated Nmethylmorphinans on Opioid Receptor Binding and Antinociception," *Journal of Medicinal Chemistry* 48, no. 15 (2005): 5052–55.
8. Eija Kalso, "Oxycodone," *Journal of Pain and Symptom Management* 29, no. 5 (2005): S47–S56.
9. Julia Riley et al., "Oxycodone: A Review of Its Use in the Management of Pain," *Current Medical Research and Opinion* 24, no. 1 (2008): 175–92.

10. Clifford J. Woolf and Maliha Hashimi, "Use and Abuse of Opioid Analgesics: Potential Methods to Prevent and Deter Non-Medical Consumption of Prescription Opioids.," *Current Opinion in Investigational Drugs* 5, no. 1 (2004): 61–66.
11. Fadia Mayyas et al., "A Systematic Review of Oxymorphone in the Management of Chronic Pain," *Journal of Pain and Symptom Management* 39, no. 2 (2010): 296–308.
12. Mariana Spetea and Helmut Schmidhammer, "Recent Advances in the Development of 14-Alkoxy Substituted Morphinans as Potent and Safer Opioid Analgesics," *Current Medicinal Chemistry* 19, no. 15 (2012): 2442–57.
13. A. E. Takemori and P. S. Portoghese, "Evidence for the Interaction of Morphine with Kappa and Delta Opioid Receptors to Induce Analgesic in Beta-Funaltrexamine-Treated Mice," *Journal of Pharmacology and Experimental Therapeutics* 243, no. 1 (1987): 91–94.
14. W. R. Martin et al., "The Effects of Morphine- and Nalorphine-Dependent Chronic Spinal Dog," *Journal of Pharmacology and Experimental Therapeutics* 197, no. 3 (1976): 517–532.
15. Brigitte L. Kieffer et al., "The Delta Opioid Receptor: Isolation of cDNA by Expression Cloning and Pharmacological Characterization," *Proceedings of the National Academy of Sciences USA* 89, no. 24 (1992): 12048–52.
16. Yan Chen et al., "Molecular Cloning and Functional Expression of a mu-Opioid Receptor from Rat Brain," *Molecular Pharmacology* 44, no. 1 (1993): 8–12.
17. Jia-Bei Wang et al., "Human mu Opiate Receptor: cDNA and Genomic Clones, Pharmacologic Characterization and Chromosomal Assignment," *FEBS Letters* 338, no. 2 (1994): 217–22.
18. David John Bennett and Gordon William Kirby, "Constitution and Biosynthesis of Capsaicin," *Journal of the Chemical Society C: Organic* 1 (1968): 442–46.
19. Joshua J. Tewksbury and Gary P. Nabhan, "Directed Deterrence by Capsaicin in Chillies," *Nature* 412 (2001): 403–4.
20. Miriam Monforte-Gonzalez et al., "Capsaicin Accumulation Is Related to Nitrate Content in Placentas of Habanero Peppers (*Capsicum chinense* Jacq.)," *Journal of the Science of Food and Agriculture* 90, no. 5 (2010): 764–68.
21. Ernst Späth and Stephen F. Darling, "Synthese des Capsaicins," *European Journal of Inorganic Chemistry* 63, no. 3 (1930): 737–43.
22. Stuart Bevan, Talisia Quallo, and David A. Andersson, "TRPV1," in *Handbook of Experimental Pharmacology: Mammalian Transient Receptor Potential (TRP) Cation Channels (vol. 1)*, edited by Bernd Nilius and Veit Flockerzi (Berlin: Springer, 2014): 207–45.
23. Michael J. Caterina et al., "The Capsaicin Receptor: A Heat-Activated Ion Channel in the Pain Pathway," *Nature* 389, no. 6653 (1997): 816–24.
24. S. Bevan and J. Yeats, "Protons Activate a Cation Conductance in a Sub-Population of Dorsal Root Ganglion Neurons," *Journal of Physiology* 433, no. 1 (1991): 145–61.

25. Makoto Tominaga et al., "The Cloned Capsaicin Receptor Integrates Multiple Pain-Producing Stimuli," *Neuron* 21, no. 3 (1998): 531–43.
26. John B. Davis et al., "Vanilloid Receptor-1 Is Essential for Inflammatory Thermal Hyperalgesia," *Nature* 405, no. 6785 (2000): 183–87.
27. M. J. Caterina et al., "Impaired Nociception and Pain Sensation in Mice Lacking the Capsaicin Receptor," *Science* 288, no. 5464 (2000): 306–13.
28. S. Bevan et al., "Capsazepine: A Competitive Antagonist of the Sensory Neurone Excitant Capsaicin," *British Journal of Pharmacology* 107, no. 2 (1992): 544–52.
29. István Borbiró, Doreen Badheka, and Tibor Rohacs, "Activation of TRPV1 Channels Inhibits Mechanosensitive Piezo Channel Activity by Depleting Membrane Phosphoinositides," *Science Signaling* 8, no. 363 (2015): 1–15.
30. Christopher H. Gibbons, Ningshan Wang, and Roy Freeman, "Capsaicin Induces Degeneration of Cutaneous Autonomic Nerve Fibers," *Annals of Neurology* 68, no. 6 (2010): 888–98.
31. Nina N. Sun et al., "Tachykinin Substance P Depletion by Capsaicin Exacerbates Inflammatory Response to Sidestream Cigarette Smoke in Rats," *Toxicology* 201, no. 1–3 (2004): 39–50.
32. Daniel K. I. Bring, "Residual Substance P Levels After Capsaicin Treatment," *Wound Repair and Regeneration* 20, no. 1 (2012): 50–60.

Credits

Fig 7.1a: Copyright © 2017 by Louise Jolly, (CC BY-SA 1.0) at https://commons.wikimedia.org/wiki/File:Opium_poppy.jpg.

Fig 7.1b: Source: https://commons.wikimedia.org/wiki/File:Opium_pod_cut_to_demonstrate_fluid_extraction1.jpg.

Chapter 8

Natural Products for Anxiety and Insomnia Treatment

Shijun Zhang, Hallie M. Blevins, Jakob C. Green, and Liu He

ANXIETY DISORDERS ARE SERIOUS MEDICAL CONDITIONS that affect about 25 million Americans annually and significantly reduce productivity. Insomnia is one of the most reported complaints among adults, along with the aging process. Insomnia is also a common problem in patients with chronic illness. A number of different classes of pharmacotherapies have been approved by the FDA to manage or treat both disorders, and this includes benzodiazepines, barbiturates, serotonin reuptake inhibitors, serotonin norepinephrine reuptake inhibitors, and antidepressants. Besides the FDA-approved pharmacotherapies, several herbal products have been traditionally used as anxiolytics.

Kava Kava

History

The ancient origins of kava drinking are known to trace back at least 3,000 years and are associated with both social and ceremonial functions. It was, and is, highly valued for its medicinal uses as a sedative, muscle relaxant, diuretic, and remedy for nervousness and insomnia.[1] Kava, which is sometimes known is *awa* or *yaqona*, is produced from kava kava, a pepper plant typically found in the South Pacific islands that belongs to the *Piper methysticum* species (see Figure 8.1). The portion used is the roots. The kava drink is traditionally consumed by many of the island cultures of the Pacific Ocean, including those of Fiji, Vanuatu, Hawaii, and Polynesia, for both social and ceremonial purposes.[1]

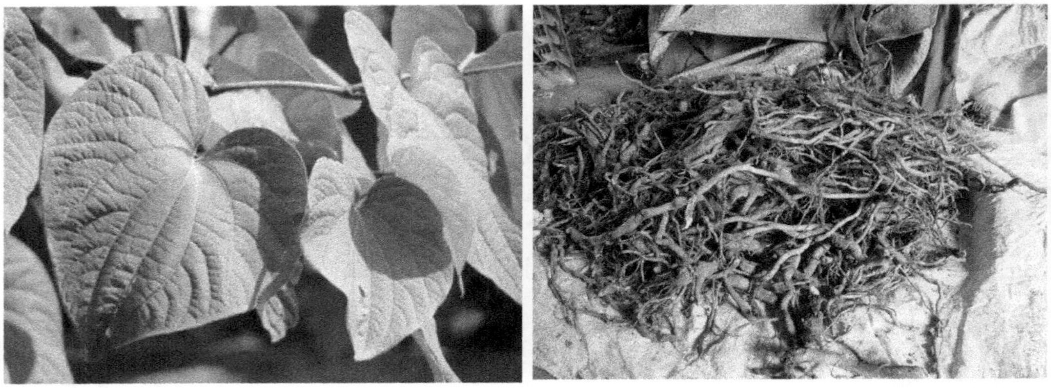

FIGURE 8.1 Images of kava kava plants and dried roots for the production of kava drink.

Dosage and Use

Currently, there is no officially established clinical dosage for kava use. It is suggested that a range of doses can be ingested, depending on the products manufactured. The total content of kavalactones has been used for the standardization of kava extracts and products. In principle, 200–250 mg of kavalactones is recommended for daily use.

Although, in general, kava is viewed as safe, there have been reports of hepatotoxicity from some cases. The World Health Organization has published recommendations for the safe use of kava products. Studies have also demonstrated that herb-drug interactions may increase kava's hepatotoxic risk, such as concurrent consumption of kava with acetaminophen (APAP).[2]

Mechanisms of Action

Studies have established that kava kava's major pharmacological effects are attributed to a group of active constituents known as kavalactones, which include the most abundant kavain, methysticin, yangonin, dihydrokavain, dihydromethysticin, and desmethyoxyyangonin (see Figure 8.2). Although numerous biological targets of kavalactones have been suggested, including monoamine oxidase-B, GABA receptors, ion channels, opioid receptors, dopamine receptors, and others, the mechanisms of action of kava as an anxiolytic still remain elusive.[3] Among the receptors, the interaction of kavain with GABA receptors has been extensively studied to show the potentiation of the functioning of the $GABA_A$ receptor.[3]

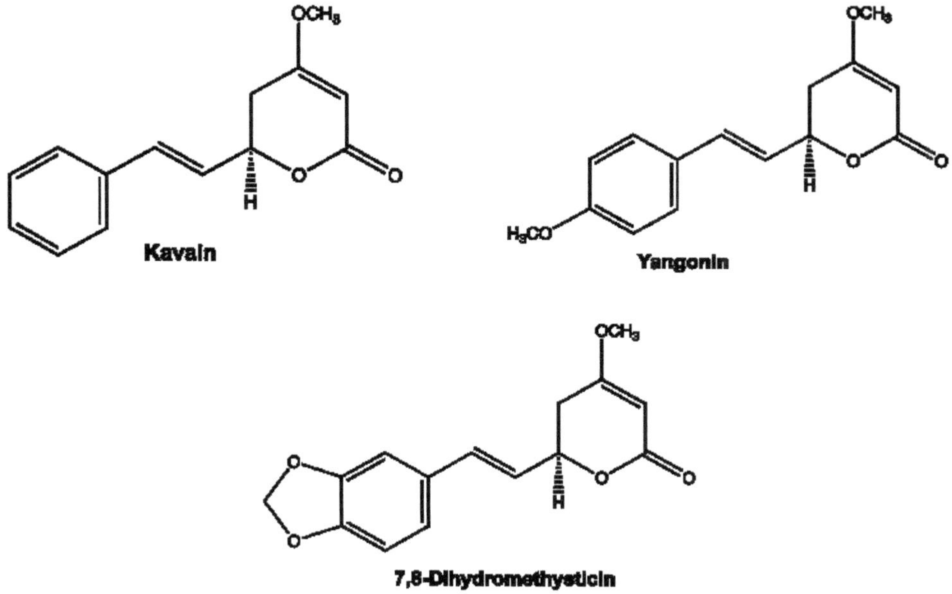

FIGURE 8.2 Representative kavalactone structures.

Valerian

History

Valerian (*Valeriana officinalis*) is a perennial and flowering herb native to North America, Asia, and Europe. It belongs to the family of *Valerianaceae* (see Figure 8.3).[4] The root of valerian is used most commonly for its sedative and hypnotic properties in patients with insomnia and less commonly as an anxiolytic. The use of this plant for medicinal purposes can trace back to the time of ancient Greece and Rome. The valerian extract has been used traditionally in Europe to manage sleeping disorders, and it has also been gaining popularity in the United States for insomnia.[4]

Extensive studies have been conducted to understand the chemical constituents of the plant. To date, two major classes of chemical compositions of valerian extracts have been isolated and characterized, and this includes sesquiterpenes of the volatile oil, represented by valeric acid and iridoids represented by valepotriates (see Figure 8.4).

Dosage and Use

The preparation of valerian extracts is available as tea, tincture, tablets, and capsules. Although there is no officially approved dosage for valerian extracts, the generally suggested dose of valerian root extract for treatment of insomnia ranges from 300 to 600 mg/day. An

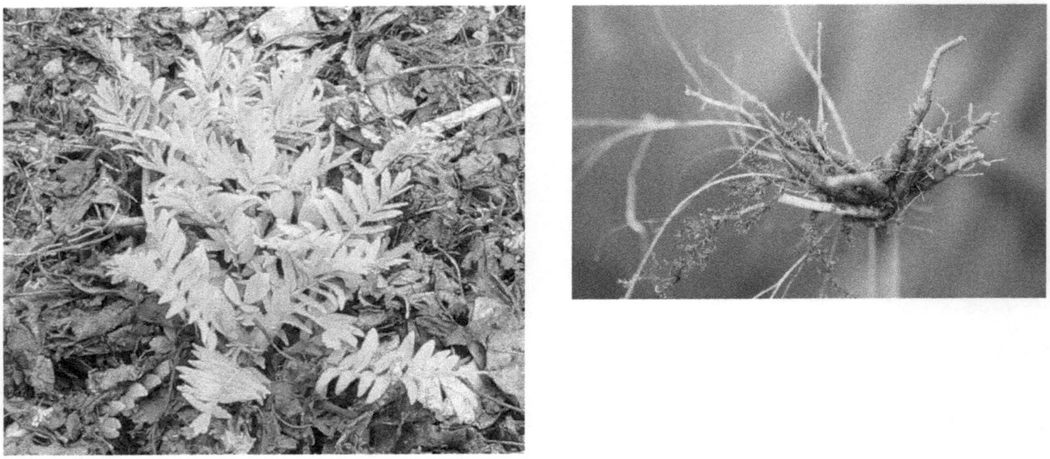

FIGURE 8.3 Images of Valerian.

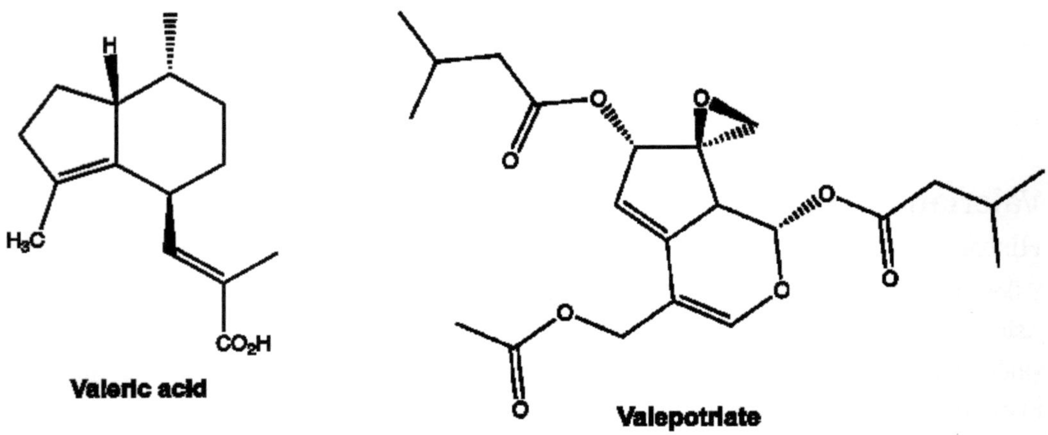

FIGURE 8.4 Chemical structures of valeric acid and valepotriate.

equivalent dose of dried herbal valerian root is 2–3 g. The product is recommended to be ingested 30 minutes to two hours before bedtime.

Mechanisms of Action

Although extensive preclinical studies have been performed to understand and characterize how valerian works pharmacologically, the MOA of valerian extracts for insomnia still remains elusive. One study showed that valerian shows binding affinity at the melatonin (ML 1 and ML 2) and serotonin (5-HT4e, 5-HT6 and 5-HT7) receptors.[5] Other studies established that valerian has a similar MOA as benzodiazepines but binds to a different subunit in the $GABA_A$ receptors.

Motherwort (*Leonurus cardiac*)

History

Motherwort (*Leonurus cardiaca*) is a perennial herb that belongs to the genus of *Leonurus* (see Figure 8.5). Motherwort likely originated from the central and northern Asia and spread to Western Europe, where its use as a medicinal herb became documented in the beginning of the 17th century.[6] This plant has been recognized as an invasive species to North America. There are 22 species in the genus of *Leonurus*, and the medicinal use of the plant is mainly represented by *L. cardiaca*. Motherwort product consists of the dried aerial part of *Leonurus cardiaca* collected during flowering season.[6]

Dosage and Use

A variety of pharmacological properties have been demonstrated for motherwort, and this includes antibacterial, antioxidant, anti-inflammatory, and heart-strengthening uses. Several clinical studies have established the sedative effects of motherwort in comparison with other products, including valerian and melatonin.[7]

Studies have identified a variety of compounds from motherwort: terpene analogs, flavonoids, phenylpropanoids, volatile oils, sterols, and tanins. The representative compounds are

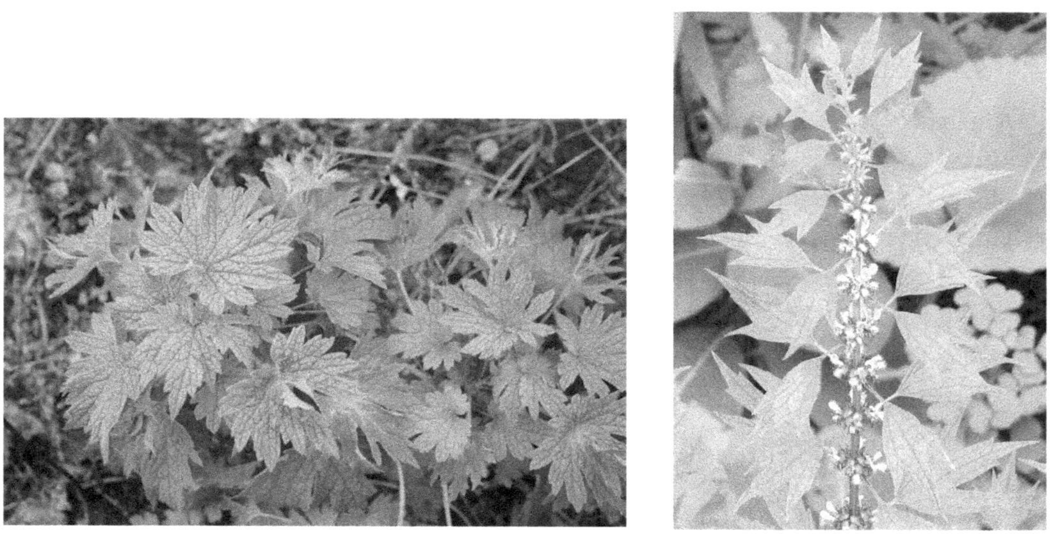

FIGURE 8.5 Images of motherwort.

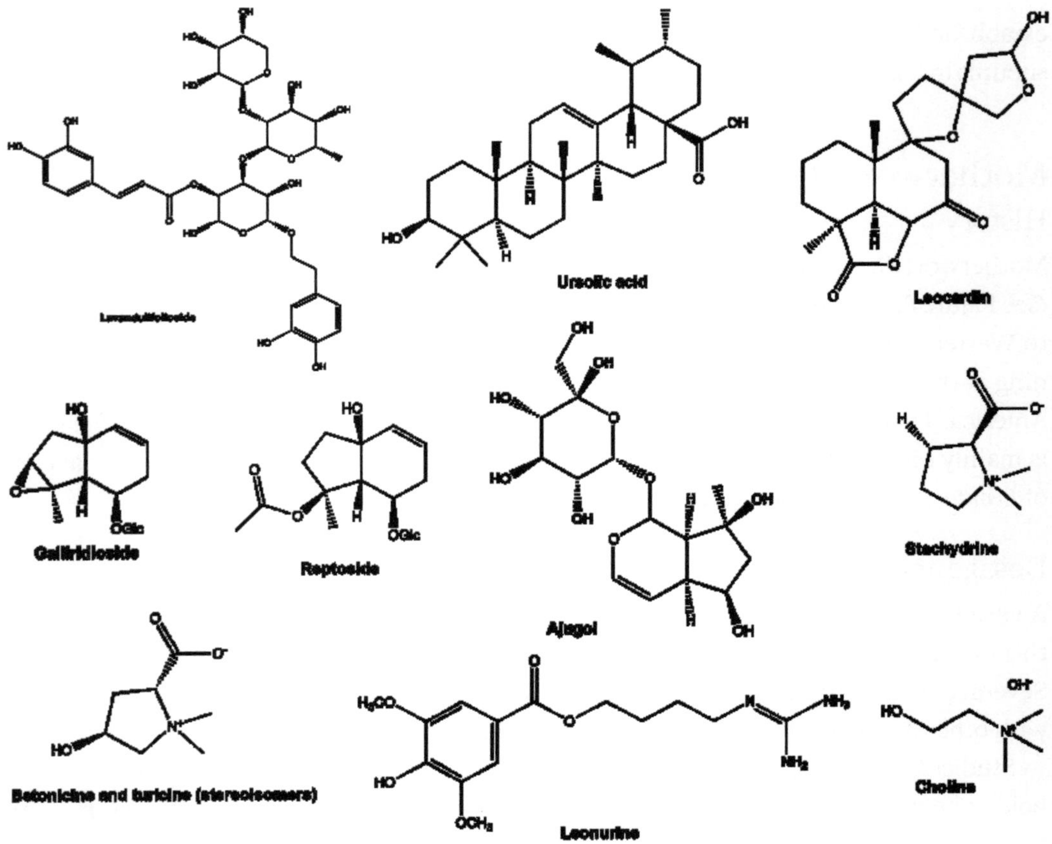

FIGURE 8.6 Chemical structures of active constituents in motherwort.

shown in Figure 8.6. For quality standardization, according to the *European Pharmacopoeia*, motherwort product should contain a minimum of 0.2 percent flavonoids.[7]

Motherwort extracts are available in the following formulations: tincture, tea, dried products in tablets, and capsules. It has been suggested that there can be beneficial effects of using motherwort extracts for the following conditions, based on traditional medicine use: alcoholism, anxiety, high blood pressure, menopausal symptoms, postpartum bleeding, cancer, heart condition, intestinal gas, itching, lack of or painful menstrual periods, shingles, and anxiety.

Mechanisms of Action

Since multiple chemical components and multiple pharmacological functions have been identified and demonstrated for motherwort, its MOA has been not fully understood and established.[7]

References

1. Angelique Showman et al., "Contemporary Pacific and Western Perspectives on ʻAwa (*Piper methysticum*) Toxicology," *Fitoterapia* 100 (2015): 56–67.
2. Sreekanth C. Narayanapillai et al., "Flavokawains A and B in Kava, Not Dihydromethysticin, Potentiate Acetaminophen-Induced Hepatotoxicity in C57BL/6 Mice," *Chemical Research in Toxicology* 27, no. 10 (2014): 1871–76.
3. Han Chow Chua et al., "Kavain, the Major Constituent of the Anxiolytic Kava Extract, Potentiates $GABA_A$ Receptors: Functional Characteristics and Molecular Mechanism," *PLoS One* 11, no. 6 (2016): 1–17.
4. Susan Hadley and Judith J. Petry, "Valerian," *American Family Physician* 67, no. 8 (2003): 1755–58.
5. Vikas Kumar, "Potential Medicinal Plants for CNS Disorders: An Overview," *Phytotherapy Research* 20, no. 12 (2006): 1023–35.
6. J. Janick, "History of Asian Horticulture Technology," *Acta Horticulturae* 620 (2003): 19–32.
7. Katarzyna Wojtyniak, Marcin Szymański, and Irena Matlawska, "*Leonurus cardiaca* L. (Motherwort): A Review of Its Phytochemistry and Pharmacology," *Phytotherapy Research* 27, no. 8 (2013): 1115–20.

Credits

Fig 8.1a: Copyright © 2007 by Forest & Kim Starr, (CC BY 3.0) at https://commons.wikimedia.org/wiki/File:Starr_070515-7054_Piper_methysticum.jpg.

Fig 8.1b: Copyright © 2018 by Taryn, (CC BY-SA 2.0) at https://www.flickr.com/photos/tarale/14090487142.

Fig 8.3a: Copyright © 2005 by Raul654, (CC BY-SA 3.0) at https://commons.wikimedia.org/wiki/File:Valeriana_officinalis.jpg.

Fig 8.3b: Copyright © 2019 by xbqs42. Reprinted with permission.

Fig 8.5a: Copyright © 2007 by Cody Hough, (CC BY-SA 3.0) at https://commons.wikimedia.org/wiki/File:Fort_Custer_Plant3.JPG.

Fig 8.5b: Copyright © 2012 by D. Gordon E. Robertson, (CC BY-SA 3.0) at https://commons.wikimedia.org/wiki/File:Motherwort.jpg.

Chapter 9

Natural Products with Immune Modulating Effects

Shijun Zhang, Hallie M. Blevins, Jakob C. Green, and Liu He

THE BASIS OF OUR BODY'S SELF-DEFENSE is the immune system. Upon pathogenic invasion or endogenous tissue damage, the immune system will be triggered to respond with inflammatory responses to eliminate the changes and maintain the homeostasis of our physiological system. Immunotherapy has been recognized as an effective strategy to manage a variety of diseases, including autoimmune diseases and cancer. In nature, there are also many medicinal plants or herbal medicines that possess such functions, and they are commonly known as tonics, immunostimulants, or adaptogens.

Ginseng

History

The name of ginseng typically refers to three species: Asian ginseng, American ginseng, and Siberian ginseng. Both Asian and American ginseng belong to the genus of *Panax*, meaning "all heal" in Greek. American and Asian ginseng are slow-growing perennial plants with fleshy roots. Although they are different species, the medicinal functions of the roots of American ginseng (*Panax quinquefolius*) and Asian ginseng (*Panax ginseng*) overlap. On the other hand, Siberian ginseng (*Eleuthrococcus senticoccus*) belongs to a different genus, in the family of Araliaceae, and is a small woody shrub (see Figure 9.1). Siberian ginseng is a relatively new addition to Western natural medicine, but it has gained popularity due to its similar medicinal functions as the well-known American and Asian ginseng.

According to the yin and yang theory, Asian ginseng's function is more yang, while American ginseng's function is more yin (see Figure 9.2). This traditional view was probably based on the

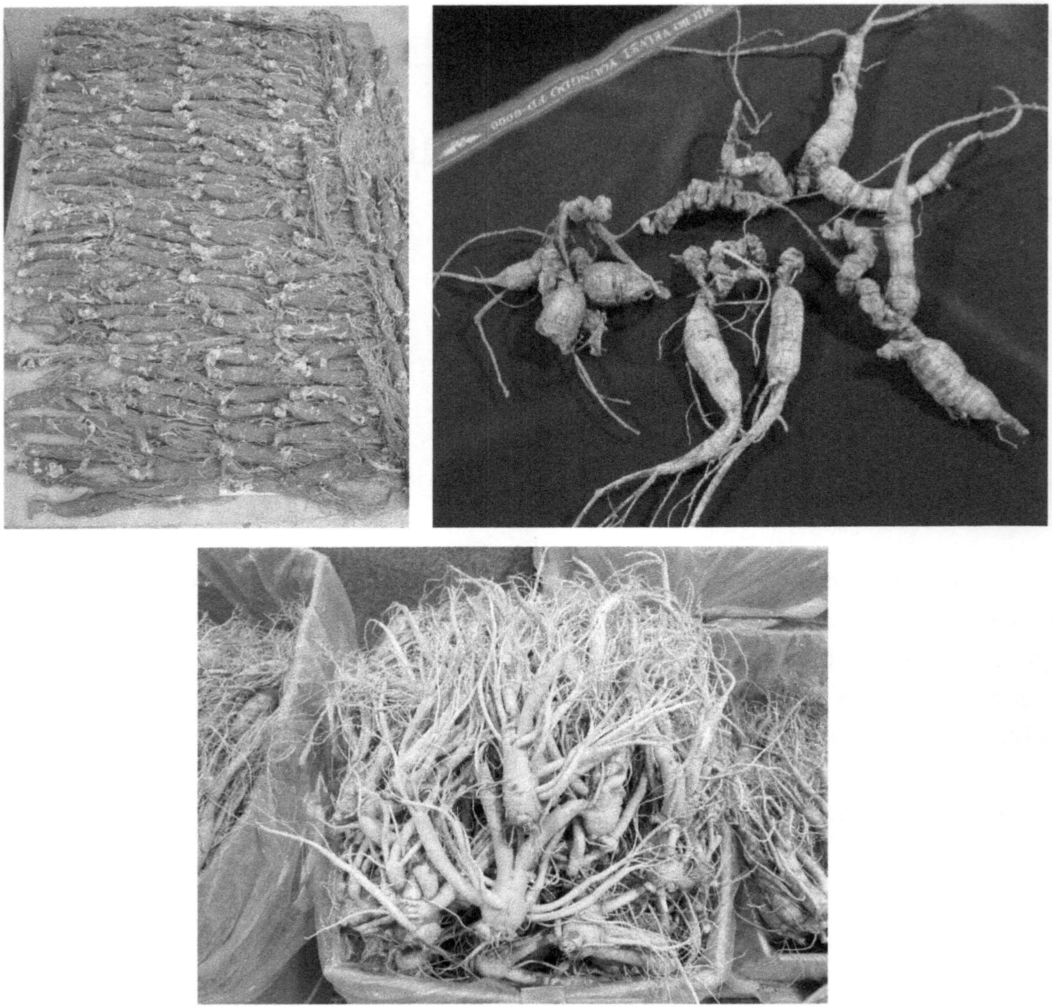

FIGURE 9.1 Images of ginseng roots.

geographic difference of these two species. Pharmacologically, the medicinal properties of ginseng are essentially determined by the presence of the secondary metabolites in the roots.

The major secondary products isolated from the roots of American and Asian ginseng are a group of ginsenosides that belong to the family of terpene saponins. Structurally, ginsenosides are glycosylated analogs of two major aglycones: panaxadiol and panaxatriol (see Figure 9.3).[1] To date, more than 30 ginsenosides have been isolated and characterized.[2][3]

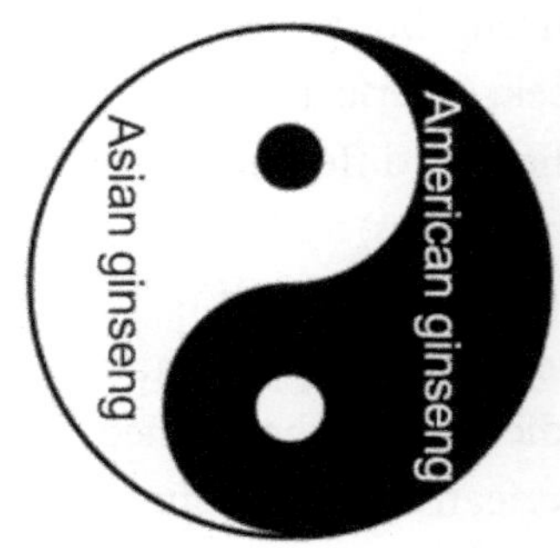

FIGURE 9.2 Yin/yang theory of ginseng pharmacology.

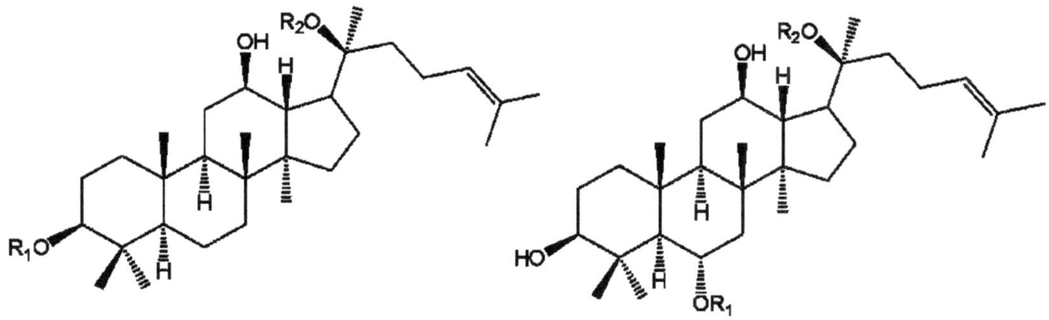

FIGURE 9.3 Chemical structures of ginsenosides from panaxadiol and panaxatriol.

The level of the ginsenosides from both species could be impacted significantly by environmental factors such as temperature, mineral nutrients, and so on. The major secondary metabolites from the roots of Siberian ginseng are an array of eleuthrosides. Although structurally different from the secondary metabolites of *Panax ginseng*, they exert similar pharmacological properties, including increasing endurance, improving memory function, increasing resistance to stressors, anti-inflammation, and neuroprotection.[4]

Ginseng products are mainly derived from the roots of the plants. The use of ginseng dates back to more than 5,000 years ago by Emperor Shen-Nong. Since then, ginseng has been widely used as a general tonic to improve general well-being worldwide. The quality control of *Panax ginseng* is based on the standardization of ginsenosides, at least 4–5 percent.

Dosage and Uses

In general, ginseng is well tolerated and safe as supplementation. There is no clinically approved dose for ginseng products. For mental function: 200 to 400 mg of a specific *Panax ginseng* extract taken once daily or in two divided doses for up to 12 weeks, or 200 to 960 mg as a single dose, has been suggested.[5]

The following beneficial effects have been observed for ginseng as a nutritional supplement: tonic for debility, insomnia, aging, increased alertness, diabetes, improved sexual function, and increased physical performance.

Mechanisms of Action

Besides being used as a general tonic, ginseng products and isolated chemical ingredients have been extensively studied as potential treatments for a variety of diseases, including human cancers, inflammatory disorders, cardiovascular diseases, and neurological disorders. In general, it is believed that the ginsenosides and eleuthrosides, the major pharmacologically active ingredients of ginseng, are responsible for most of the observed pharmacological activities of ginseng. Given the complex nature of the chemical compositions of ginseng, multiple mechanisms have been suggested for ginseng's medicinal functions:

- Immune modulation: Studies have shown that ginseng can modulate the proliferation of immune cells as well as the level of different cytokines.
- Neuroprotection: Studies have demonstrated that ginseng can regulate the level of neurotransmitters and transcriptors.[6]
- Cardioprotection: Regulation of signaling molecules such as NO and glucose metabolism have been suggested as contributing factors for the protective activities.
- Cancer: Ginseng has been shown to regulate cellular signaling pathways that control apoptosis and proliferation.[7][8]

Echinacea

History

Echinacea is a genus of eleven species in the family of Asteraceae and they are commonly known as coneflowers. Echinacea are perennial plants with large and showy composite flowers. The mostly used three species of echinacea for phytomedicine are *E. purpurea*, *E. pallida*, and *E. angustifolia* (see Figure 9.4).[9] Echinacea is one of the most used medicinal plants by Native Americans in the Midwest for wound healing and infection. The current use of echinacea is mainly for common cold, infection, and upper respiratory infection.[10][11][12][13]

Dosage and Uses

Echinacea has shown beneficial effects for common colds, flu-like infections, and upper respiratory infections.[10][11][12][13] Echinacea has shown effects in reducing the duration and severity of common colds.

Mechanisms of Action

Several classes of chemical constituents have been isolated and identified from echinacea products. This includes alkylamides, caffeic acid derivatives, polyalkynes, polyalkenes, and polysaccharides (see Figure 9.5).[14][15][16] Studies from in vitro and in vivo disease models have demonstrated the immunostimulatory and anti-inflammatory effects of echinacea.[17][18][19][20][21][22][23][24][25][26][27][28][29][30] The observed immunostimulatory effects have been associated with the increased phagocytosis of macrophages and increased mobility of leukocytes.[17] Increased cytokine production and natural killer cell activity have also been observed upon application of echinacea.[19][21][22] Inhibition of cyclooxygenase and 5-lipoxygenase were also observed from in vitro studies.[26][27][30] Furthermore, activation of

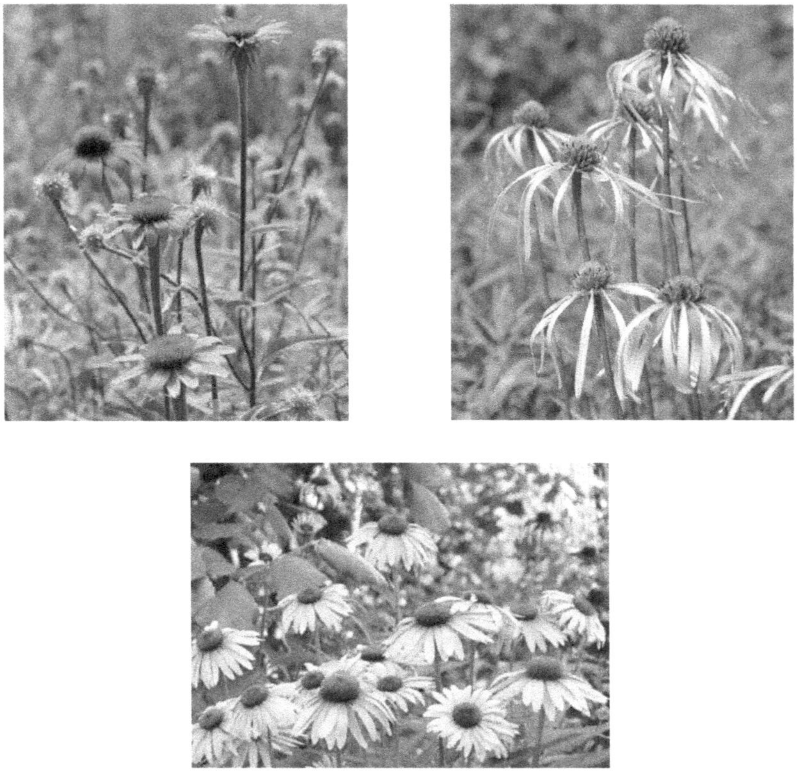

FIGURE 9.4 Images of *E. purpurea*, *E. pallida*, and *E. augustifolia*.

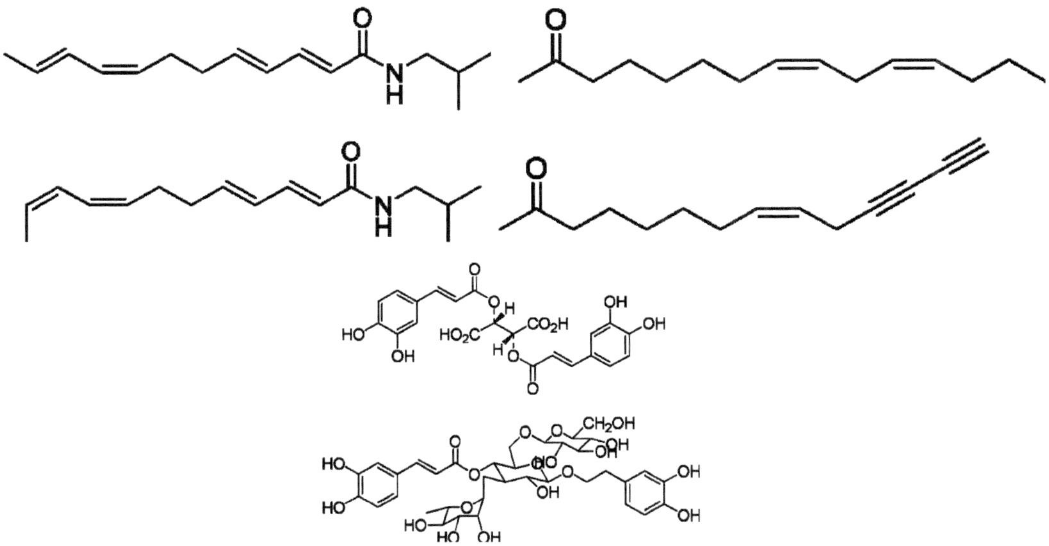

FIGURE 9.5 Representative chemical constituents of echinacea.

the cannabinoid system by echinacea has been reported, suggesting a contribution to psychoactive activity and immunostimulatory activity.[31] It is believed that the complex nature of the chemical ingredients in echinacea are responsible for the noted multiple pharmacological properties of this herbal medicine.

Astragalus

History

Astragalus is a large genus with more than 2,000 species in the family Fabaceae. The species of *Astragalus membranaceus* is one of the most commonly used astragalus for medicinal purposes. Astragalus is one of the most important Chinese herbal medicines, and its use dates back to the time of Emperor Shen-Nong (200 BC). The Chinese name of astragalus, *huangqi*, reflects the yellowish appearance of its roots (see Figure 9.6). Traditionally, astragalus is used in Chinese medicine for night sweats, diarrhea, anorexia, edema, and energy tonics.[32][33] The medicinal portion of this plant is its roots.

Dosage and Uses

Although *Astragalus membranaceus* has been used for thousands of years in traditional Chinese medicine, there is no officially approved dosage for astragalus use. Astragalus is typically used with other herbs in a single decoction. The dosage ranges from 9 to 30 g, depending on the status of patients.[34]

Astragalus has been suggested to have beneficial effects for upper respiratory infection, common cold, infection, and hepatitis.[33][35][36][37]

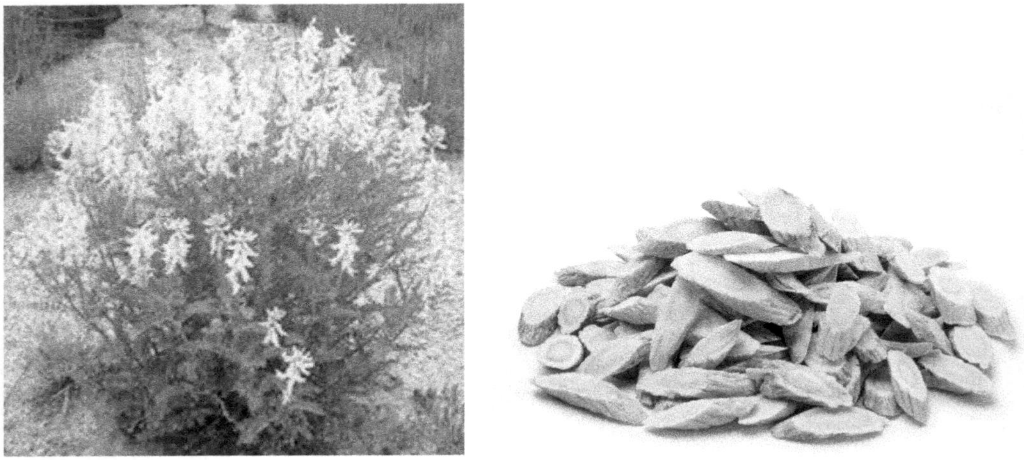

FIGURE 9.6 Images of *Astragalus membranaceus* and the roots.

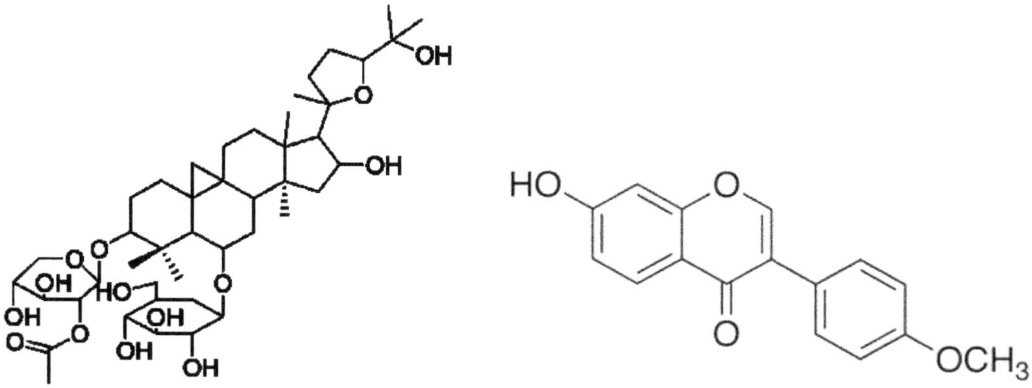

FIGURE 9.7 Chemical structures of formononetin and astragaloside I.

Mechanisms of Action

To date, more than 200 chemical ingredients have been isolated from *Astragalus membranaceus*. Among these compounds, three major classes of compounds have been well characterized as the principle ingredients of *Astragalus membranaceus*, namely, terpene saponins, flavonoids, and polysaccharides (see Figure 9.7).[38] Other chemical components include phytosterol, sterol, fatty acids, amino acids, coumarin, and trace elements.[33][39][40][41][42][43][44][45]

The following pharmacological properties have been demonstrated for astragalus in preclinical studies:

- Immunomodulating effects: This could be related to its ability to increase immune cell functions, the production of cytokines, and increasing the proliferation of T- and B-lymphocytes.[46][47]
- Antioxidant and anti-inflammatory effects: Studies suggested that the saponins and flavonoids in astragalus could be responsible for such activities via regulation of the endogenous antioxidant system and regulation of signaling pathways.[48][49][50]
- Anticancer effects: The results are mainly from in vitro studies of various human cancer cell lines. Astragalus extracts have shown effects to regulate cell cycle and immune functions.[51][52][53]

References

1. Jin Young Seo et al., "Effect of a Fermented Ginseng Extract, BST204, on the Expression of Cyclooxygenase-2 in Murine Macrophages," *International Immunopharmacology* 5, no. 5 (2005): 929–36.

2. Xiaomin Wang et al., "Determination of Ginsenosides in Plant Extracts from *Panax ginseng* and *Panax quinquefolius* L. by LC/MS/MS," *Analytical Chemistry* 71, no. 8 (1999): 1579–84.
3. H. Yu et al., "Purification and Characterization of New Special Ginsenosidase Hydrolyzing Multiglycisides of Protopanaxadiol Ginsenosides, Ginsenosidase Type I," *Chemical and Pharmaceutical Bulletin (Tokyo)* 55, no. 2 (2007): 231–35.
4. Changxiao Liu and Pei Gen Xiao, "Recent Advances on Ginseng Research in China," *Journal of Ethnopharmacology* 36, no. 1 (1992): 27–38.
5. Sergiy Oliynyk and Seikwan Oh, "Actoprotective Effect of Ginseng: Improving Mental and Physical Performance," *Journal of Ginseng Research* 37, no. 2 (2013): 144–66.
6. Wolf-Dieter Rausch et al., "Neuroprotective Effects of Ginsenosides," *Acta Neurobiologiae Experimentalis* 66, no. 4 (2006): 369–75.
7. Chi-Chih Cheng et al., "Molecular Mechanisms of Ginsenoside Rh2-Mediated G1 Growth Arrest and Apoptosis in Human Lung Adenocarcinoma A549 Cells," *Cancer Chemotherapy and Pharmacology* 55, no. 6 (2005): 531–40.
8. Hideyuki Nakata et al., "Inhibitory Effects of Ginsenoside Rh2 on Tumor Growth in Nude Mice Bearing Human Ovarian Cancer Cells," *Japanese Journal of Cancer Research* 89, no. 7 (1989): 733–40.
9. Joanne Barnes et al., "Echinacea Species (*Echinacea angustifolia* (DC.) Hell., *Echinacea pallida* (Nutt.) Nutt., *Echinacea purpurea* (L.) Moench): A Review of Their Chemistry, Pharmacology and Clinical Properties," *Journal of Pharmacy and Pharmacology* 57, no. 8 (2005): 929–54.
10. Wolfram Grimm and Hans-Helge Müller, "A Randomized Controlled Trial of the Effect of Fluid Extract of *Echinacea purpurea* on the Incidence and Severity of Colds and Respiratory Infections," *American Journal of Medicine* 106, no. 2 (1999): 138–43.
11. Klaus Linde et al., "Echinacea for Preventing and Treating the Common Cold," *Cochrane Database of Systematic Reviews* 1 (2006): CD000530.
12. Marlies Karsch-Völk et al., "Echinacea for Preventing and Treating the Common Cold," *Cochrane Database of Systematic Reviews* 2, no. 2 (2014): CD000530.
13. Andreas Schapowal, Peter Klein, and Sebastian Johnston, "Echinacea Reduces the Risk of Recurrent Respiratory Tract Infections and Complications: A Meta-Analysis of Randomized Controlled Trials," *Advances in Therapy* 32, no. 3 (2015): 187–200.
14. Vinti Goel et al., "Alkylamides of *Echinacea purpurea* Stimulate Alveolar Macrophage Function in Normal Rats," Int*ernational Immunopharmacology* 2, no. 2–3 (2002): 381–87.
15. Jürg Gertsch et al., "Echinacea Alkylamides Modulate TNF-Alpha Gene Expression via Cannabinoid Receptor CB2 and Multiple Signal Transduction Pathways," *FEBS Letters* 577, no. 3 (2004): 563–69.

16. Magali Laasonen et al., "Simultaneous Analysis of Alkamides and Caffeic Acid Derivatives for the Identification of *Echinacea purpurea*, *Echinacea angustifolia*, *Echinacea pallida*, and *Parthenium integrifolium* Roots," *Planta Medica* 68, no.6 (2002): 572–74.
17. R. Bauer, et al., Immunologische in-vivo und in-vitro Untersuchungen mit Echinacea Extracten," *Arzneimittel Forschung* 38 (1988): 276–81.
18. Roger A. Burger et al., "Echinacea-Induced Cytokine Production by Human Macrophages," *International Journal of Immunopharmacology* 19, no. 7 (1997): 371–79.
19. Darryl M. See et al., "In Vitro Effects of Echinacea and Ginseng on Natural Killer and Anti-Body-Dependent Cell Cytotoxicity in Healthy Subjects and Chronic Fatigue Syndrome or Acquired Immunodeficiency Syndrome Patients," *Immunopharmacology* 35, no. 3 (1997): 229–35.
20. Nathan L. Currier, M. Sicotte, and Sandra C. Miller, "Deleterious Effects of *Echinacea purpurea* and Melatonin on Myeloid Cells in Mouse Spleen and Bone Marrow," *Journal of Leukocyte Biology* 70, no. 2 (2001): 274–76.
21. Nathan L. Currier and Sandra C. Miller, "Natural Killer Cells from Aging Mice Treated with Extracts from *Echinacea purpurea* Are Quantitatively and Functionally Rejuvenated," *Experimental Gerontology* 35, no. 5 (2000): 627–39.
22. Nathan L. Currier and Sandra C. Miller, "*Echinacea purpurea* and Melatonin Augment Natural-Killer Cells in Leukemic Mice and Prolong Life Span," *Journal of Alternative and Complementary Medicine* 7, no. 3 (2001): 241–51.
23. Gertsch et al., "Echinacea Alkylamides Modulate TNF-Alpha Gene Expression."
24. A. Tubaro et al., "Anti-Inflammatory Activity of a Polysaccharidic Fraction of *Echinacea angustifolia*," *Journal of Pharmacy and Pharmacology* 39, no. 7 (1987): 567–69.
25. Giuseppina Mattace Raso et al., "In-Vivo and In-Vitro Anti-Inflammatory Effect of *Echinacea purpurea* and *Hypericum perforatum*," *Journal of Pharmacy and Pharmacology* 54, no. 10 (2002): 1379–83.
26. L. J. Clifford et al., "Bioactivity of Alkamides Isolated from *Echinacea purpurea* (L.) Moench," *Phytomedicine* 9, no. 3 (2002): 249–53.
27. B. Muller-Jakic et al., "In Vitro Inhibition of Cyclooxygenase and 5-Lipoxygenase by Alkamides from *Echinacea* and *Achillea* Species," *Planta Medica* 60, no. 1 (1994): 37–40.
28. S. Merali et al., "Antifungal and Anti-Inflammatory Activity of the Genus *Echinacea*," *Pharmaceutical Biology* 41, no. 6 (2003): 412–20.
29. Anita Matthias et al., "*Echinacea* Alkylamides Modulate Induced Immune Responses in T-Cells," *Fitoterapia* 79, no. 1 (2008): 53–58.
30. Shannon E. Binns, Bernard R. Baum, and John T. Arnason, "A Taxonomic Revision of the Genus *Echinacea* (Heliantheae; Asteraceae)," *Systematic Botany* 27 (2002): 610–32.
31. Karin Woelkart et al., "The Endocannabinoid System as a Target for Alkamides from *Echinacea angustifolia* Roots," *Planta Medica* 71, no. 8 (2005): 701–705.

32. Harriet Beinfeield and Efrem Korngold, "The Cauldron of Chinese Herbs," in *Between Heaven and Earth: A Guide to Chinese Medicine* (New York: Ballantine, 1991), 265–321.
33. Hong-Yen Hsu, *Oriental Materica: A Concise Guide* (Long Beach, CA: Oriental Healing Arts Institute, 1986).
34. Roy Upton et al., *American Herbal Pharmacopoeia: Botanical Pharmacognosy–Microscopic Characterization of Botanical Medicines* (Boca Raton, FL: CRC Press, 2011).
35. Y.D. Zhang et al., "Effects of Astragalus (ASI, SK) on Experimental Liver Injury (in Chinese)," *Yao Xue Xue Bao* 27, no. 6 (1992): 401–6.
36. Cheng-Xiu Li et al., "The Protective Effects of Traditional Chinese Medicine Prescription, Han-Dan-Gan-Le, on CCl4-Induced Liver Fibrosis in Rats," *American Journal of Chinese Medicine* 26, no. 3 (1998): 325–32.
37. Wen L. Yuan et al., "Effect of *Astragalus membranaceus* on Electric Activities of Cultured Rat Beating Heart Cells Infected with Coxsackie B-2 Virus," *Chinese Medical Journal (English)* 103, no. 3 (1990): 177–82.
38. Xia Q. Ma et al., "Chemical Analysis of Radix Astragali (Huangqi) in China: A Comparison with its Adulterants and Seasonal Variations," *Journal of Agricultural and Food Chemistry* 50, no. 17 (2002): 4861–66.
39. Weici Tang and Gerhard Eisenbrand, *Chinese Drugs of Plant Origin: Chemistry, Pharmacology, and Use in Traditional and Modern Medicine* (Beijing: Springer-Verlag, 1992), 191–97.
40. Tang and Eisenbrand, *Chinese Drugs of Plant Origin.*
41. Mistuo Miyazawa and Hiromu Kameoka, "Volatile Flavor Components of Astragali Radix (*Astragalus membranaceus* Bunge)," *Agricultural and Biological Chemistry* 51, no. 11 (1987): 3153–54.
42. A. Subarnas, Y. Oshima, and H. Hikino, "New Constituents of *Astragalus mongholicus*," *Planta Medica* 57, no. 6 (1991): 590.
43. H. Zheng, Z. Dong, and J. She, *Modern Study of Traditional Chinese Medicine* (Beijing: Xue Yuan Press, 1997).
44. Ke C. Huang, *The Pharmacology of Chinese Herbs* (Boca Raton, FL: CRC Press, 1999).
45. Simon Mills and Kerry Bone, *Principles and Practice of Phytotherapy: Modern Herbal Medicine* (Edinburgh: Churchill Livingstone, 2000).
46. Yan Jiao et al., "Influence of Flavonoid of *Astragalus membranaceus*'s Stem and Leaves on the Function of Cell Mediated Immunity in Mice (in Chinese)," *Chinese Journal of Integrated Traditional and Western Medicine* 19, no. 6 (1999): 356–58.
47. Bao-Mei Shao et al., "A Study on the Immune Receptors for Polysaccharides from the Roots of *Astragalus membranaceus*: A Chinese Medicinal Herb," *Biochemical and Biophysical Research Communications* 320, no. 4 (2004): 1103–11.

48. Dehong Yu et al., "Isoflavonoids from *Astragalus mongholicus* Protect PC12 Cells from Toxicity Induced by L-glutamate," *Journal of Ethnopharmacology* 98, no. 1–2 (2005): 89–94.
49. De-Hong Yu et al., "Protection of PC12 Cells Against Superoxide-Induced Damage by Isoflavonoids from *Astragalus mongholicus*," *Biomedical and Environmental Sciences* 22, no. 1 (2009): 50–54.
50. Shizuo Toda and Yoshiaki Shirataki, "Inhibitory Effects of Astragali Radix, a Crude Drug in Oriental Medicines, on Lipid Peroxidation and Protein Oxidative Modification by Copper," *Journal of Ethnopharmacology* 68, no. 1–3 (1999): 331–33.
51. Shung-Te Kao et al., "The Chinese Medicine Bu-Zhong-Yi-Qi-Tang Inhibited Proliferation of Hepatoma Cell Lines by Inducing Apoptosis via G0/G1 Arrest," *Life Sciences* 69, no. 13 (2001): 1485–96.
52. Di Na et al., "Astragalus Extract Inhibits Destruction of Gastric Cancer Cells to Mesothelial Cells by Anti-Apoptosis," *World Journal of Gastroenterology* 15, no. 5 (2009): 570–77.
53. William Chi Shing Choand Kwok Nam Leung. "In Vitro and In Vivo Immunomodulating and Immunorestorative Effects of *Astragalus membranaceus*," *Journal of Ethnopharmacology* 113, no. 1 (2007): 132–41.

Credits

Fig 9.1a: Copyright © 2005 by Shizhao, (CC BY-SA 2.0) at https://commons.wikimedia.org/wiki/File:Red_ginseng.JPG.
Fig 9.1b: Copyright © 2013 by John Carl Jacobs, (CC BY-SA 4.0) at https://commons.wikimedia.org/wiki/File:American_Ginseng_3.jpg.
Fig 9.1c: Copyright © 2010 by Eugene Kim, (CC BY 2.0) at https://www.flickr.com/photos/eekim/5152038565.
Fig 9.4a: Copyright © 2013 by Eric Hunt, (CC BY-SA 4.0) at https://commons.wikimedia.org/wiki/File:Echinacea_purpurea_Grandview_Prairie.jpg.
Fig 9.4b: Copyright © 2019 by Eric Hunt, (CC BY-SA 4.0) at https://commons.wikimedia.org/wiki/File:Echinacea_pallida_(8).jpg.
Fig 9.4c: Copyright © 2007 by Dy-e, (CC BY-SA 3.0) at https://commons.wikimedia.org/wiki/File:Echinacea_angustifolia.jpg.
Fig 9.6a: Copyright © 2007 by Doronenko, (CC BY-SA 3.0) at https://commons.wikimedia.org/wiki/File:Astragalus_membranaceus.jpg.
Fig 9.6b: Copyright © 2019 Depositphotos/koosen.

Chapter 10

Natural Products with Anti-Inflammatory Effects

Shijun Zhang, Hallie M. Blevins, Jakob C. Green, and Liu He

INFLAMMATORY RESPONSES ARE PART OF THE immune response upon detection of invasion or tissue damage. It is one of our body's self-defense mechanisms. However, chronic inflammation is typically detrimental and leads to a variety of inflammatory disorders. Pharmacotherapies such as steroids and NSAIDS have been well established and approved to manage inflammation-related symptoms. Besides the well-established and FDA-approved pharmacotherapies, many herbal plants have also traditionally been used for this purpose.

Turmeric

History

Turmeric (*Curcuma longa*) is rhizomatous of the ginger family, Zingiberaceae, and is native to tropical South Asia, including India and China.[1] Turmeric is a perennial plant with trumpet-shaped and yellow flowers. Turmeric is one of the popular food coloring ingredients in the Indian culinary culture and is the main ingredient in Indian curry. The history of medicinal use of turmeric dates back about 5,000 years, and it was a principal healing agent in Ayurveda and Chinese medicine. Turmeric has long been known for its effects on a variety of ailments, including inflammatory disorders, digestive and liver problems, skin disease, and wounds. The portion used for medicinal purposes is the root of turmeric (Figure 10.1).[1]

Dosage and Uses

Turmeric spices contain around 3 percent curcumin, compared to 95 percent curcumin in extracts. The amount of curcumin content in the product has been used as standardization for quality control. Human clinical trial studies established that curcumin at 8 g/day is safe and up

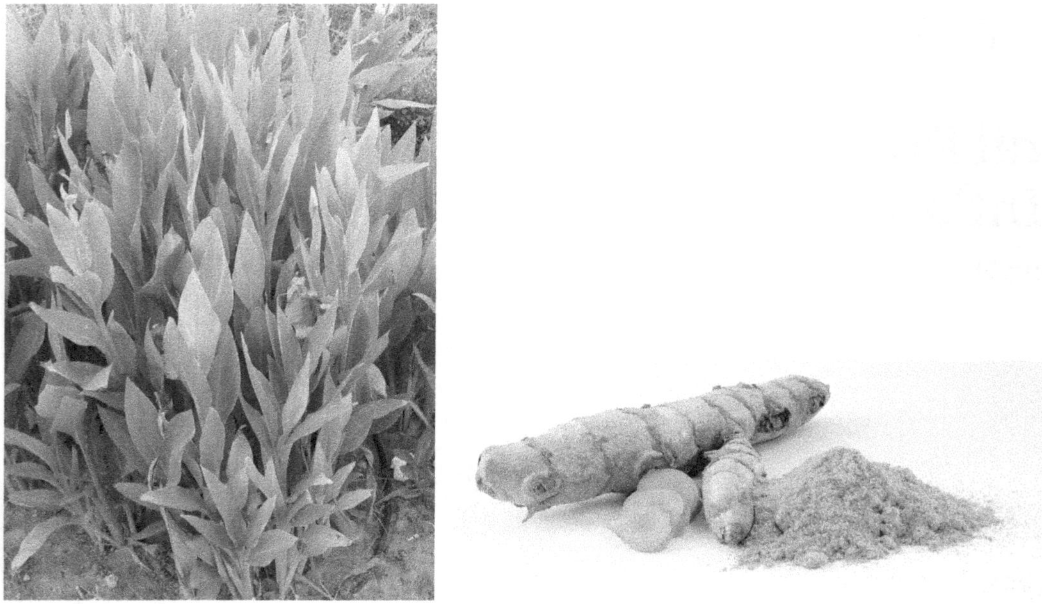

FIGURE 10.1 Images of turmeric and its root under processing.

to 12 g/day can be tolerated. Although a high dose of curcumin is consumed, only low levels of curcumin, around μM concentration, can be achieved in circulation. This is mainly due to its low bioavailability and metabolism.

Curcumin has been tested for a variety of diseases in clinical trials. However, no conclusive outcomes have been reached yet. The following have been suggested as potential indications for curcumin use: cancer, cardiovascular disease, arthritis, inflammatory disorders, and Alzheimer's disease.

Mechanisms of Action

Several curcuminoids from turmeric, including curcumin, demethoxycurcumin, and bisdemethoxycurcumin, have been identified and extensively studied for their contributions to the observed pharmacological properties of turmeric (see Figure 10.2). Among the identified curcuminoids, curcumin (diferuloylmethane) is widely accepted as the major constituent that is responsible for turmeric's pharmacological functions. In 1949, curcumin was first shown to have antibacterial activity. Since then, extensive in vitro and in vivo studies have established that curcumin shows anticancer, anti-inflammatory, anti-infectious, and neuroprotective properties.[2] Consequently, a diverse list of cellular signaling and molecular targets have been suggested for curcumin, and this includes protein kinases, enzymes, cytokines, and transcription factors. Curcumin has also shown effects to block protein

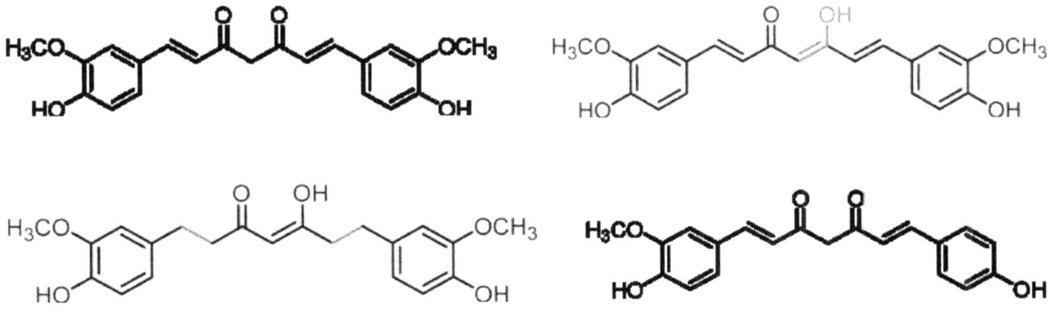

FIGURE 10.2 Representative chemical structures of curcuminoids.

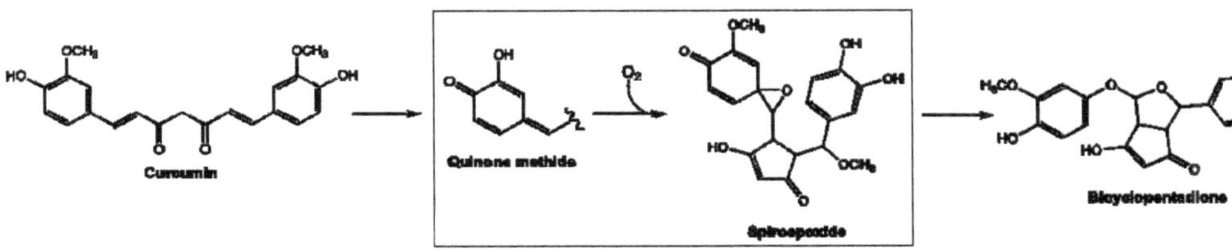

FIGURE 10.3 Metabolism of curcumin.
Curcumin's active intermediates, quinone methide and spiroepoxide, modulate protein function by adducting covalently to the inflammatory protein, IKK β.[3]

aggregations that are involved in neurodegenerative disorders.[2] Although curcumin has been recognized as one of nature's most powerful healers, concerns have also been raised for its molecular promiscuity.

The promiscuity of curcumin could relate to its structural nature of being a Michael addition acceptor. Studies have also identified metabolites of curcumin that can form covalent adducts with macromolecules (see Figure 10.3).

Willow Bark

History

The story of the discovery of aspirin stretches back to the time of Hippocrates (400 BC), when bark from willow trees was used as a pain reliever and antipyretic.[4][5] Willow trees are deciduous trees native to Europe, Asia, and North America. The most well-known willow trees are white willow (*Salix alba*), black willow (*Salix nigra*), crack willow (*Salix fragilis*), purple willow (*Salix purpurea*), and weeping willow (*Salix babylonica*). Willow bark has traditionally been used in China and Europe to treat pain, headache, and inflammatory conditions.[4][5] The first clinical report of willow bark was in 1763 to treat malarial fever.[4][5]

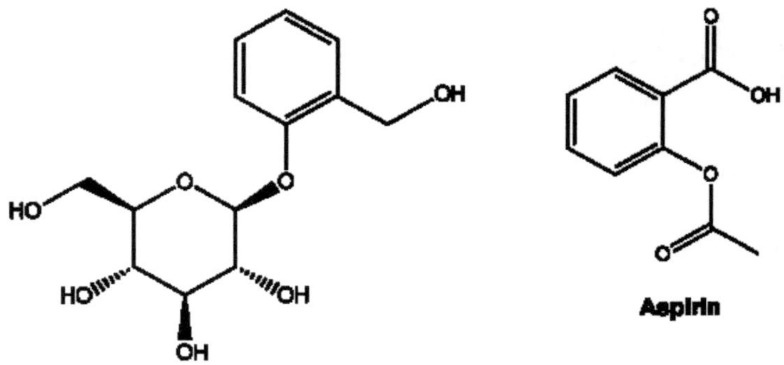

FIGURE 10.4 Chemical structures of salicin and aspirin.

Currently, willow bark is used for medicinal purposes, usually including a combination of the bark from white, purple, and crack willows.

Dosage and Uses

Willow bark is available as capsules that contain the dried willow bark powders or tincture. Typically the products are standardized based on the content of salicin. The recommended dose for pain relief is 120–240 mg of salicin a day. Willow bark has been recommended for lower back pain, arthritis, and other inflammatory symptoms.

Mechanisms of Action

One of the identified ingredients from willow bark is salicin, and it is generally believed that the analgesic and anti-inflammatory effects of willow bark are attributed to salicin. This is probably due to the structural similarity of salicin with aspirin (see Figure 10.4) and the well-established antipyretic effects of aspirin. However, studies to compare the level of salicylic acid, the metabolite of both salicin and aspirin, after salicin and aspirin ingestion suggested that a daily dose of salicin is not sufficient to produce the observed analgesic effects. Flavonoids and polyphenols have also been identified from willow bark, and they may contribute to the anti-inflammatory and analgesic effects of willow bark.[6]

Ginkgo Biloba

History

Ginkgo biloba, also known as ginkgo, is one of the most ancient plants and has been considered the living fossil of the Ginkgophyta division. Originating in China, the tree is now widely cultivated worldwide. Ginkgo trees have unique fan-shaped leaves and are dioecious (see

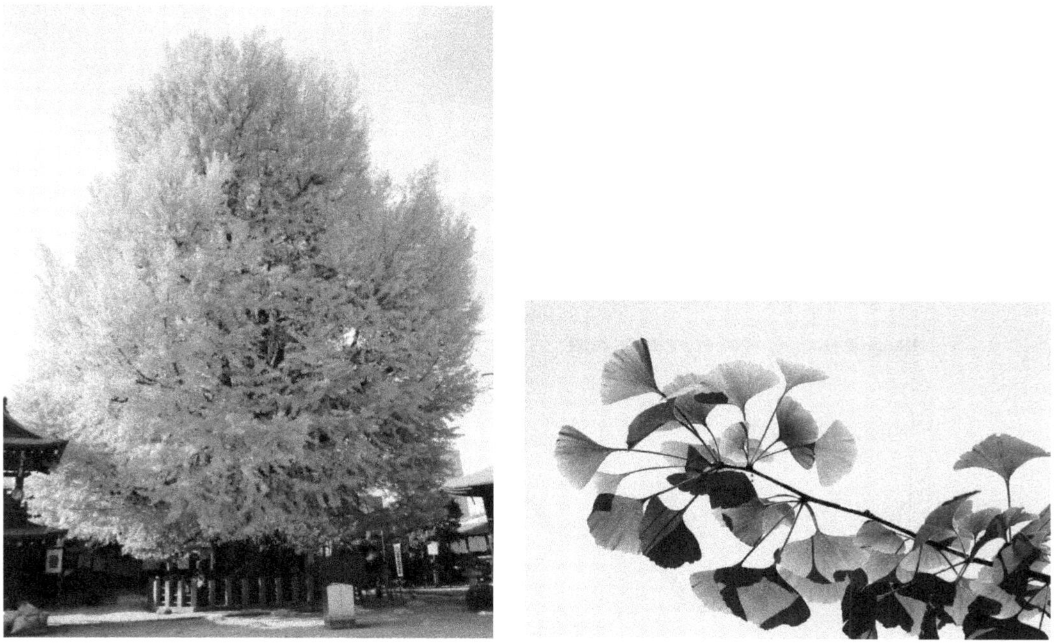

FIGURE 10.5 Images of ginkgo tree and fan-shaped leaves.

Figure 10.5). In the fall season, the tree has beautiful yellow foliage. *Ginkgo biloba* extracts have been used for centuries as a traditional Chinese medicine to treat a variety of disorders, such as heart disease, asthma, vertigo, and cognitive problems. Ginkgo extracts are mainly derived from the leaves of the tree.[7]

Extensive studies have been conducted to isolate and identify the chemical constituents of ginkgo extracts. Three main classes of compounds have been identified and well characterized: terpene lactones, flavone glycosides, and proanthocynanidines. Terpene lactones are represented by ginkgolides (A, B, and C) and bilobalides. Flavone glycosides are represented by quercetin, ginkgetin, and catechin (see Figure 10.6).[8]

Dosage and Uses

Ginkgo extract is available as capsules, tablets, liquid extracts, and dried leaves/tea. The German Commission E recommends 120 to 240 mg of extract two to three times daily for cerebral insufficiency. Dosages of ginkgo as high as 720 mg/day have been used in clinical trials for dementia, memory, and circulatory disorders.[9]

The German Commission E approved *Ginkgo biloba* for treating impairments in memory, concentration, attention, and mood; vertigo; and vascular tinnitus.

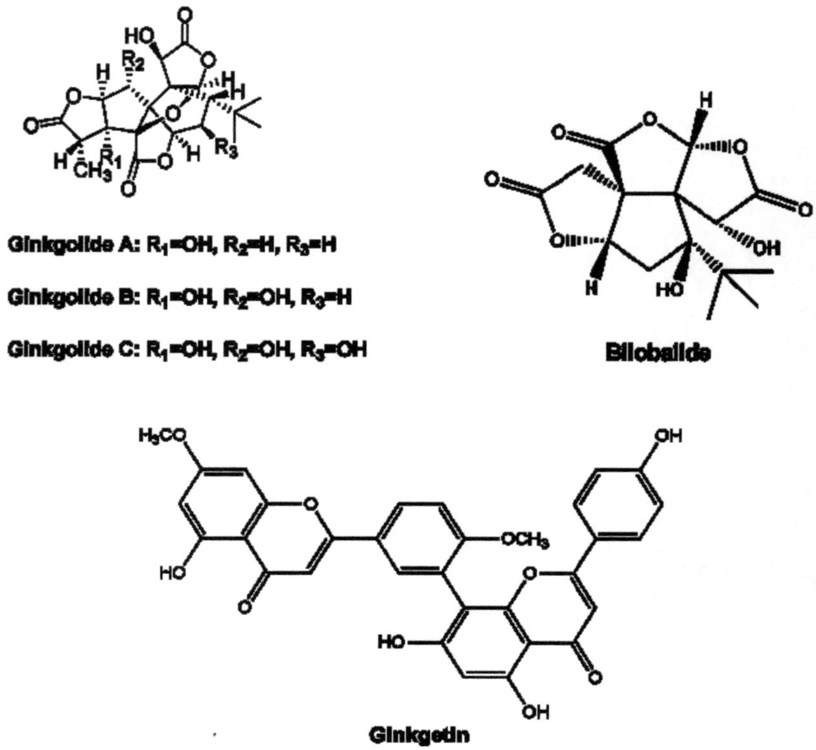

FIGURE 10.6 Representative structures of ginkgolides, bilobalides, and flavonoids.

Ginkgo extracts have been tested for use in treating cancer, circulatory disorders, psychiatric disorders, and inflammatory disorders. However, none of these indications have been approved.[10][11]

Mechanisms of Action

Although significant advances have been achieved to understand mechanistically how ginkgo extracts exert the observed pharmacological functions, the exact mechanisms of action of ginkgo extracts still remain elusive. Based on studies from in vitro and in vivo disease models, the following mechanisms have been proposed to explain the beneficial effects of ginkgo extracts:

Antioxidant effects: Ginkgo extracts have shown effects as free radical scavengers. Free radicals play important roles in producing oxidative stress, lipid peroxidation, and DNA damage. Therefore, the free radical scavenging effects of ginkgo extracts could contribute to the protective functions.[9]

Mitochondria regulation: Mitochondria is the main organelle that produces most of the needed energy for normal physiology. Mitochondria are also the main source of ROS. Studies have shown that ginkgo extracts can regulate mitochondrial dysfunction through multiple mechanisms, such as respiration, mitochondria DNA, mitochondrial apoptosis, mitochondria membrane potential, and intramitochondrial Ca homeostasis.[10]

Anti-inflammatory effects: Ginkgo extracts have been shown to inhibit intercellular adhesion molecule 1, interleukin 1, and myeloperoxidase, consequently leading to anti-inflammatory effects. The proanthocynanidines have shown effects to block nucleocytoplasmic translocation and the release of high-mobility group box 1 (HMGB1) protein, which acts as a damage-associated molecular pattern molecule.

Other mechanisms have also been suggested, such as anti-platelet-activating factor, regulation of mitogen activated protein kinases, Ca homeostasis, and neurotransmitter system modulation.[11]

References

1. Mehdi Sharifi-Rad et al., "Plants of the Genus *Zingiber* as a Source of Bioactive Phytochemicals: From Tradition of Pharmacy," *Molecules* 22, no. 12 (2017): 2145.
2. Sigma-Aldrich, "Turmeric, Curcumin," Plant Profiler, accessed April 28, 2019, https://www.sigmaaldrich.com/life-science/nutrition-research/learning-center/plant-profiler/curcuma-longa.html.
3. Rebecca L. Edwards et al., "The Anti-Inflammatory Activity of Curcumin Is Mediated by Its Oxidative Metabolites," *Journal of Biological Chemistry* 292, no. 52 (2017): 21243–52.
4. Michael J. R. Desborough and David M. Keeling, "The Aspirin Story – From Willow to Wonder Drug," *British Journal of Haematology* 177, no. 5 (2017): 647–83.
5. Maria Rosa Montinari, Sergio Minelli, and Rafaelle De Caterina, "The First 3500 Years of Aspirin History from Its Roots – A Concise Summary," *Vascular Pharmacology* 113 (2019): 1–8.
6. Mohamed Khayyal et al., "Mechanisms Involved in the Anti-Inflammatory Effect of a Standardized Willow Bark Extract," *Drug Research* 55, no. 11 (2005): 677–87.
7. Bruce J. Diamond et al., "*Ginkgo biloba* Extract: Mechanisms and Clinical Indications," *Archives of Physical Medicine and Rehabilitation* 81, no. 5 (2000): 668–78.
8. Laura L. Boles Ponto and Susan K. Schultz, "*Ginkgo biloba* Extract: Review of CNS Effects," *Annals of Clinical Psychiatry* 15, no. 2 (2003): 109–19.
9. Chun Shi et al., "*Ginkgo biloba* Extract in Alzheimer's Disease: From Action Mechanisms to Medical Practice," *International Journal of Molecular Sciences* 11, no. 1 (2010): 107–23.
10. Georgianne Valli and Elsa-Grace V. Giardina, "Benefits, Adverse Effects and Drug Interactions of Herbal Therapies with Cardiovascular Effects," *Journal of the American College of Cardiology* 39, no. 7 (2002): 1083–95.
11. Rubin Bressler, "Herb-Drug Interactions: Interactions Between *Ginkgo biloba* and Prescription Medications," *Geriatrics* 60, no. 4 (2005): 30–33.

Credits

Fig 10.1a: Copyright © 2013 by Aravind Sivaraj, (CC BY-SA 3.0) at https://commons.wikimedia.org/wiki/File:Turmeric_plants_at_the_Heritage_Park_in_Abu_Dhabi,_UAE.JPG.
Fig 10.1b: Copyright © 2014 by Simon A. Eugster, (CC BY-SA 3.0) at https://commons.wikimedia.org/wiki/File:Curcuma_longa_roots.jpg.
Fig 10.5a: Copyright © 2016 by 立花左近, (CC BY-SA 3.0) at https://commons.wikimedia.org/wiki/File:Big_Ginkgo_Tree_in_Hida_Kokubun-ji.jpg.
Fig. 10.5b: Source: https://pixabay.com/photos/ginkgo-gingko-biloba-leaves-bokeh-4195732/.

Chapter 11

Natural Products for Infectious Diseases Treatment

Aaron E. May, Heather A. Pendergrass, and Julia A. Hotinger

Infectious diseases are brought about by pathogenic species, including bacteria, fungi, parasites, and viruses. Infectious diseases can be spread by a variety of methods, including person-to-person contact, ingestion of contaminated food, and insect/animal bites. The successful treatment of infectious diseases has been a large driving force in the increased lifespan of humans over the last century. Before the discovery of penicillin, the leading causes of death in the United States were influenza, pneumonia, tuberculosis, and heart disease.[1] The leading causes of death have now been replaced with heart disease, cancer, and accidents.[2]

Many plants and bacteria produce small-molecule natural products that combat infectious diseases.[3][4] This process is often for the direct benefit of the producing organism. For example, many *Streptomyces* bacterial strains produce antibiotics to kill their bacterial competition in order to obtain more nutrients.[5] These natural products can be harnessed and used by humans to treat a variety of illnesses and conditions, including infectious diseases.

This chapter contains a variety of examples of small molecules from plants and bacteria being used to combat infectious diseases. These selections have been chosen to highlight the breadth of infectious diseases that can be treated, as well as the diversity and variety of natural products that are made by plants and microbial sources.

Fighting Bacterial Pathogens: The Discovery and Use of Beta-Lactam Antibiotics

The discovery of antibiotics is attributed to Alexander Fleming in 1929.[6] While studying the Gram-positive bacterium *Staphylococcus* on agar plates, Fleming noticed a contaminating mold growing on a plate. This mold, *Penicillium notatum*, was causing cell lysis of *Staphylococcus*, leading

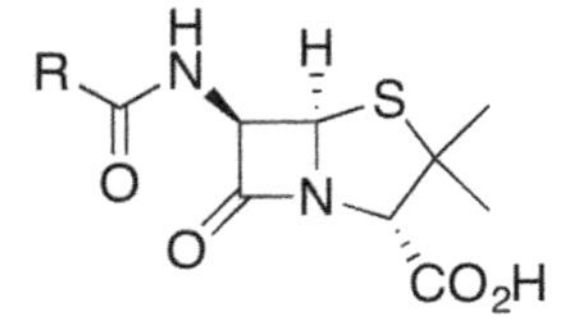

Penicillin	R =
G	benzyl
V	phenoxymethyl
X	p-hydroxybenzyl

FIGURE 11.1 Naturally occurring penicillins.

Fleming to postulate that the mold had antibiotic activity. Fleming showed that cultures of *P. notatum* had antibiotic activity, and he named these antibiotics penicillins (see Figure 11.1). Although the structure and mechanism of action of the penicillins were not known at the time, Fleming's studies showed that penicillins were effective against a variety of Gram-positive bacteria (*Staphylococcus, Pneumococcus,* and *Streptococcus*) but not effective against Gram-negatives.

A significant amount of time passed before the penicillins were used in animal and human studies. In 1940, Florey used penicillin to treat rats and mice, and *S. aureus* infections were treated with penicillin in humans in 1941.[7][8] Penicillins were used throughout World War II to treat infections, and the Nobel Prize was awarded in 1945 for the discovery of penicillin and its use in treating infectious diseases.[9] The beta-lactam structure of penicillin was proven by X-ray crystallography in 1949.[10]

Penicillin acts by reacting with penicillin-binding proteins (PBPs), enzymes that catalyze the cross-linking of the peptidoglycan layer of the cell wall (see Figure 11.2).[11] Since Gram-positive bacteria have an exposed peptidoglycan layer, they are significantly more susceptible to penicillins than Gram-negatives, which have their peptidoglycan layer embedded within an inner and outer cell membrane.

PBPs catalyze peptidoglycan cross-linking by using their active-site serine to attack the carbonyl of the penultimate D-alanine of the pentapeptide chain on N-acetylmuramic acid (see Figure 11.3). This forms a tetrahedral intermediate that breaks down and expels the terminal alanine, making a PBP-Ala ester. This PBP ester reacts with the amine of diaminopimelic acid to form a cross-link, regenerating the PBP catalyst. This cross-linking reaction

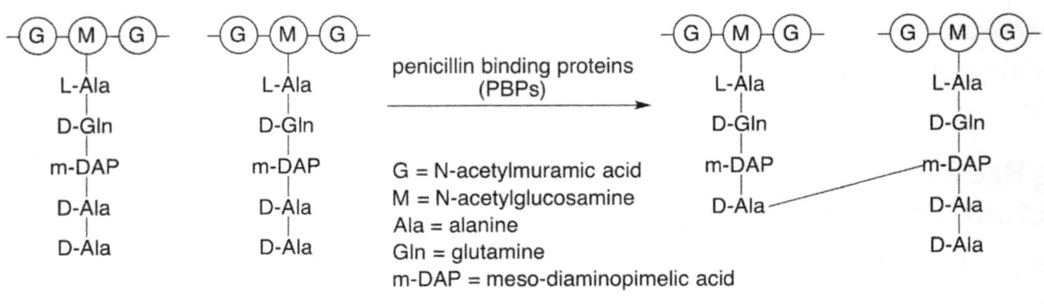

FIGURE 11.2 Peptidoglycan crosslinking catalyzed by penicillin binding proteins.

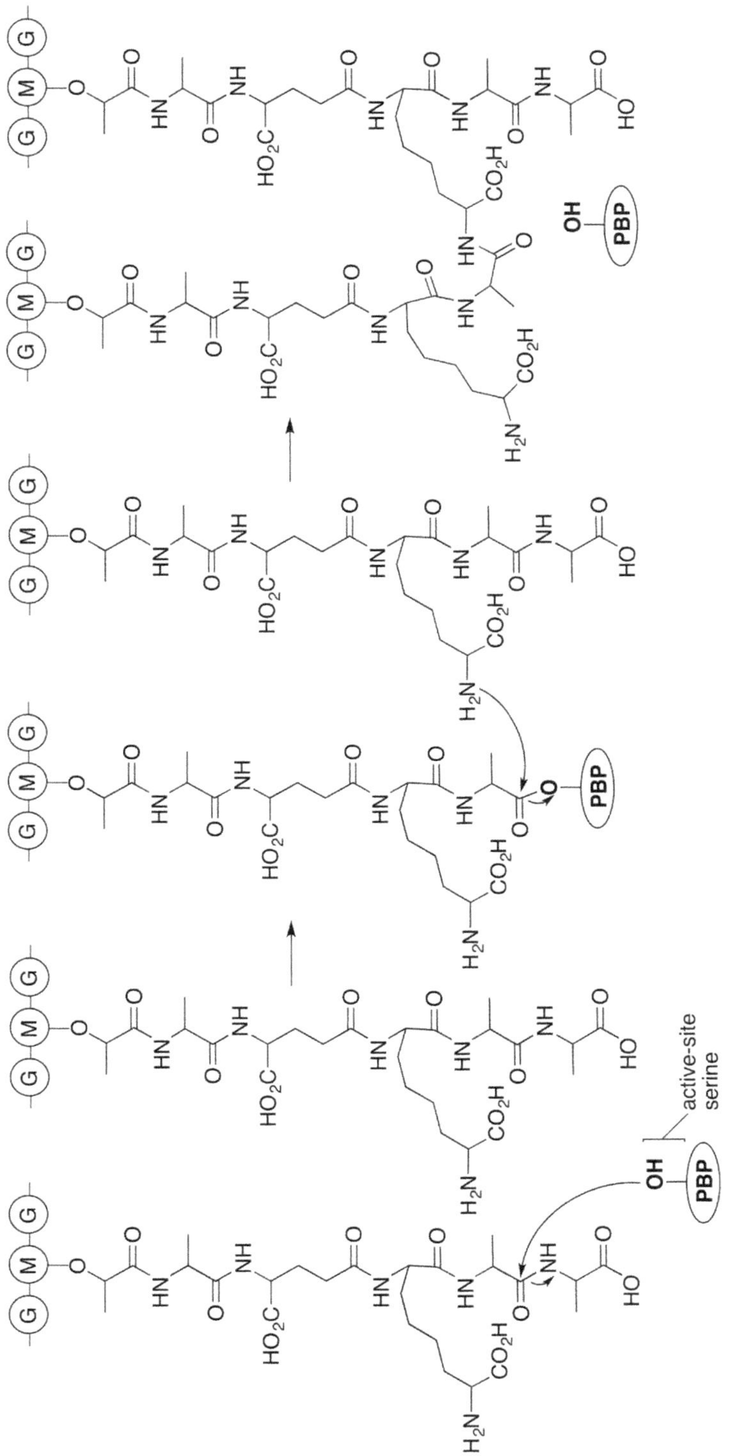

FIGURE 11.3 Mechanism of PBP-catalyzed cross-linking.

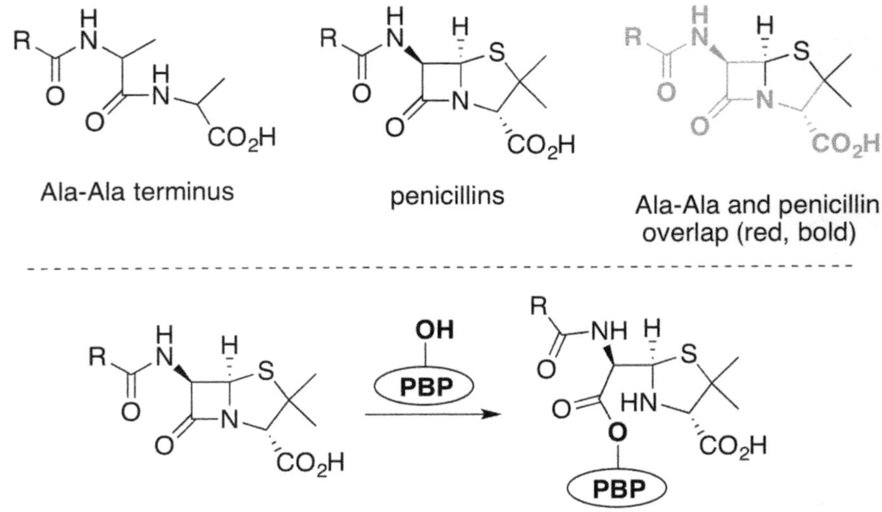

FIGURE 11.4 Overlap of Ala-Ala terminus with penicillins, and reaction of penicillins with PBPs.

is necessary to reinforce the cell wall, and interrupting this process results in a weakened cell wall and nonviable cells.

Penicillins are antibiotics because of their ability to react with PBPs, which keeps cells from forming a viable cell wall. They do so by structurally mimicking the terminal Ala-Ala linkage of the pentapeptide (see Figure 11.4). PBPs react with penicillins at the beta-lactam, opening the beta-lactam and producing a stable ester with penicillins. Penicillins are referred to as suicide inhibitors, because one molecule of penicillin will remain bound to and deactivate one PBP. Without enough unbound PBPs, the cell wall cannot be created, and the bacterial population will fail to grow.

Bacteria can become resistant to penicillins by producing PBPs that have a lower affinity for penicillins.[12] Bacteria can also become resistant to beta-lactams by producing enzymes called beta-lactamases.[13] These enzymes react with penicillins by the same mechanism as PBPs, but the ester formed by the active site serine on the penicillin is susceptible to hydrolysis (see Figure 11.5). This process regenerates the beta-lactamase, allowing it to deactivate multiple molecules of penicillin. The ring-opened penicillin is no longer capable of reacting with PBPs.

Cephalosporins were the first beta-lactams to be discovered that were partially resistant to beta-lactamases. In 1960, methicillin was discovered.[14] This agent was highly resistant to beta-lactamases. The acronym MRSA (methicillin-resistant *Staphylococcus aureus*) refers to *Staphylococcus* that encodes a PBP (PBP2a) that binds poorly to beta-lactams but still efficiently performs cell wall crosslinking.[15]

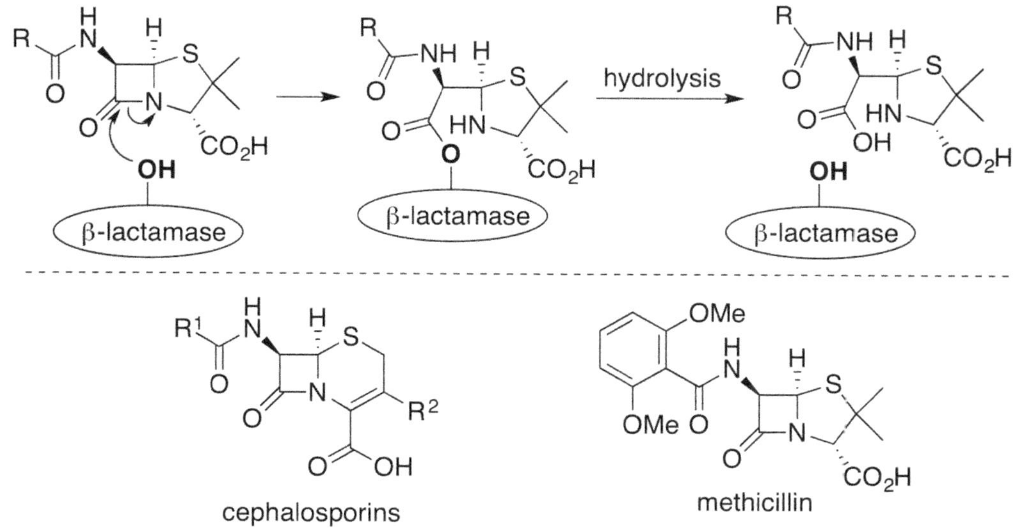

FIGURE 11.5 Hydrolysis by beta-lactamases (top). Cephalosporins and methicillin are resistant to beta-lactamases (bottom).

With suicide substrates for beta-lactamases, resistance to penicillins can be mitigated. Clavulanic acid, sulbactam, tazobactam, and avibactam are all agents that have been used to inhibit beta-lactamases and thus allow antibiotic beta-lactams to last longer in vivo and more efficiently target PBPs (see Figure 11.6).[16] The most recent beta-lactam antibiotic approved by the FDA was ceftaroline fosamil in 2010.[17][18] Resistance to this agent has already been discovered, highlighting the difficulty in producing agents that will remain effective in the fight against bacterial pathogens.[19]

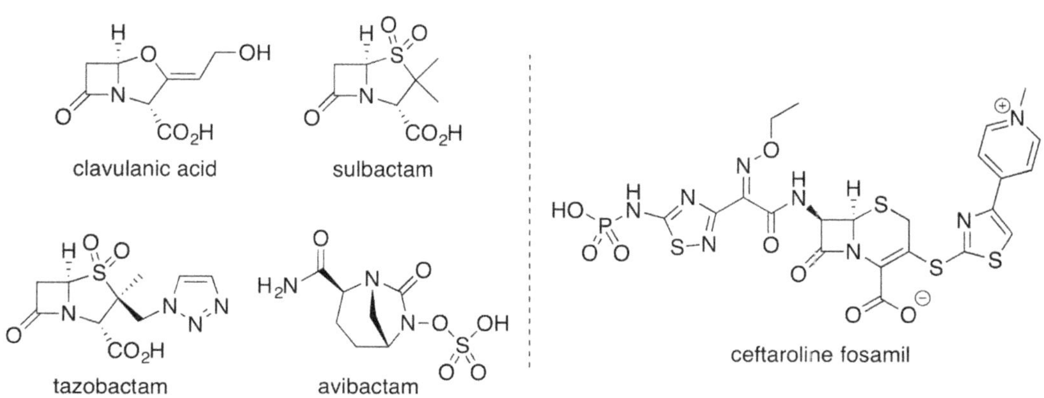

FIGURE 11.6 Structures of beta-lactamase inhibitors (left). Structure of ceftaroline fosamil (right).

Antimalarials: Combating Human Parasites

Malaria is a mosquito-borne infectious disease that infects over 200 million people per year, killing roughly 400,000 annually.[20] Malaria is caused by the parasite *Plasmodium*, with *P. falciparum* accounting for approximately 75 percent of infections and *P. vivax* accounting for 20 percent.[21] Malaria is transmitted specifically by the bite of an infected female *Anopheles* mosquito. The transmission cycle of malaria involves being infected by a mosquito, followed by liver and blood infection. Carriers of malaria can then provide the parasite to a mosquito, which then subsequently infects a new host.[22]

The death rate from malaria has dropped by about half in the last 20 years due to a combination of strategies, including the use of insecticides, mosquito nets, and the usage of other parasites that kill larval mosquitos.[23][24] The treatment of malaria with small-molecule natural products has also been critical in saving lives.

Plasmodium feeds on and grows within red blood cells. The parasite digests hemoglobin inside its food vacuoles, which produces free heme as a byproduct. Heme is slightly toxic and is normally converted into hemozoin, a dimeric crystalline and nontoxic form of heme.[25] The conversion of heme into hemozoin is performed by the enzyme heme polymerase.[26] If heme polymerase is inhibited, then free heme will build to toxic levels and kill *Plasmodium* parasites.

Cinchona alkaloids are produced by the bark of trees in the *Cinchona* family. There are 25 species of *Cinchona*, and they are native to South America. *Cinchona* alkaloids inhibit heme polymerase, which creates a toxic environment to *Plasmodium*. Cinchona alkaloids include quinine and quinidine (see Figure 11.7).[27] Although neither of these agents is in common use today against malaria, they did form the template for the effective agents chloroquine and mefloquine. Each of these quinolone alkaloids contains a basic nitrogen. This is important, because the food vacuoles of *Plasmodium* are acidic. An uncharged alkaloid can penetrate the food vacuole but remains inside after protonation, increasing the local concentration of the agents.

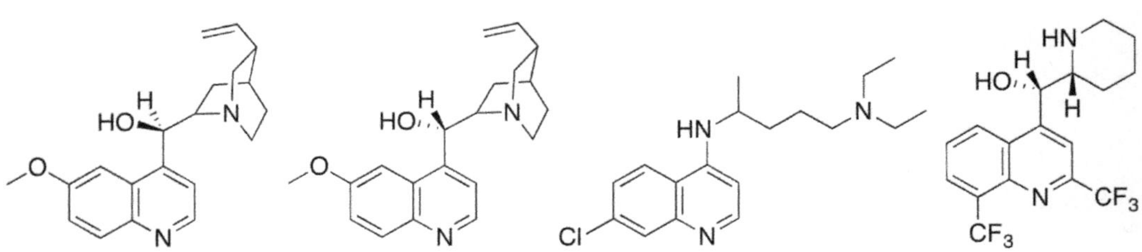

FIGURE 11.7 Quinoline alkaloids used to treat malaria.

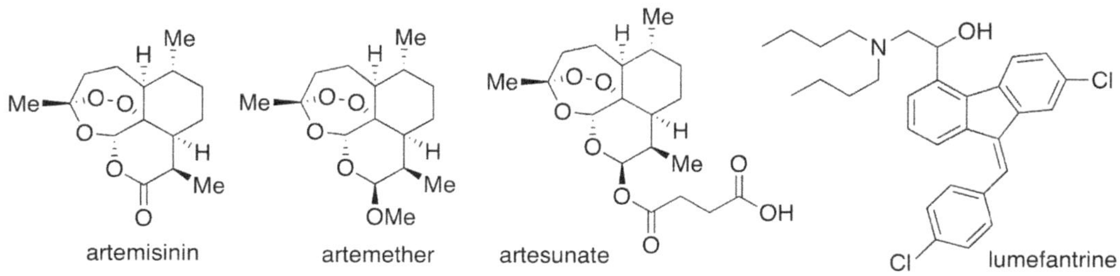

FIGURE 11.8 Structures of artemisinins and lumefantrine.

Artemisinin is an antimalarial drug produced by the plant *Artemisia annua* and was first isolated in 1972 (see Figure 11.8).[28] This peroxide-containing molecule is believed to react with heme to produce a free radical intermediate that is toxic to *Plasmodium*.[29] Semisynthesis of artemisinin is performed to make the drugs artesunate and artemether, which each are more stable and have improved properties compared to artemisinin itself.[30]

The artemisinin class of drugs is used clinically in combination with the antimalarial lumefantrine.[31] This agent has an unclear mode of action, but the combination of the two antimalarials is particularly effective. A major reason for using both agents is that for resistance to occur, the *Plasmodium* would have to become resistant to both agents simultaneously, which has not yet been observed.

Quorum Sensing Inhibition: Keeping Bacteria Blind

Quorum sensing (QS) is a process used by bacteria to control gene expression in response to cell density.[32] Small molecules called autoinducers are produced by bacteria and allow a bacterial population to sense how many neighboring cells are present (see Figure 11.9).[33] QS is used to control a variety of critical functions in pathogenesis, including the formation of biofilms and the expression of antibiotic resistance genes.

QS inhibition research is interested in keeping pathogenic bacteria from coordinating their virulence mechanisms and preventing them from expressing their antibiotic resistance genes.[34] QS inhibitors would either prevent infection from occurring or allow existing antibiotics to be more effective. An example of a natural product QS inhibitor is the molecule known as furanone A, which was isolated from the algae *Delisea pulchra*. This furanone was shown to react with Las, which is a promoter responsible for the activation of QS.

Furanone A was used as a template for the synthetic furanone named C-30. This agent had no antibiotic activity itself but was able to significantly increase the effectiveness of the antibiotic tobramycin against biofilms.[35] It did so by keeping the QS-controlled antibiotic resistance genes against tobramycin from being expressed. This process could serve as a

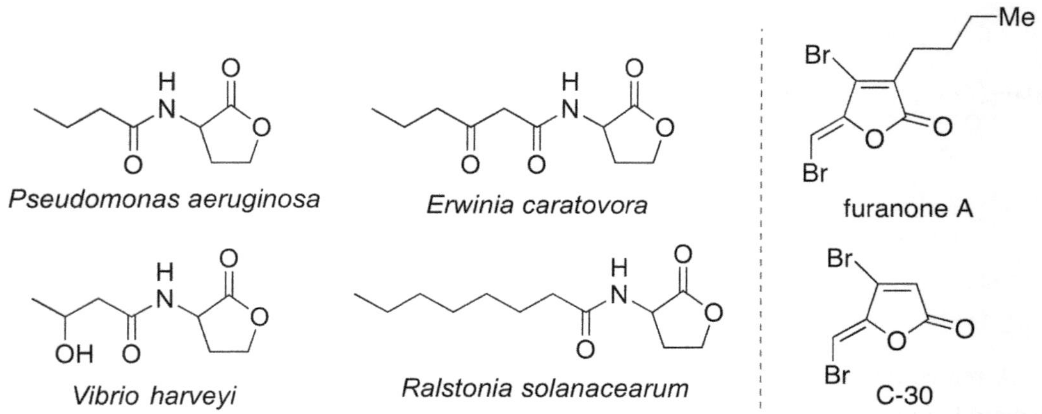

FIGURE 11.9 Quorum sensing signaling molecules by bacterial type (left). Quorum sensing inhibitors (right).

roadmap for allowing our existing pool of antibiotics to remain effective for longer periods of time.

Type III Secretion System Inhibition: Disarming Gram-Negative Pathogens

Many Gram-negative pathogenic bacteria use what is called a Type III Secretion System (TTSS) to infect eukaryotic host cells.[36] The TTSS functions as a molecular syringe to inject pathogenic proteins, called effectors, into the eukaryotic host cell. These effectors reprogram the host cells for purposes beneficial to the pathogen, including suppressing the immune response.[36]

Several natural product TTSS inhibitors have now been discovered, including many from the soil bacteria *Streptomyces*, and also from various plants.[37][38][39][40] A key question about natural products is the question of why the natural products are being made in the first place. For a traditional antibiotic, this is an easy question to answer: the bacteria are making them as self-defense compounds to kill their competitors. Since TTSS inhibitors themselves are not antibiotics but only keep infections from occurring, their role in nature is slightly more complicated.

An interesting recent example of how a TTSS inhibitor may be being used to prevent infection is in beewolf digger wasps. These wasps cultivate *Streptomyces* on their antennae.[41] During the formation of larval cocoons, *Streptomyces* is incorporated into them by the adult wasps. It was discovered that *Streptomyces* used by these wasps produced the natural product piericidin A, which is a traditional antibiotic against Gram-positive bacteria but is also a TTSS inhibitor against Gram-negatives (see Figure 11.10).[38] This result suggests that nature

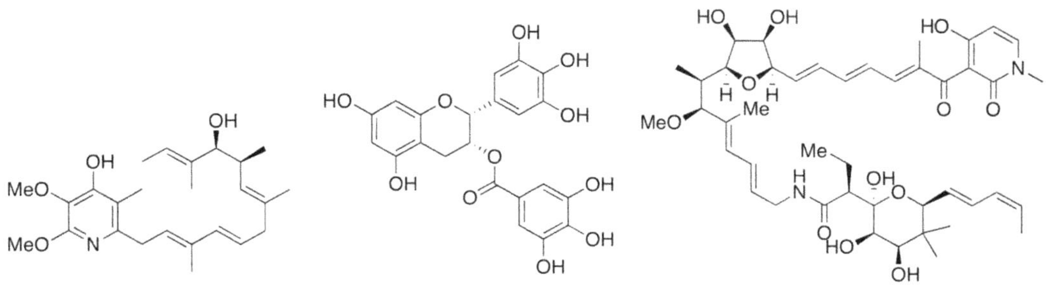

piericidin A epigallocatechin-3-gallate aurodox

FIGURE 11.10 Selected examples of natural product Type III Secretion System Inhibitors.

has been using a TTSS inhibition strategy, and that bacteria may be engaging in symbiotic relationships with insects and/or animals.

Many TTSS inhibitors have recently been discovered from plants, including the molecule epigallocatechin-3-gallate (EGCG) from green tea.[42][43] The use of tea in traditional medicine has long been established, and EGCG is likely a critical component of its activity. Many plants are preyed upon by Gram-negative pathogens that use a TTSS, such as *Pseudomonas syringae*.[44][45] Plants provide an intriguing option in the discovery of new TTSS inhibitors.

TTSS inhibition is still a relatively new field, as the first TTSS inhibitor was discovered in 2002.[46] In the following years, a variety of small molecules have been discovered that inhibit the TTSS, but the most progress and best activity have come from natural products.[47] Omura showed that the natural product aurodox was capable of protecting mice from an otherwise lethal dose of *Citrobacter rodentium*.[40] This is an exciting result, and it suggests that TTSS inhibitors could be used prophylactically.

Natural products have played an important role in how infectious diseases are treated and have been a major reason behind the significantly increased lifespans observed over the last 100 years. Nevertheless, there is still much to learn about strategies that nature may be using to fight or prevent infection. Harnessing such knowledge will determine whether or not this success can be built upon.

References

1. "Historical Data, 1900-1998," Centers for Disease Control and Prevention, National Center for Health Statistics, National Vital Statistics. https://www.cdc.gov/nchs/nvss/mortality_historical_data.htm.
2. Sherry L. Murphy et al., "Mortality in the United States, 2017. NCHS Data Brief, no. 328" (Hyattsville, MD: National Center for Health Statistics, 2018).

3. Marwa Donia and Mark T. Hamann, "Marine Natural Products and Their Potential Applications as Anti-Infective Agents," *Lancet Infectious Diseases* 3, no. 6 (2003): 338–48.
4. Mohd Shahid et al., "Plant Natural Products as a Potential Source for Antibacterial Agents: Recent Trends," *Antiinfective Agents in Medicinal Chemistry* 8, no. 3 (2009): 211–25.
5. Keith F. Chater, "Recent Advances in Understanding *Streptomyces*," *F1000 Research* 5 (2016): 2795.
6. Alexander Fleming, "On the Antibacterial Action of Cultures of a Penicillium, with Special Reference to Their Use in the Isolation of B. influenzae," *British Journal of Experimental Pathology* 10, no 3 (1929): 226–36.
7. E. Chain et al., "Penicillin as a Chemotherapeutic Agent," *Lancet* 236, no. 6104 (1940): 226–28.
8. E. P. Abraham et al., "Further Observations on Penicillin," *Lancet* 238, no. 6155 (1941): 177–89.
9. "The Nobel Prize in Physiology or Medicine 1945," The Nobel Prize. https://www.nobelprize.org/prizes/medicine/1945/summary.
10. D. C. Hodgkin, "The X-Ray Analysis of the Structure of Penicillin," *Advancement of Science* 6, no. 22 (1949): 85–89.
11. Eric Sauvage et al., "The Penicillin-Binding Proteins: Structure and Role in Peptidoglycan Biosynthesis," *FEMS Microbiology Reviews* 32, no. 2 (2008): 234–58.
12. Andre Zapun, Carlos Contreras-Martel, and Thierry Vernet, "Penicillin-Binding Proteins and β-Lactam Resistance," *FEMS Microbiology Reviews* 32, no. 2 (2008): 361–85.
13. G. A. Jacoby and A. A. Medeiros, "More Extended-Spectrum Beta-Lactamases," *Antimicrobial Agents and Chemotherapy* 35, no. 9 (1991): 1697–1704.
14. R. Knox, "A New Penicillin (BRL 1241) Active Against Penicillin-Resistant *Staphylococci*," *British Medical Journal* 2, no. 5200 (1960): 690–93.
15. Daniel Lim and Natalie C J. Strynadka, "Structural Basis for the β Lactam Resistance of PBP2a from Methicillin-Resistant *Staphylococcus aureus*," *Nature Structural and Molecular Biology* 9, no. 11 (2002): 870–76.
16. Sarah M. Drawz and Robert A. Bonomo, "Three Decades of Beta-Lactamase Inhibitors," *Clinical Microbiology Reviews* 23, no. 1 (2010): 160–201.
17. Joseph B. Laudano, "Ceftaroline Fosamil: A New Broad-Spectrum Cephalosporin," *Journal of Antimicrobial Chemotherapy* 66, no. S3 (2011): 1–8.
18. Celine Vidaillac, Steven N. Leonard, and Michael J. Rybak, "In Vitro Activity of Ceftaroline Against Methicillin-Resistant *Staphylococcus aureus* and Heterogeneous Vancomycin-Intermediate *S. aureus* in a Hollow Fiber Model," *Antimicrobial Agents and Chemotherapy* 53, no. 11 (2009): 4712–17.
19. Scott Wesley Long et al., "PBP2a Mutations Causing High-Level Ceftaroline Resistance in Clinical Methicillin-Resistant *Staphylococcus aureus* Isolates," *Antimicrobials Agents and Chemotherapy* 58, no. 11 (2014): 6668–74.

20. "Malaria," Newsroom, World Health Organization. https://www.who.int/en/news-room/fact-sheets/detail/malaria.
21. Elizabeth A. Ashley, Aung Pyae Phyo, and Charles J. Woodrow, "Malaria," *Lancet* 391, no. 10130 (2018): 1608–21.
22. Shahid M. Khan and Andrew P. Waters, "Malaria Parasite Transmission Stages: An Update," *Trends in Parasitology* 20, no. 12 (2004): 575–80.
23. "This Year's World Malaria Report at a Glance," World Health Organization. https://www.who.int/malaria/media/world-malaria-report-2018/en.
24. Ulrike Fillinger and Steve W. Lindsay, "Larval Source Management for Malaria Control in Africa: Myths and Reality," *Malaria Journal* 10, no. 1 (2011): 353.
25. Amit V. Pandey et al., "Hemozoin Formation in Malaria: A Two-Step Process Involving Histidine-Rich Proteins and Lipids," *Biochemical and Biophysical Research Communications* 308, no. 4 (2003): 736–43.
26. Albert C. Chou and Coy D. Fitch, "Control of Heme Polymerase by Chloroquine and Other Quinoline Derivatives," *Biochemical and Biophysical Research Communications* 195, no. 1 (1993): 422–27.
27. David J. Sullivan, "Cinchona Alkaloids: Quinine and Quinidine," in *Treatment and Prevention of Malaria: Antimalarial Drug Chemistry, Action and Use* edited by Henry M. Staines and Sanjeeve Krishna (Berlin: Springer Business and Media, 2012), 45–68.
28. C. Faurant, "From Bark to Weed: The History of Artemisinin," *Parasite* 18, no. 3 (2011): 215–18.
29. S. R. Meshnick et al., "Iron-Dependent Free Radical Generation from the Antimalarial Agent Artemisinin (Qinghaosu)," *Antimicrobial Agents and Chemotherapy* 37, no. 5 (1993): 1108–14.
30. Yupin Suputtamongkol et al., "A Comparison of Oral Artesunate and Artemether Antimalarial Bioactivities in Acute Falciparum Malaria," *British Journal of Clinical Pharmacology* 52, no. 6 (2001): 655–61.
31. Kayla R. Stover, Travis King, and Jessica Robinson, "Artemether-Lumefantrine: An Option for Malaria," *Annals of Pharmacotherapy* 46, no. 4 (2012): 567–77.
32. Jeroen S. Dickschat, "Quorum Sensing and Bacterial Biofilms," *National Product Reports* 27, no. 3 (2010): 343–69.
33. Kristina M. Smith, Yigong Bu, and Hiroaki Suga, "Induction and Inhibition of *Pseudomonas aeruginosa* Quorum Sensing by Synthetic Autoinducer Analogs," *Chemistry and Biology* 10, no. 1 (2003): 81–89.
34. Thomas Bovbjerg Rasmussen et al., "Screening for Quorum-Sensing Inhibitors (QSI) by Use of a Novel Genetic System, the QSI Selector," *Journal of Bacteriology* 187, no. 5 (2005): 1799–814.
35. Morten Hentzer et al., "Attenuation of *Pseudomonas aeruginosa* Virulence by Quorum Sensing Inhibitors," *EMBO Journal* 22, no. 15 (2003): 3803–15.

36. G. R. Cornelis and F. Van Gijsegem, "Assembly and Function of Type III Secretory Systems," *Annual Review of Microbiology* 54 (2000): 735–74.
37. Tracy C. Holmes et al., "Molecular Insights into the Biosynthesis of Guadinomine: A Type III Secretion System Inhibitor," *Journal of the American Chemical Society* 134, no. 42 (2012): 17797–806.
38. Miles C. Duncan et al., "An NF-κB-Based High-Throughput Screen Identifies Piericidins as Inhibitors of the *Yersinia pseudotuberculosis* Type III Secretion System," *Antimicrobial Agents and Chemotherapy* 58, no. 2 (2014): 1118–26.
39. Roger G. Linington et al., "Caminosides B-D, Antimicrobial Glycolipids Isolated from the Marine Sponge *Caminus sphaeroconia*," *Journal of Natural Products* 69, no. 2 (2006): 173–77.
40. Kyota Kimura et al., "A Small-Molecule Inhibitor of the Bacterial Type III Secretion System Protects Against In Vivo Infection with *Citrobacter rodentium*," *Journal of Antibiotics (Tokyo)* 64, no. 2 (2011): 197–203.
41. Johannes Kroiss et al., "Symbiotic Streptomycetes Provide Antibiotic Combination Prophylaxis for Wasp Offspring," *Nature Chemical Biology* 6, no. 4 (2010): 261–63.
42. Lun K. Tsou, Jacob S. Yount, and Howard C. Hang, "Epigallocatechin-3-Gallate Inhibits Bacterial Virulence and Invasion of Host Cells," *Bioorganic and Medicinal Chemistry* 25, no. 11 (2017): 2883–87.
43. Norobu Nakasone et al., "Epigallocatechin Gallate Inhibits the Type III Secretion System of Gram-Negative Enteropathogenic Bacteria Under Model Conditions," *FEMS Microbiology Letters* 364, no. 13 (2017): fnx111.
44. Xiu-Fang Xin and Shen Yang He, "*Pseudomonas syringae* pv. Tomato DC3000: A Model Pathogen for Probing Disease Susceptibility and Hormone Signaling in Plants," *Annual Review of Phytopathology* 51, no. 1 (2013): 473–98.
45. Qiaoling Jin et al., "Type III Protein Secretion in *Pseudomonas syringae*," *Microbes and Infection* 5, no. 4 (2003): 301–10.
46. Roger G. Linington et al., "Caminoside A, an Antimicrobial Glycolipid Isolated from the Marine Sponge *Caminus sphaeroconia*," *Organic Letters* 4, no. 23 (2002): 4089–92.
47. Aaron Elijah May and Chaitan Khosla, "Discovery and Mechanism of Type III Secretion System Inhibitors," *Israel Journal of Chemistry* 53, no. 8 (2013): 577–87.

Chapter 12

Antiviral Natural Products

Aaron E. May, Julia A. Hotinger, and Heather A. Pendergrass

Viruses are infectious agents that can only replicate inside the living cells of another organism. They typically contain a single type of nucleic acid (either DNA or RNA) and a protein coat.[1] A virus can be enclosed in an envelope that contains lipids, proteins, and carbohydrates. Viruses do not have the machinery required to create their own protein and multiply their own nucleotides and instead require the host's ribosome and replication machinery to create new proteins and DNA/RNA strands.[2]

Viruses cause a variety of diseases, including hepatitis, influenza, measles, polio, rabies, ebola, and human immunodeficiency virus (HIV). Viruses such as influenza use mammalian cells as hosts (see Figure 12.1). They can attach to host epithelial cells, and they enter the cell via endocytosis.[3] The virus breaks apart inside the host, revealing RNA that can enter the nucleus. In the nucleus, RNA polymerase replicates the viral RNA. Viral proteins can then be made, which assemble into new viral particles, which can then leave the cell and reach a new host. It is through this process that the virus proliferates and causes new infections.

Other viruses specialize in infecting bacterial cells and are referred to as bacteriophages. These viruses inject their nucleotide sequences into host cells (see Figure 12.2).[4] These nucleotides are typically either linear or circular double-stranded DNA. This DNA can be incorporated into host genomes and replicated. This process is referred to as the lysogenic cycle. Environmental stresses can cause the phage DNA that has been incorporated into the genome to break free and produce more phage particles within the host cell. Infected cells can then lyse, releasing new phages into the environment. This process is called the lytic cycle.

Generally speaking, it is more difficult to create new and effective antivirals than it is to create antibiotics, since antivirals can also interfere with host cellular machinery. Antiviral agents can work in a variety of ways.[5] Some may target specific viral proteins, keeping new viruses from

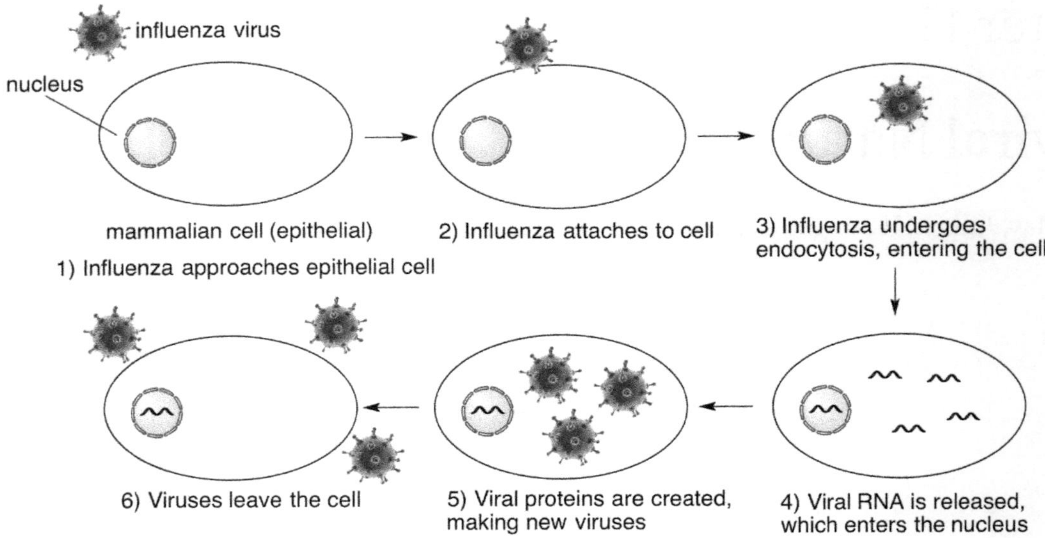

FIGURE 12.1 Viral cycle of influenza.

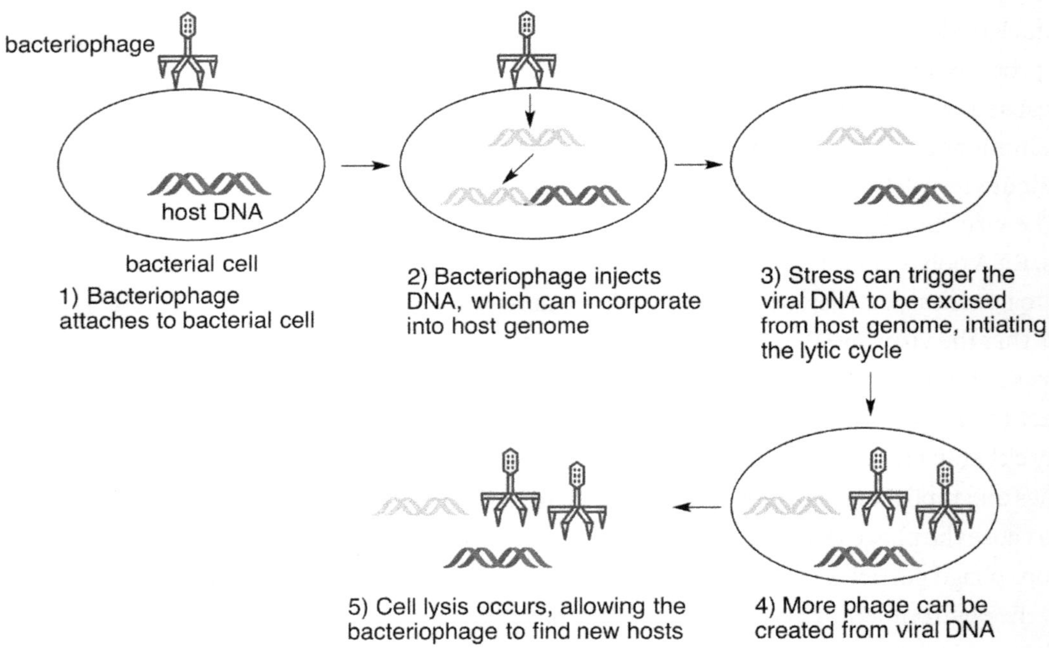

FIGURE 12.2 Viral cycle of bacteriophages.

assembling.[6] Others may interfere with viral entry or adherence. Antivirals may also function by interfering with RNA polymerase.[7] Many antiviral agents are prodrugs and contain purine or pyrimidine analogs. These molecules act as antimetabolites by interfering with normal metabolism. They may bind to a critical enzyme but be unable to be processed, tying up the enzyme and keeping it from performing its function.

Antiviral Nucleotides

An early example of an antiviral natural product is vidarabine, also known as Ara-A, or adenine arabinoside (see Figure 12.3).[8] This molecule was isolated in the 1950s from the Caribbean sea sponge *Cryptotheca crypta*. Ara-A is an analog of adenosine and exhibits antiviral activity by two unique mechanisms. Ara-A is a prodrug and is phosphorylated by kinases at the 5' position to produce the diphosphate Ara-ADP. This molecule inhibits ribonucleotide reductase, which is the enzyme that produces deoxyribonucleotides.[9] Since these molecules are the building blocks of DNA, the lack of supply leads to a lack of DNA assembly. Ara-ATP is also formed by kinases by phosphorylation of the 5' position, and this molecule is an inhibitor of DNA polymerase.[10] The combination of the lack of DNA building blocks and inhibition of DNA polymerase makes an effective antiviral agent. A major drawback of vidarabine is the requirement that it be given intravenously. It also is a teratogen, meaning it can cause birth defects.

Modern synthetic nucleoside and nucleotide antiviral analogs include acyclovir, ganciclovir, and cidofovir (see Figure 12.4).[11] Acyclovir is based off the guanosine scaffold and is used as an orally active nucleoside against herpes simplex virus. Acyclovir is phosphorylated in the cell by thymidine kinase but is incapable of forming DNA chains, since it is missing the 3' hydroxyl group of the deoxyribose sugar necessary for cross-linking.[12] Acyclovir is thus capable of reacting with a growing DNA chain, but does not allow it to be extended further.

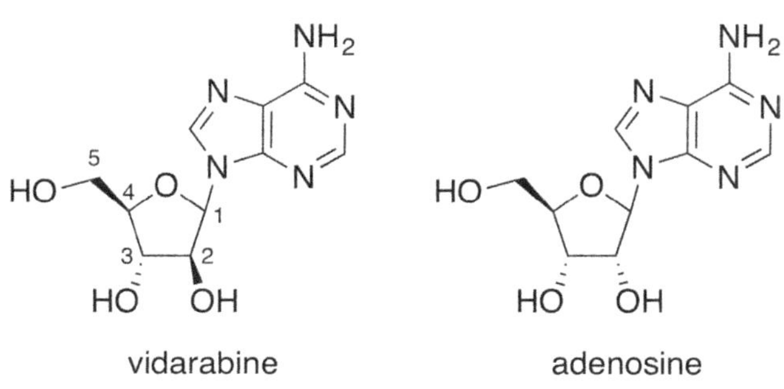

FIGURE 12.3 Vidarabine and adenosine.

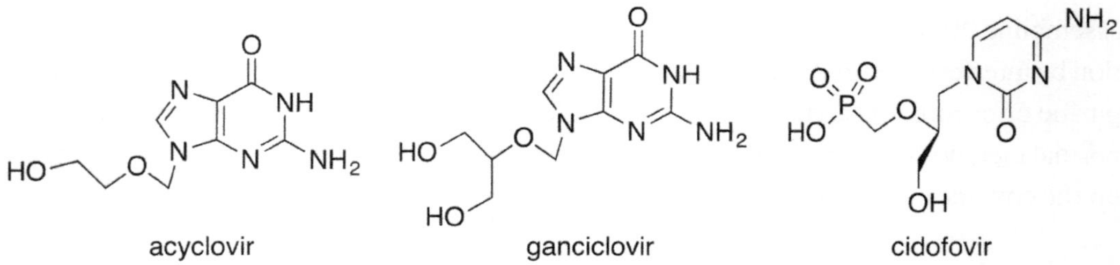

FIGURE 12.4 Modern synthetic nucleotide and nucleoside analogs.

Ganciclovir is used against cytomegalovirus (CMV) and is phosphorylated by a kinase that is encoded by the CMV DNA sequence.[13] Phosphorylated ganciclovir is an inhibitor of DNA polymerase. Cidofovir is also used to treat CMV and does not require additional phosphorylation.[14] It also is an inhibitor of DNA polymerase.

Disrupting Viral Coating—Castanospermine

Viruses are typically coated in proteins that provide shape or rigidity to hold the DNA or RNA cargo of the virus. Interfering with the assembly of this coating is a strategy to reduce or inhibit viral replication. Castanospermine is a natural product isolated from *Castanospermum australe* that inhibits the Dengue virus by inhibiting the function of two structural proteins (see Figure 12.5).[15] The first is the E protein, which is a surface protein that is associated with viral entry, and the second is the prM protein, which is a membrane protein involved in forming a glycoprotein sphere around the genomic DNA. Castanospermine functions as an alpha-glucosidase inhibitor, which prevents prM from being glycosylated and maturing to an effective viral coating. The structure of castanospermine resembles glucose, allowing it to bind and interfere with normal glucosidase function.

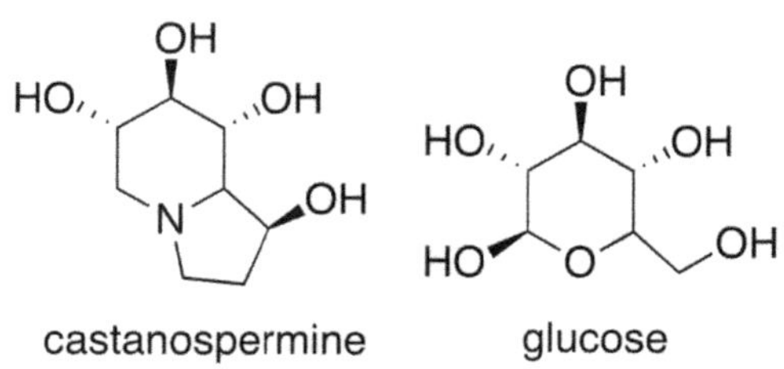

FIGURE 12.5 Structure of the natural product glucosidase inhibitor castanospermine and comparison with glucose.

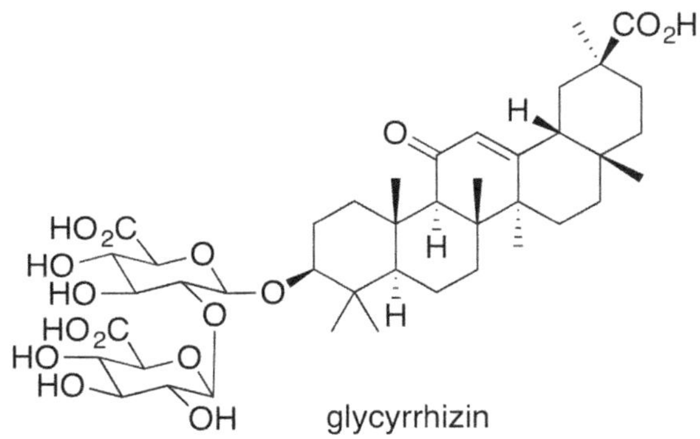

FIGURE 12.6 Structure of glycyrrhizin.

Broad Spectrum Antiviral—Glycyrrhizin

Glycyrrhizin is a natural product isolated from the root of *Glycyrrhiza glabra*, also known as licorice (see Figure 12.6). This natural product is associated with a wide variety of antiviral activity, and licorice has been used therapeutically for over 1,000 years.[16] Glycyrrhizin has been used to treat hepatitis B and C in humans and can reduce liver inflammation and necrosis.[17] It has also been shown to inhibit HIV replication.[18]

Mice receiving glycyrrhizin via IP were capable of surviving a tenfold LD_{50} dose of influenza A2.[19] In a test of murine herpes encephalitis, IP-dosed glycyrrhizin reduced viral replication by over 50 percent.[20] The mechanism of action for the activity of glycyrrhizin is not entirely clear, but it may in part be due to disruption of adherence of viral particles to their target cells. Glycyrrhizin is also correlated with modulating immune signaling pathways, which may contribute to some of the observed biological activity.[21]

Fighting the Flu—Shikimic Acid as a Starting Point for Tamiflu

Natural products often serve as antiviral drugs, but they can also be used as a template or starting material for the production of new synthetic drugs. The conversion of a natural product to a new chemical entity is referred to as semisynthesis.[22] Shikimic acid is a natural product first isolated in 1885 from the oriental plant *Illicium religiosum* (see Figure 12.7). The biosynthetic route to produce shikimic acid is referred to as the shikimic acid pathway. This process is performed by nonmammalian life forms (e.g., plants, bacteria, fungi) to produce shikimic acid, which is further converted into the amino acids tyrosine, tryptophan, and phenylalanine.[23]

Shikimic acid is also used as a starting material for the chemical synthesis of the antiviral agent oseltamivir phosphate, or Tamiflu®.[24] After replicating inside the host epithelial cell,

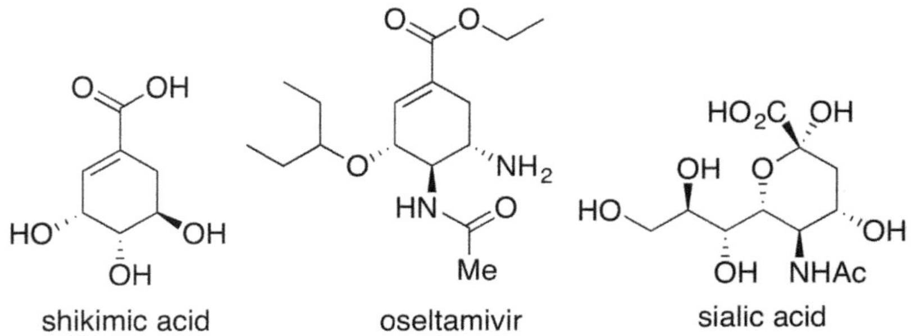

FIGURE 12.7 Shikimic acid, oseltamivir, and sialic acid.

the flu virus exits the cell. To break free of the cell, it must be released by receptors on the cell surface that are holding onto it. These receptors contain sialic acid, and neuraminidase is the enzyme on the surface of the flu virus that cleaves it. This cleavage causes releasing of the virus so that it can continue to proliferate in new hosts.[25] Oseltamivir functions as a mimic of sialic acid and binds to the active site of the neuraminidase.[26] This keeps the virus from breaking free from the cell, thus reducing the amount of virus that can proliferate.

Activating Latent HIV—Prostratin and Bryostatin

A cure for HIV has not yet been realized. A particular problem is that HIV is capable of remaining in a dormant or latent state within resting CD4+ cells.[27] These cells are referred to as latent HIV reservoirs. Treatment of HIV infection with highly active antiretroviral therapy (HAART) targets the actively replicating virus but not the latent HIV.[28] An idea for curing HIV infection is to simultaneously activate latent HIV reservoirs while also treating the active infection in the hopes of eliminating the virus entirely.[29]

Prostratin is a natural product isolated from the bark of *Homalanthus nutans* (see Figure 12.8).[30] Some of the early studies performed with this molecule suggested that it could activate latent HIV.[31] Prostratin is an activator of protein kinase C (PKC), a family of enzymes responsible for a large number of cell signaling cascades in mammals.[32] Drugs modulating PKCs have been tested for a variety of conditions, including cancer, diabetic neuropathy, and Alzheimer's disease.[33]

The most potent PKC-activating natural products are the bryostatins. These molecules were isolated from the marine organism *Bugula neritina*.[34] Brysostatin-1 has been shown to activate latent HIV in resting CD4+ cells at concentrations of 1,150 picograms/mL.[35][36] A phase I clinical trial of bryostatin-1 was performed on patients with HIV while also undergoing HAART.[37] It was found that no statistically significant activation of latent HIV occurred and that PKC activity was not significantly changed. Serum concentrations of bryostatins

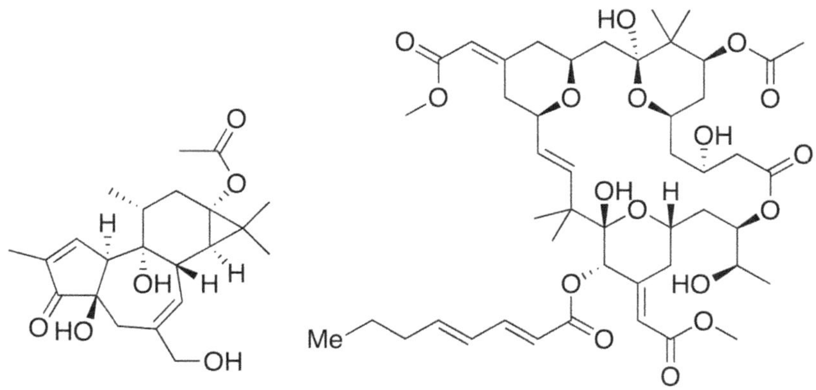

prostratin bryostatin

FIGURE 12.8 Structures of natural product protein kinase C activators prostratin and bryostatin.

were low, less than 50 picograms/mL at the highest dose tested, suggesting that significantly more of the drug would be needed to achieve a therapeutic effect.

Natural products have been critical in fighting diseases caused by viruses. As the field of antivirals moves forward, it is important that new natural products be discovered. A key goal in this regard should be the identification of new viral target proteins or enzymes. This will undoubtedly require the creation of new assays for assessing the viability of the new targets.

References

1. Anton S. Petrov and Stephen Harvey, "Structural and Thermodynamic Principles of Viral Packaging," *Structure* 15, no. 1 (2007): 21–27.
2. Bernard N. Fields, "How Do Viruses Cause Different Diseases?" *JAMA* 250, no. 13 (1983): 1754–56.
3. Juan Fontana and Alasdair C. Steven, "Influenza Virus-Mediated Membrane Fusion: Structural Insights from Electron Microscopy," *Archives of Biochemistry and Biophysics* 581 (2015): 86–97.
4. Ryland Fletcher Young, "Bacteriophage Lysis: Mechanism and Regulation," *Microbiological Reviews* 56, no. 3 (1992): 430–81.
5. Kelly Melville, Thalia Rodriguez, and Hana M. Dobrovolny, "Investigating Different Mechanisms of Action in Combination Therapy for Influenza," *Frontiers in Pharmacology* 9 (2018): 1207.
6. J. F. Marcos et al., "Inhibition of a Plant Virus Infection by Analogs of Melittin," *Proceedings of the National Academy of Sciences USA* 92, no. 26 (1995): 12466–69.
7. Ching-Hsiu Tsai et al., "Antiviral Therapy Targeting Viral Polymerase," *Current Pharmaceutical Design* 12, no. 11 (2006): 1339–55.

8. Richard J. Whitley et al., "Pharmacology, Tolerance, and Antiviral Activity of Vidarabine Monophosphate in Humans," *Antimicrobial Agents and Chemotherapy* 18, no. 5 (1980): 709–15.
9. E. Colleen Moore and Seymour S. Cohen, "Effects of Arabinonucleotides on Ribonucleotide Reduction by an Enzyme System from Rat Tumor," *Journal of Biology Chemical* 242, no. 9 (1967): 2116–18.
10. W. E. Müller et al., "Mode of Action of 9-β-D-Arabinofuranosyladenine on the Synthesis of DNA, RNA, and Protein In Vivo and In Vitro," *Cancer Research* 35, no. 8 (1975): 2160–68.
11. Roy F. Chemaly et al., "In Vitro Comparison of Currently Available and Investigational Antiviral Agents Against Pathogenic Human Double-Stranded DNA Viruses: A Systematic Literature Review," *Antiviral Research* 163 (2019): 50–58.
12. Gertrude B. Elion, "The Biochemistry and Mechanism of Action of Acyclovir," *Journal of Antimicrobial Chemotherapy* 12, no. SB (2012): S9–17.
13. Thomas Matthews and Richard Boehme, "Antiviral Activity and Mechanism of Action of Ganciclovir," *Reviews of Infectious Disease* 10, no. S3 (1988): S490–94.
14. Julie B. Kendle and Patty Fan-Havard, "Cidofovir in the Treatment of Cytomegaloviral Disease," *Annals of Pharmacotherapy* 32, no. 11 (1998): 1181–92.
15. Kevin Whitby et al., "Castanospermine, a Potent Inhibitor of Dengue Virus Infection In Vitro and In Vivo," *Journal of Virology* 79, no. 14 (2005): 8698–706.
16. Cristina Fiore et al., "Antiviral Effects of Glycyrrhiza Species," *Phytotherapy Research* 22, no. 2 (2008): 141–48.
17. Hiromitsu Kumada, "Long-Term Treatment of Chronic Hepatitis C with Glycyrrhizin [stronger neo-minophagen C (SNMC)] for Preventing Liver Cirrhosis and Hepatocellular Carcinoma," *Oncology* 62, no. S1 (2002): 94–100.
18. Hideki Nakashima et al., "A New Anti-Human Immunodeficiency Virus Substance, Glycyrrhizin Sulfate; Endowment of Glycyrrhizin with Reverse Transcriptase-Inhibitory Activity by Chemical Modification," *Japanese Journal of Cancer Research* 78, no. 8 (1987): 767–71.
19. T. Utsunomiya, M. Kobayashi, R. B. Pollard, and F. Suzuki, "Glycyrrhizin, an Active Component of Licorice Roots, Reduces Morbidity and Mortality of Mice Infected with Lethal Doses of Influenza Virus," *Antimicrobial Agents and Chemotherapy* 41 (1997): 551-56.
20. T. Sekizawa, K. Yanagi, and Y. Itoyama, Y. "Glycyrrhizin Increases Survival of Mice with Herpes Simplex Encephalitis," *Acta Virology* 45, no. 1 (2001): 51–54.
21. Jia-Ying Tan et al., "Glycyrrhizin Affects Monocyte Migration and Apoptosis by Blocking HMGB1 Signaling," *Molecular Medicine Reports* 17, no. 4 (2018): 5970–75.
22. Zongru Guo, "The Modification of Natural Products for Medical Use," *Acta Pharmaceutica Sinica B* 7, no. 2 (2017): 119–36.
23. Hiroshi Maeda and Natalia Dudareva, "The Shikimate Pathway and Aromatic Amino Acid Biosynthesis in Plants," *Annual Review of Plant Biology* 63 (2012): 73–105.

24. Garima Rawat, Priyanka Tripathi, and R. K. Saxena, "Expanding Horizons of Shikimic Acid: Recent Progresses in Production and Its Endless Frontiers in Application and Market Trends," *Applied Microbiology and Biotechnology* 97, no. 10 (2013): 4277–87.
25. Yulia Shtyrya, Larisa V. Mochalova, and Nicolai V. Bovin, "Influenza Virus Neuraminidase: Structure and Function," *Acta Naturae* 1, no. 2 (2009): 26–32.
26. Anne Moscona, "Neuraminidase Inhibitors for Influenza," *New England Journal of Medicine* 353 (2005): 1363–73.
27. Richard A. Koup, "A New Latent HIV Reservoir," *Nature Medicine* 7 (2001): 404–5.
28. Reuben Granich et al., "Highly Active Antiretroviral Treatment as Prevention of HIV Transmission: Review of Scientific Evidence and Update," *Current Opinion in HIV and AIDS* 5, no. 4 (2010): 298–304.
29. Youry Kim, Jenny L. Anderson, and Sharon R. Lewin, "Getting the 'Kill' into 'Shock and Kill': Strategies to Eliminate Latent HIV," *Cell Host Microbe* 23, no. 1 (2018): 14–26.
30. Kirk Gustafson et al., "A Nonpromoting Phorbol from the Samoan Medicinal Plant *Homalanthus nutans* Inhibits Cell Killing by HIV-1," *Journal of Medicinal Chemistry* 35, no. 11 (1992): 1978–86.
31. Joseph Kulkosky et al., "Prostratin: Activation of Latent HIV-1 Expression Suggests a Potential Inductive Adjuvant Therapy for HAART," *Blood* 98, no. 10 (2001): 3006–15.
32. Yasutomi Nishizuka, "The Molecular Heterogeneity of Protein Kinase C and Its Implications for Cellular Regulation," *Nature* 334, no. 6184 (1988): 661–65.
33. Charleata A. Carter and Cynthia J. M. Kane, "Therapeutic Potential of Natural Compounds That Regulate the Activity of Protein Kinase C," *Current Medicinal Chemistry* 11, no. 21 (2004): 2883–902.
34. George R. Pettit et al., "Isolation and Structure of Bryostatin 1," *Journal of the American Chemical Society* 104, no. 24 (1982): 6846–48.
35. C. Korin Bullen et al., "New Ex Vivo Approaches Distinguish Effective and Ineffective Single Agents for Reversing HIV-1 Latency In Vivo," *Nature Medicine* 20, no. 4 (2014): 425–29.
36. Gregory M. Laird et al., "Ex Vivo Analysis Identifies Effective HIV-1 Latency-Reversing Drug Combinations," *Journal of Clinical Investigation* 125, no. 5 (2015): 1901–12.
37. Carolina Gutiérrez et al., "Bryostatin-1 for Latent Virus Reactivation in HIV-Infected Patients on Antiretroviral Therapy," *AIDS* 30, no. 9 (2016): 1385–92.

Credits

Fig. 12.1a: Copyright © 2015 Depositphotos/Den.Barbulat.
Fig. 12.1a: Copyright © 2015 Depositphotos/davooda.
Fig, 12.2a: Copyright © 2016 Depositphotos/YershovOleksandr1.
Fig. 12.2b: Copyright © 2019 Depositphotos/nadia1992.

Chapter 13

Natural Products for Cardiovascular Diseases Treatment

Daniel Afosah, Shravan Morla, Carissa Campbell, and Umesh R. Desai

Introduction

Cardiovascular diseases remain the leading cause of mortality worldwide, and according to estimates, these diseases accounted for more than 17 million deaths in 2016.[1] In addition to prescription medicines, herbal preparations are utilized by numerous patients for management of their cardiovascular diseases, a practice that must have originated in ancient times. Current studies point to an increased reliance on alternate, plant-based treatment options by more than 15 million people in the United States.[2] This can be attributed to factors including the rising cost of conventional drugs and the belief that herbal preparations are natural and hence have the least propensity to cause adverse effects.

Herbal medicines have been used to manage several cardiovascular diseases, such as hypertension, atherosclerosis and thrombosis, cardiac failure, and angina pectoris. The use of most of these herbal preparations is mainly based on anecdotal evidence. Yet some of these have been evaluated using in vitro and in vivo assays. A select few herbal products have been evaluated in clinical studies. It is important to mention that some cardiovascular drugs in use today have herbal origins, the most prominent being digoxin, reserpine, and acetylsalicylic acid.

There are, however, some critical challenges that need to be addressed regarding the use of herbal/natural products for cardiovascular diseases, and for all diseases in general. This is especially important because of their increasing popularity. The most notable of these concerns is the safety and efficacy of these preparations, especially in children and pregnant and lactating women. Some herbs have very toxic effects, and unfortunately the data, especially clinical, for many of these herbal preparations are not available or adequate.[3] Standardization issues for these herbal preparations also exist, and there are varied reports regarding discrepancies in phytochemical composition and content. Also, in cases of overdose, appropriate actions to counteract severe effects for most of these agents remain unknown.[4] Another major issue with use of herbal preparations for cardiovascular diseases is the potential for herb-herb and herb-drug interactions, which can have unknown and dire consequences. This is particularly important because many people using herbal preparations for cardiovascular diseases use prescription medications concomitantly.

Nevertheless, herbal preparations find great use in the management of cardiovascular diseases, and significant research efforts are necessary to ascertain their efficacy and safety, elucidate their mechanisms of action, and standardize preparations. The following sections highlight particular herbal/natural preparations that have use in the management of cardiovascular diseases.

Congestive Heart Failure

Congestive heart failure (CHF) is a disease characterized by the heart's failure to adequately pump blood, resulting in the retention of fluid in tissues and organs. Heart failure is caused by a wide range of factors, which include other heart conditions, genetic defects, and systemic disease.[5] The principal signs of the disease are shortness of breath, fatigue, and edema,[6] and diagnosis of the disease is fundamentally clinical, arrived at on the basis of patients' medical history and physical examination.[6][7] However, laboratory tests on patient samples can also help in reaching a diagnosis. Currently, more than 25 million people suffer from heart failure worldwide, and owing to an increase in the aging population, CHF prevalence is on an upward trend.[8] For instance, in the United States, CHF is the leading cause of hospitalization for adults 65 years and above.[9] The American College of Cardiology Foundation and the American Heart Association classify heart failure into four stages based on disease severity.[7] Stage A encompasses at-risk patients who have no heart disease or symptoms. Stage B patients show structural heart disease but do not present with symptoms. Stages C and D represent patients who show structural heart defects with history of disease symptoms and patients with advanced disease requiring specialized medical treatment, respectively. Current treatment options for congestive heart failure include the use of angiotensin-converting enzyme inhibitors and angiotensin receptor blockers, diuretics, beta blockers, and digoxin, a cardiac glycoside obtained from plant sources.[7] In advanced stages of the disease, defibrillators are used to maintain heartbeat.[10] Digoxin, which is obtained from the *Digitalis spp.*, commonly known as foxglove, is still used today for the management of CHF.[11] Additionally, supplementation with coenzyme Q10, a natural product, is becoming popular as research reveals its association with and benefits in CHF.[12] These two natural products are described in detail below.

Coenzyme Q10

Coenzyme Q10 (CoQ10) is a highly lipophilic molecule that resembles vitamin K in structure.[13] CoQ10 exists in two forms, the oxidized form, ubiquinone, and the more bioavailable reduced form, ubiquinol.[14] This molecule, which was first isolated from beef mitochondria in 1957, is found in many organisms, ranging from aerobic bacteria to plants and mammals.[15][16][17] In humans, it is present as an energy source for mitochondria throughout the tissues in the body, with the heart, kidneys, and liver having the highest concentrations due to the higher rates of metabolism in these organs.[15] With aging, CoQ10 biosynthesis declines, which can result in deficiencies.[18] CoQ10 is important for the production of ATP and functions as a cofactor in oxidative phosphorylation in mitochondria, mediating electron transfer in the electron transport chain (ETC) from complex 1 (NADH coenzyme Q reductase) to complex 3 (cytochrome bc1 complex), and from complex 2 (succinate dehydrogenase) to complex 3.[12] Being important for the production of ATP, CoQ10 plays vital roles in high energy–requiring cells, including cardiac cells. In addition to being important for cellular function and energy, it has also been shown to have antioxidant, free radical scavenging, and vasodilation effects.[17] These are all important for cardiac health, and low CoQ10 levels have been linked to cardiac diseases including heart failure.[13][19] In fact, research shows that CoQ10 is a predicting factor of CHF, and long-term therapy has been demonstrated to improve the conditions of patients with heart failure.[12][19][20] CoQ10 deficiency is also associated with mitochondrial diseases, neurogenerative disorders, diabetes, and cancer, and improvements in some of these disorders are achieved with administration of CoQ10.[15][21] CoQ10 has been demonstrated to be beneficial in doxorubicin toxicity, mitral valve prolapse syndrome, and even in Meniere-like syndrome (acute sudden deafness).[19]

CoQ10 can be obtained from food; generally diets consisting of meat, fish, nuts, and certain oils are considered to be rich in CoQ10, while diets consisting of mainly dairy, vegetables, fruit, and cereal contain lower amounts.[22] Plant sources of CoQ10 include broccoli, cauliflower, and spinach. However, only about 2–5 mg of CoQ10 is obtained from food, and hence CoQ10 supplementation is required in cases of deficiency. CoQ10 is produced in large scale using microorganisms, mainly bacteria and yeast,[16] for the preparation of supplements,

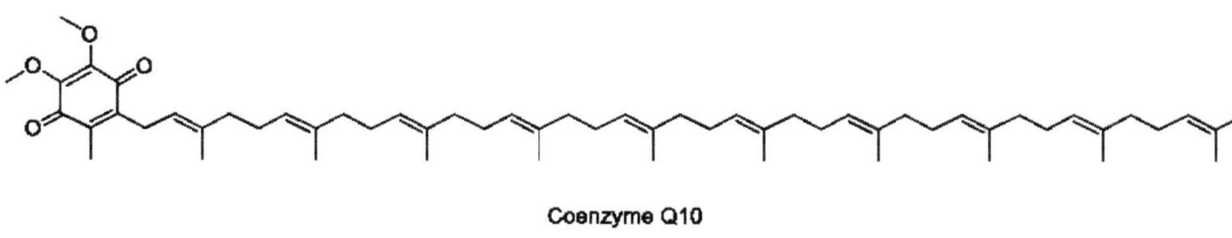

FIGURE 13.1 Structure of coenzyme Q10.

which are available as suspensions, tablets, soft gelatin capsules, IV, and oil suspensions.[14] The liquid dosage forms are generally more bioavailable compared to the other dosage forms.

Dosage and Toxicity

CoQ10 is well tolerated and has been shown to be very safe as a supplement, with very minor side effects associated with its use. These adverse effects include itching and gastrointestinal disturbances. However, being structurally similar to vitamin K, CoQ10 has potential procoagulant effects and has been reported to decrease the anticoagulant effect of warfarin. Statins have also been shown to reduce blood CoQ10 levels.[23] In humans, a daily intake of 12 mg/kg/day is suggested, with up to 100-fold this amount thought to be within the safety limit.[17] No signs of genotoxicity have been observed in animals, and studies also indicate that the lethal dose in rats is in excess of 5 g/kg.[17] Recent clinical trials show that CoQ10 supplementation is beneficial in heart failure.[24] A meta-analysis involving 14 randomized controlled clinical trials with 2,149 patients showed a decrease in mortality and improvement in exercise capacity in heart failure patients using CoQ10.[25] Some research indicates that in order to have an effect on cardiovascular health, a daily intake in the range of 30–1,200 mg for a period of eight weeks is required.[26]

Foxglove Species

Foxglove refers to the about 20 species of the genus *Digitalis*, from the family Plantaginaceae. It is a biennial plant that originated in Europe but is now found worldwide due to its being an invasive species. The plant, which stands 3–4 feet high, is often found growing in sandy, acidic soils along rocky coasts and in shaded, wooded areas. The plant has serrated, wrinkled leaves; wide and long purple, pink, or white flowers with characteristic spots and markings; and roots that can be described as knotty and fibrous. The most studied species of digitalis are *Digitalis purpurea* and *Digitalis lanata*. *Digitalis purpurea* was first illustrated and described by Leonhart Fuchs, a German botanist, in 1542 and was named *Digitalis* due to its fingerlike appearance.[27] Foxglove is present in many folklores, literature, and even art. Vincent van Gogh's *Portrait of Dr. Gachet* depicts a homeopathic doctor holding the flower of a foxglove plant, and it is thought that Van Gogh used foxglove for medicinal purposes.[28]

The use of foxglove for the treatment of cardiac disease was documented in the 18th century by William Withering; however, there are reports indicating that the Romans used foxglove for heart failure much earlier.[29] Foxglove has been added into juices, syrups, and ointments to treat various ailments such as epilepsy, ulcers, dropsy, and wounds. Foxglove has also been studied for possible use in the treatment/management of cancer.[30][31] The bioactive phytochemical constituents of digitalis are the cardiac glycosides, also known as cardiotonic glycosides. These compounds have a sugar moiety attached to a steroidal

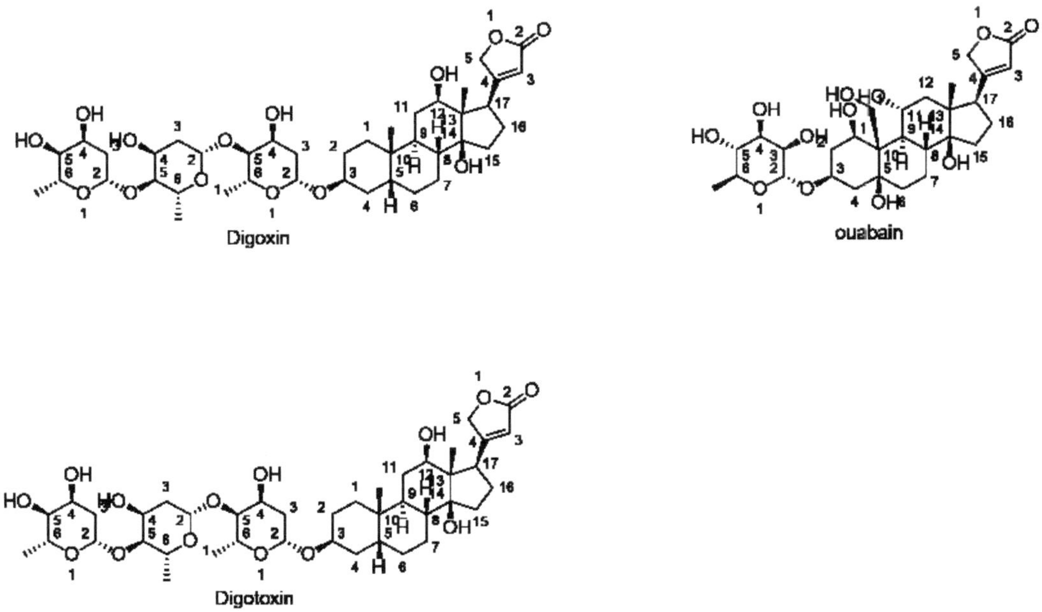

FIGURE 13.2 Structures of foxglove components.

nucleus, thought to be the pharmacophore, with the most commonly encountered sugars being glucose, galactose, mannose, rhamnose, and digitalose.[32] The steroidal core is also connected to a lactone group at position 17, which is important for pharmacological activity and is used to characterize the glycosides.[31][32] Cardiac glycosides that have a five-membered lactone ring are known as cardenolides and are the most prominent digitalis phytochemicals, whilst those connected to a six-membered lactone ring are known as bufodienolides.[31]

Cardiac glycosides exert their pharmacological activity by inhibiting membrane-bound Na+/K+-ATPase. This causes increased intracellular Na+ and a corresponding elevation in Na+/Ca2+ exchange. Intracellular calcium levels are elevated as a result, which ultimately results in increased myocardial contraction.[33] The most well-known and well-studied cardiac glycosides are digoxin, digitoxin, and ouabain, with digoxin being the most widely used digitalis derivative. Digoxin is available as tablets, injectables, elixirs, and capsules. In addition to cardiac glycosides, steroidal compounds including saponins and sterols, phenolic compounds such as flavonoids and phenylethanoic acids, and polysaccharides are present.[34] As with many plants, seasonal changes have an impact on the phytochemical constituents of digitalis plants.

Dosage and Toxicity and Clinical Studies

A number of clinical trials point to the benefits of cardiac glycosides in the management of congestive heart failure, manifesting as decreased hospitalizations and decreased disease progression or worsening.[35][36] The dosing of digitalis and digitalis-derived drugs vary between patients and is usually titrated according to age, lean body weight, and renal function. However, digitalis extracts and cardiac glycosides have narrow therapeutic windows and can cause poisoning if use is not well monitored.[32][37] Due to this, serum digoxin levels should not exceed 1 ng/mL;[33] however, digoxin toxicity has been observed even within the therapeutic range of 0.5–0.9 ng/mL. Toxicity to cardiac glycosides manifests as bradycardia; gastrointestinal symptoms, including nausea, vomiting, abdominal pain, and diarrhea; weakness; heart block; ventricular fibrillation; tachycardia; and xanthopsia, or yellow, blurred vision.[38] The narrow therapeutic window of cardiac glycosides has led to their substitution with other therapeutic agents for the management of congestive heart failure. A number of drug-drug interactions involving digitalis have been reported. Among these are interactions between digitalis and antiarrhythmic drugs, with Amiodarone and dronedarone increasing digoxin serum levels and quinidine decreasing the elimination of digoxin, as well as preventing its transport across epithelial membranes.[35][37] Macrolide antibiotics also inhibit digoxin metabolism. Since cardiac glycosides are excreted renally, diuretics may also potentiate incidence of digitalis toxicity by interfering with the glomerular filtration rate.[39] On the other hand, decreased serum digoxin levels are observed with rifampicin and phenytoin, which induce p-glycoprotein.[40] Cardiac glycosides are not contraindicated in pregnancy or lactation and have been used to treat fetal tachycardia.[41] However, they should be avoided in patients with atrioventricular node block and Wolff-Parkinson-White syndrome.[40]

Hypertension

Hypertension, or high blood pressure, is a long-term medical condition in which the blood pressure in the arteries is persistently greater than normal. Recent studies have found that one in every four adults in the United States has hypertension.[42] It is an asymptomatic condition and hence can be difficult to diagnose. It is estimated that about 32 percent of the population with hypertension are unaware of their hypertensive state.[43] If untreated, it can lead to severe consequences, including renal failure, coronary disease, cardiac failure, and even stroke. Primary hypertension, or essential hypertension, as seen in about 95 percent of hypertension cases, has no identified cause and is usually attributed to a combination of genetic, environmental, and lifestyle factors. Secondary hypertension, occurring in about 5 percent of patients, has a definite cause and can be due to Cushing's syndrome, Conn's syndrome, sleep apnea, diabetes mellitus, obesity, and other conditions.

Lifestyle changes play an important role in the management of hypertension. Increasing fruit and vegetable intake, reducing alcohol consumption, regular exercise, cessation of smoking, and limiting caffeine intake can all assist in managing hypertension. Specific advice on

TABLE 13.1 Pharmacological Classes of Antihypertensive Drugs

Type	Example
α-adrenergic receptor blockers	Doxazosin
Angiotensin converting enzyme inhibitors	Captopril
Angiotensin II receptor antagonists	Losartan
β-blockers	Propranolol
Calcium channel blockers	Verapamil
Centrally acting agents	Clonidine
Direct acting vasodilators	Hydralazine
Diuretics	Chlorothiazide
Renin inhibitors	Aliskiren

reducing the amount of salt in food is given to hypertensive patients, as some studies have shown that reducing salt intake can reduce hypertension by 5/3 mm Hg.[44] High salt intake, however, is not linked to the cause of hypertension.

In most patients, however, lifestyle changes alone are not sufficient for disease management, and antihypertensive drugs are required. There are multiple antihypertensive drugs currently available on the market, and successful treatment of hypertension with limited side effects is now possible. There are about nine major pharmacological classes of antihypertensives based on their mechanism of action (see Table 13.1).[45]

Historically, people have also used herbal remedies to treat hypertension. Many of these herbal remedies have been studied by researchers, and the active ingredients in a few of these preparations are now being marketed as antihypertensives in many regions of the world. Some of the widely used herbal extracts with antihypertensive effects are highlighted below.

Rauwolfia Serpentina and Related Alkaloids

Rauwolfia serpentina is a shrub belonging to the Apocynaceae family and is native to tropical and subtropical regions of the world.[46] It is mostly grown in the deciduous forests of India, Burma, Bangladesh, Sri Lanka, and Malaysia. The earliest descriptions of the plant (also known as *sarpagandha* and *chandrika*) were found in Indian manuscripts dating back to 1000 BC, where its usefulness in the treatment of snake and insect bites, malaria,

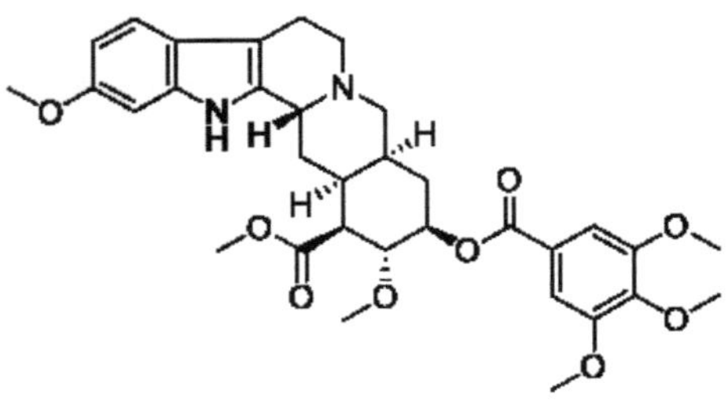

FIGURE 13.3 Structure of reserpine.

abdominal pain, dysentery, and hypertension was mentioned.[47] Considering its popularity for the treatment of hypertension, an Indian physician, Rustom Jal Vakil, conducted a clinical trial using 50 patients.[48] According to this study, significant decreases in systolic and diastolic blood pressure were observed in 85 percent and 81 percent of the patients, respectively. Following the publication of this work in the *British Medical Journal* in 1949, physicians all over the world started using *Rauwolfia* for the treatment of hypertension. Many studies have reported the efficiency of *Rauwolfia serpentina* in the treatment of hypertension.

The chemistry and pharmacology of *Rauwolfia serpentina* have been extensively studied.[49] Indole alkaloids present in the plant are asserted to be responsible for its pharmacological action in reducing blood pressure levels. More than 50 different indole alkaloids have been isolated from the plant,[50] the most abundant being reserpine, ajmaline, serpentine, serpentinine, ajmalicine, and yohimbine.[51] The concentrations of these alkaloids depend on the part of the plant from which they are isolated and the geographical location of the plant. All parts of the *Rauwolfia serpentina* are known to contain the active ingredients; however, they are concentrated in the bark of the root. Among the alkaloids present, reserpine is the principal alkaloid known for hypotensive effects. It is a white-to-yellow powder with a bitter taste.[52] It is also odorless, insoluble in water, and freely soluble in acetic acid. The amount of reserpine in the plant has been found to be in the range of 0.03–0.14 percent.[52]

Reserpine exerts an antihypertensive effect by binding to vesicular monoamine transporters (VMATs) in the presynaptic neurons.[53] VMAT1 (found in the neuroendocrine cells of the peripheral nervous system) and VMAT2 (mostly found in the brain) are responsible for the transport of norepinephrine, dopamine, serotonin, and dopamine into vesicles, which release these neurotransmitters into the synapse. Reserpine blocks intracellular neurotransmitters from binding to VMATs, ultimately leading to no or slight release of neurotransmitters into the synapse. In 1955, reserpine was approved by the FDA for the treatment of hypertension, tachycardia, and thyrotoxicosis. Rauwiloid, another *Rauwolfia serpentina* alkaloid, also possesses antihypertensive properties; however, it has a lower efficacy compared to reserpine.[54] Other phytochemicals that have been found in *Rauwolfia serpentina* include flavonoids, tannins, vitamins including ascorbic acid, riboflavin and thiamine, and minerals.[55]

Because of its effect on the nervous system, *Rauwolfia* has been studied for the treatment of mental disorders, including anxiety, autism, migraines, schizophrenia, and insomnia.[56] *Rauwolfia* is known to cause many side effects, including sedation, lethargy, hypotension, nausea, vomiting, abdominal cramping, gastric ulceration, nightmares, bradycardia, angina-like symptoms, bronchospasm, skin rash, itching, galactorrhea, breast enlargement, and sexual dysfunction. About 5–15 percent of patients had nasal congestion.[52] Prolonged use of *Rauwolfia* can cause depression.[57] Parkinson's-like symptoms and convulsions are seen when extremely high doses are taken.

The use of reserpine as a solo drug has declined since its association with depression; however, it is now given in combination with thiazide diuretics to reduce mortality in patients with hypertension. In a recent study to evaluate the safety of antihypertensive preparations containing *Rauwolfia*, it was found that these preparations were generally safe for use, though some patients reported side effects, including nasal congestion and fatigue.[58]

Stephania Tetrandra

Stephania tetrandra S. Moore (han-fang-chi) is a Chinese herb used for the treatment of hypertension. The root of han-fang-chi was known to be prescribed as an analgesic and a diuretic in the late 1500s by the Chinese physician Li Shih-Chen.[59] Its antihypertensive effects are described in the Chinese herbology, *Compendium of Materia Medica*, and are also listed in the Chinese pharmacopeia. Tetrandrine, a bisbenzyltetrahydroisoquinoline alkaloid isolated from the root of han-fang-chi, is thought to be the major active ingredient responsible for the antihypertensive activity.[60] However, studies show that an extract of the plant containing only 7 percent tetrandrine is equipotent with tetrandrine in reducing the blood pressure of hypertensive rats, which points to the presence of other antihypertensive compounds.[61] The first pharmacological and toxicological study demonstrating the antihypertensive and cardiodepressant effects of tetrandrine was published in 1937. Tetrandrine acts as an antagonist at L- and T-calcium channels and exerts an antihypertensive effect by allosterically blocking the Ca^{2+} ion channels.[62][63] A number of animal studies point to effectiveness of tetrandrine as an antihypertensive agent.[64][65] Tetrandrine, however, has very low bioavailability, which has hindered its development, and several efforts have been applied to improve its bioavailability. Tetrandrine is also found to influence multiple signaling pathways, other than the Ca^{2+} ion channels, and studies show that it possesses anti-inflammatory,[66] anticancer,[67] antioxidant,[68] antidiabetic,[69] and antimicrobial[70] properties. Tetrandrine is also known to possess hypnotic activity.[71] It has been studied under clinical trials for the treatment of silicosis, but its poor bioavailability resulted in development being halted.

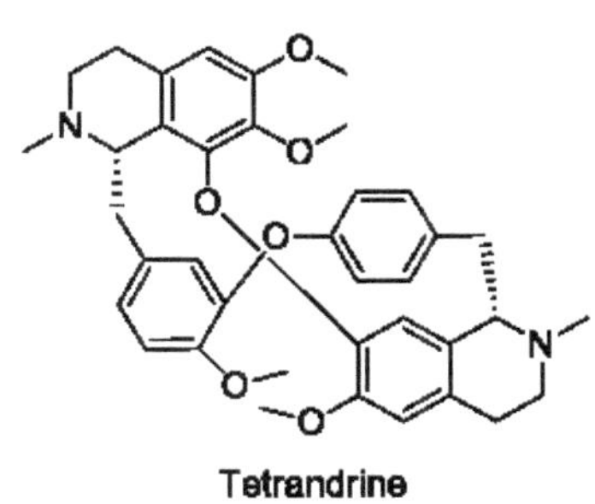

FIGURE 13.4 Structure of tetrandrine.

Lingusticum Wallichii

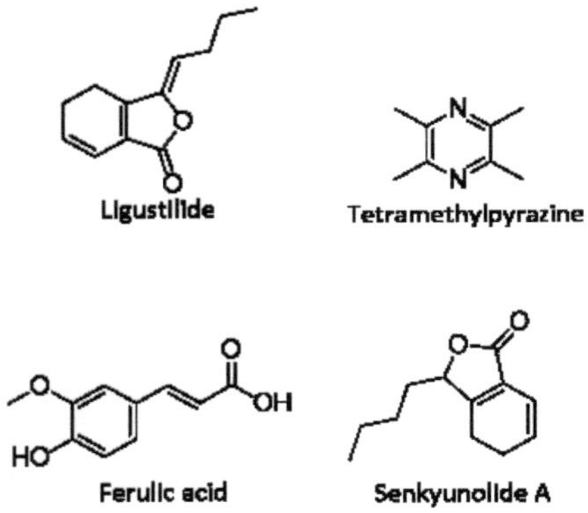

FIGURE 13.5 Structures of *Lingusticum wallichii* components.

Lingusticum wallichii, also known as *Ligusticum chuanxiong*, is a plant belonging to the Umbelliferae family. It is mainly grown in China and is also included in the *Compendium of Materia Medica* for its medicinal use.[72] Chemically, it is composed of essential oils, alkaloids, phenolic acids, phthalide lactones, and flavonoids, but ligustilide, tetramethylpyrazine, ferulic acid, and senkyunolide A are the main components responsible for its pharmacological actions.[72] Extracts of the rhizome of *Lingusticum wallichii* have been shown to have a vasorelaxation and antihypertensive effect in spontaneously hypertensive rats.[73] It also showed a decrease in the portal pressure in portal hypertensive rats. Additionally, *Ligusticum wallichii* fosters improvement of blood flow, inhibition of platelet aggregation, and vascular relaxation.

Tetramethylpyrazine (TMP), a biologically active component originally derived from *Ligusticum wallichii*, has been used widely in China for the treatment of angina pectoris and cerebral ischemic syndromes. The antihypertensive effects of TMP have been demonstrated using rat models of hypertension.[74] Pharmacological studies showed that vasodilation induced by TMP involved the opening of potassium channels.[75] Another biologically active component, ferulic acid, has shown hypotensive effects in spontaneously hypertensive rats.[76]

Uncaria Rhynchophylla

The genus *Uncaria*, belonging to the family Rubiaceae, is mostly distributed in tropical regions, including Southeast Asia, Africa, and eastern South America.[77] Of the 34 species belonging to the genus, 19 are found to be of use for their medical values. They are found to have antioxidant,[78] antidiabetic,[79] antimicrobial,[80] anti-inflammatory,[81] immunostimulant,[82] anticancer,[83] antidepressant,[84] and antihypertensive effects.[85]

Uncaria rhynchophylla, in particular, is known for its antihypertensive effects. The stems and hooks of the plant are prepared as a decoction and it is included in the traditional medicinal formulation Gou-Teng (Choto-san in Japanese).[86] Extracts of the plant have been shown to exert antihypertensive effects in rats, reducing systolic blood pressure significantly.[87] Its pharmacological activity has been attributed to the presence of active compounds, predominantly indole alkaloids, rhynchophylline and isorhynchophylline. Both rhynchophylline and isorhynchophylline are found to block the release of calcium from L-type Ca^{2+} channels and induce hypotensive effects in rats.[88] Extracts of *Uncaria rhynchophylla* also possess vasodilatory effects, which contribute to its antihypertensive properties.[89]

Veratrum

Veratrum is a genus of flowering herbs belonging to the family of Liliacea or Melanthiacea.[90] Different species of the genus are grown throughout the northern hemisphere. In China, the roots and rhizomes of several *Veratrum* species (Li-lu) have been used to treat aphasia, dysentery, jaundice, scabies, and chronic malaria for centuries.[91] In North America, *Veratrum viride* (green false hellebore) and *Veratrum album* (white false hellebore) gained the attention of pharmaceutical companies in the 19th century for their hypotensive effect.

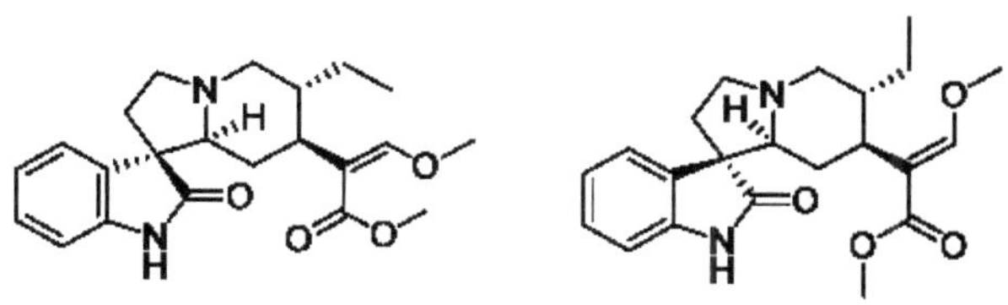

FIGURE 13.6 Structures of *Uncaria rhynchophylla* components.

A diverse spectrum of steroidal alkaloids, more than 100, were extracted from *Veratrum* plants. These steroidal alkaloids belong to two major classes: cyclopentanophenanthrene or solanum alkaloids and c-nor-d-homosteroidal alkaloids.[92] Following the promising efficacy of *Veratrum* in different animal models and human patients, several pharmaceutical companies introduced *Veratrum*, both in crude and purified form, into the market for treatment of hypertension.[93] Veratrum alkaloids exerted a hypotensive effect by binding to the sodium ion channels.[94] Upon binding, the sodium channel remains in an open state, delaying repolarization of the cellular membrane and causing rapid onset. Their binding is found to be reversible, thereby leading to a short duration of action.

As a result of their rapid onset, overdosing led to several cases of *Veratrum* poisoning. Atropine was used as an antidote and is the first line of choice to treat hypotension and bradycardia caused by *Veratrum* poisoning.[95] However, the use of *Veratrum* alkaloids was eventually abandoned, as better-tolerated and more effective pharmaceutical agents were developed to treat hypertensive emergencies.[96]

Atherosclerotic and Thrombotic Disorders

Atherosclerosis is the major underlying cause of arterial diseases and involves the buildup of lipids and fibrous materials in the arteries. Together with thrombotic disorders, it results in life-threatening acute coronary syndromes and stroke and is the major cause of morbidity and premature mortality worldwide.[97] Abnormal plasma lipid levels have long been known to play a role in atherosclerosis[98] and are thought to drive the development of atherosclerosis. In particular, elevated plasma cholesterol, LDL cholesterol, and apolipoproteins have been found in patients presenting with atherosclerosis. Other risk factors for atherosclerosis include smoking, hypertension, and hyperglycemia. In recent years, the role of inflammation and immunity in atherosclerosis has become evident, and the disease is now regarded as a chronic inflammatory disease.[99][100] Atherosclerotic plaques have been found to contain inflammatory cells, and a recent clinical study shows that targeting inflammation alone is beneficial in atherosclerosis.[101] The low-grade inflammation associated with atherosclerosis is initiated by plasma accumulation of oxidized LDL, which causes the release of inflammatory mediators including interleukins, adhesion molecules, and C-reactive protein.[102] Oxidized LDL has been found in animal and human atherosclerotic lesions and is recognized as a clinical marker of plaque inflammation.[103] This highlights the role that oxidative stress plays in atherosclerosis, and findings show that vascular oxidative stress is a promoter of atherosclerosis.[104] Rupture of an atherosclerotic plaque promotes platelet aggregation and the formation of a thrombus, which upon detachment into circulation can have fatal consequences. A multipronged approach that encompasses lipid lowering and anti-inflammatory, antioxidant, and antiplatelet aggregation strategies will be beneficial in preventing and treating atherosclerosis and thrombosis. Current therapy for atherosclerosis and thrombosis involves the use of lipid-lowering drugs, such as the statins, fibrates and bile acid sequestrants, antiplatelet aggregation drugs such as aspirin and clopidogrel, and anticoagulants such as the heparins and direct oral anticoagulants.[105]

The use of herbal preparations for atherosclerotic and thrombotic disorders dates back to ancient times, and studies have revealed that the chemical compounds in these medicinal plants possess lipid-lowering, anti-inflammatory, anticoagulant, and antioxidative properties.[106][107] Some of these are described in detail below.

Willow Bark

Willow bark refers to whole or fragmented dried bark of various *Salix* species of the family Salicaceae. These include *Salix alba*, *Salix nigra*, *Salix fragilis*, *Salix daphnoides*, and *Salix purpurea*. Willow bark has been in use for thousands of years for the treatment of fever pain and inflammatory conditions.[108][109] Compounds found in willow bark include the phenolic glycosides: salicin, acetylsalicin, salicortin, picein, triandrin, and their derivatives, such as salicyl alcohol and salicylic acid esters. Willow bark preparations are standardized based on these compounds and should contain not less than 1.5 percent, expressed as salicin.[110] Greater than 80 percent of salicin in willow bark is absorbed upon ingestion and is metabolized to salicylic acid.[111] Acetylsalicylic acid, one of the most important nonsteroidal anti-inflammatory drugs (NSAIDs) and the most widely used drug, is salicin-based.[109] Other compounds, including the flavonoids, taxifolin and catechin, and tannins, have been identified in willow bark in significant amounts, and these have been shown to have significant pharmacological activity as well.[110][112][113] In fact, polyphenolic compounds make up a significant fraction of willow phytochemicals.[108] The phytochemical constituents of willow

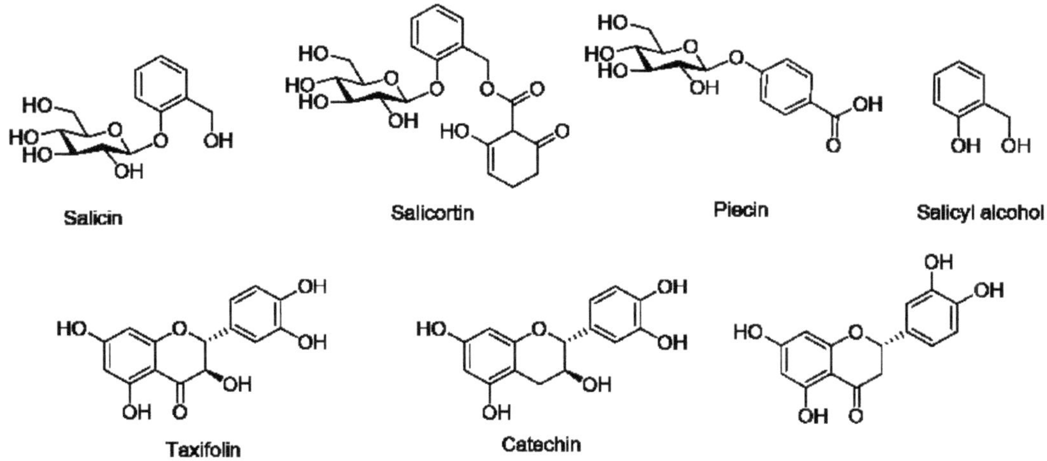

FIGURE 13.7 Structures of willow bark components.

bark change during the year, with the highest amount found in its dormant stages, which span fall to spring.[114] Willow bark preparations are available as extracts, which contain up to 50 percent salicin;[111] powders; and tablets. The antiatherosclerotic and antithrombotic activities of willow are due to anti-inflammatory, antioxidant, and antiplatelet activity, which are described in more detail below.

Anti-Inflammatory Effects

In vivo and in vitro studies indicate that willow bark extract interferes with NF-κB activation and the release of proinflammatory mediators.[110][115][116] Additionally, willow bark extracts inhibit cyclooxygenase-2.[117] Interestingly, in vitro studies comparing various extracts show that nonsalicin extracts have potent anti-inflammatory activity that greatly exceeds that of the salicin extracts.[108] For instance, eriodictyol shows potent anti-inflammatory activity in vitro, significantly inhibiting TNF-α-induced ICAM-1 expression.[118] It is, however, worth mentioning that active metabolites of salicin are not accounted for in these studies.

Antioxidant Activity

Willow extracts are rich in polyphenolic compounds, which have antioxidant activities. Extracts have been demonstrated to scavenge reactive oxygen species, resulting in significant antioxidant activity.[119] For instance, in in vivo studies using rabbits, willow extract increased antioxidant enzyme activity, resulting in a corresponding decrease in markers of oxidative stress.[120]

Antiplatelet Aggregation

Willow extracts also exert antiplatelet aggregation activity, and in a clinical trial, willow bark extract showed significantly better activity compared to placebo in preventing platelet aggregation.[121]

Dosage, Toxicity, and Interactions

Willow bark preparations are generally considered safe; however, they should be avoided in cases of asthma, peptic ulcer, glucose-6-phosphate deficiency, pregnancy, and lactation.[110] The dosage of willow bark extracts varies according to the preparation, and a daily dose of 120–240 mg total salicin is recommended.[108] The dry aqueous extract is given at 480–600 mg twice daily, whilst the powdered herbal substance is given at 260–500 mg three times a day.[110] Allergic reactions such as rashes, urticaria, and gastrointestinal disturbances, including nausea, vomiting, abdominal pain, diarrhea, and dyspepsia, have been reported with the use of willow bark extracts. Willow bark extract also has the potential for bleeding risk when coadministered with anticoagulants such as warfarin and should be used with caution with these drugs.[110] Care should also be taken when administering willow extract with antiplatelet drugs and NSAIDs.[110]

Hawthorn

Hawthorn refers to all plants of the *Crataegus* genus, a member of the Rosaceae family, which comprises over 1,000 species.[122] This thorny shrub, with characteristic bright green leaves, white flowers, and red berries containing a few seeds, is found in East Asia, Europe, and eastern North America.[123][124] In addition to being a source of food, hawthorn has been used for its medicinal properties since the first century. To date, over 20 species have been used for medicinal purposes for diseases in the cardiovascular, digestive, and excretory systems.[123] Almost 200 phytochemical constituents of hawthorn have been identified, and these include flavonoids, oligomeric proanthocyanidines, terpenoid glycosides, triterpene acids, organic acids, sterols, cardioactive amines, and lignans.[122][124][125] Flavonoids and oligomeric proanthocyanidines are the major groups of bioactive compounds and have historically been used in standardizing hawthorn preparations. The leaves, flowers, and roots have marginal variations in their phytochemical constituents and are all used for medicinal purposes.[125][126] Interspecies and seasonal variations in the content and composition of hawthorn phytochemicals have also been reported.[122][127] The most studied hawthorn species is *Crataegus pinnatifida*, from which over 150 chemical constituents have been identified.[128] Hawthorn extracts have been shown to prevent the development of atherosclerosis in in vitro and in vivo models,[129] and this is thought to be due to the correction of dyslipidemia and antioxidant activity, as well as the inhibition of thromboxane A2 (TXA2) activity.[122][130]

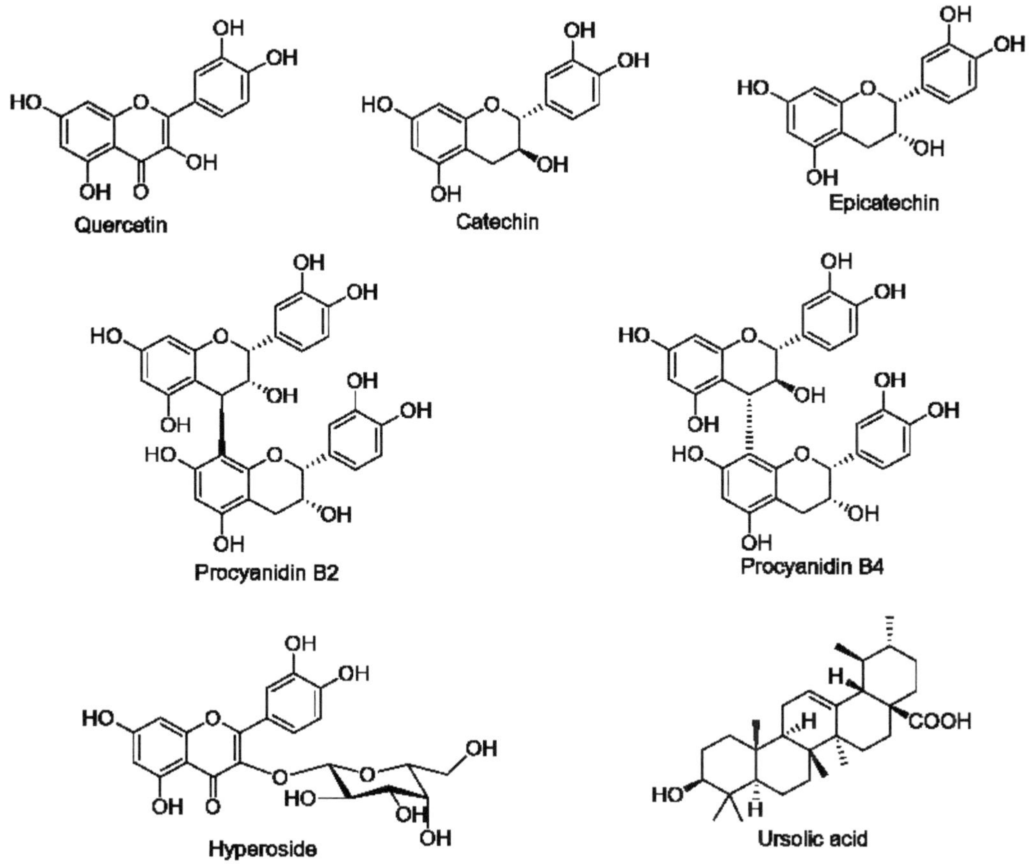

FIGURE 13.8 Structures of hawthorn components.

Hypolipidemic Activity

In several studies, hawthorn has been found to decrease serum levels of total cholesterol, LDL cholesterol, and triglycerides in hypercholesterolemic and atherosclerotic animals.[122] Various chemical components of hawthorn, including total flavonoids present in the leaves and the isolated compounds hyperoside and ursolic acid, have been demonstrated to be responsible for these antihyperlipidemic effects,[128] which have been demonstrated in mouse, rat, and rabbit models.[129][131] Mechanisms thought to account for the antihyperlipidemic effects include depression of hepatic cholesterol synthesis, enhancement of LDL-receptor activity, regulation of lipoprotein lipase expression, and downregulation of caspase-3 gene expression, among others.[126]

Antioxidant Activity

Extracts of hawthorn have been shown to possess antioxidant activities.[132] In vivo studies reveal that they exert a protective effect on oxidative stress in atherosclerotic rats.[133] This activity is thought to be due to the oligomeric proanthocyanidines and flavonoid constituents of hawthorn.

Antiplatelet Aggregation Properties

Studies also indicate that components of hawthorn extracts, in particular terpene and flavone constituents, exert antiplatelet aggregation properties and inhibit thrombus formation by interfering with ADP-induced platelet aggregation.[134][135][136]

Dosage, Toxicity, and Studies in Humans

Daily doses ranging from 160 to 1,800 mg of hawthorn extracts have been administered.[130] Hawthorn is reported to have very low toxicity and very minor side effects associated with use at therapeutic doses. These side effects include headache, rash, gastrointestinal disturbances, and sweating.[125][130][137] There is, however, not enough data to support the use of hawthorn in pregnancy and lactation, and so it should be avoided. A few clinical trials have demonstrated the ability of the plant to correct dyslipidemia and reduce oxidative stress. In one of such studies, significantly reduced total cholesterol, serum triglycerides, LDL cholesterol, apolipoprotein B, and lipid peroxidate malonic dialdehyde were observed following the administration of a preparation containing hawthorn.[123] Another study showed that the extract was effective in lowering serum lipids in patients with NYHA stage II heart failure with hyperlipidemia.[123]

Vaccinium Myrtillus

Vaccinium myrtillus, commonly known as bilberry, is a shrub from the family Ericaceae. Originally found in northern Europe, it now grows in North America and Asia and prefers moderate conditions of shade and humidity.[138] It has small bluish-black edible fruits that typically have multiple seeds. The fruits are commercially available in the fresh, frozen, and dried forms and are used as a source of food. Besides serving as a source of food, bilberry has great use for medicinal purposes, and the leaves and stems have also been used as herbal teas. Bilberry is most noted for its use for the improvement of vision, but antioxidant, anti-inflammatory, antimicrobial, and lipid- and glucose-lowering effects have been reported. These properties indicate the value of the plant in the treatment of cardiovascular diseases, cancer, infection, and diabetes, among others.[138] Numerous compounds have been identified from different parts of *Vaccinium myrtillus*, some of which have been shown to be responsible for these medicinal benefits. More than 100 phenolic compounds have

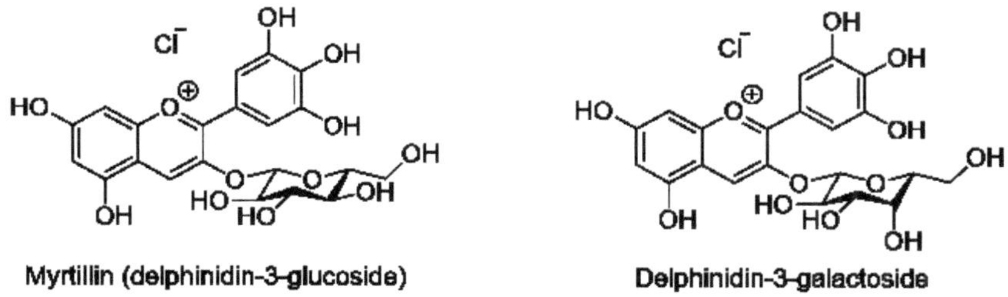

FIGURE 13.9 Structures of *Vaccinium myrtillus* components.

been identified from the plant,[139] with studies showing that the leaves are a richer source of these compounds than the fruits.[140]

The anthocyanins are the principal phytochemicals of bilberry and are predominantly found in the berry, particularly the skin,[138][139] giving bilberry fruits their characteristic color.[141] These compounds are water soluble and have an anthocyanidine core attached to sugars, including glucose, galactose, xylose, arabinose and rhamnose.[142] The anthocyanins have potent antioxidant activity, and about 15 of them have been isolated and characterized from *Vaccinium myrtillus*.[143] The anthocyanin content and profile of *Vaccinium myrtillus* are known to vary from plant to plant and to be affected by factors including seasonal variations, geographical location, genetic factors, light intensity, temperature, and processing,[139][141][144] and anthocyanin contents of up to about 1 g per 100 g of fresh fruit and 7.5 g per 100 g of dry fruit have been found, with the most abundant being myrtillin (delphinidin-3-glucoside) (17%) and delphinidine-3-galactoside (14%).[145][146]

Other compounds, including flavonols, tannins, ellagitannins, vitamin C, and phenolic acids, have been found in bilberry.[142] Bilberry has been shown to possess significant antiatherosclerotic activity, stemming from antioxidant, anti-inflammatory, and lipid-lowering properties. In a study involving mice, anthocyanin-rich extract of bilberry was shown to alter the expression of atherosclerosis-related genes in the aorta.[147] In another study involving hamsters, it was shown that the juice decreased the deposition of lipids at least fourfold.[148]

Antioxidant Activity

The anthocyanins contribute significantly to the antioxidant properties of bilberry. In vitro and in vivo models have been used to demonstrate the antioxidant properties of bilberry and also to show the correlation of this property to its antiatherosclerotic effect. Bilberry extracts prevented lipid peroxidation in vitro, with a positive correlation observed between antioxidant activity and polyphenol content and structural diversity of the anthocyanin-derived pigments of the extracts.[149] Using human cell lines, it has been shown that bilberry anthocyanins exert cellular antioxidant activity even at very low concentrations.[146][150] In rabbits, bilberry extracts led to decreased levels of live AST and ALT, indicating a reduction in oxidative stress.[151] In a clinical trial, a decrease in the level of oxidized peroxide was observed with administration of 40 g per day of *Vaccinium myrtillus* powder.[152]

Anti-Inflammatory Activity

Bilberry has been shown to possess anti-inflammatory activity. In vitro suppression of NF-κB activity following treatment with bilberry derived anthocyanidines was observed.[153] A clinical trial involving 300 mg/d anthocyanin supplementation for three weeks resulted in decreased levels of IL-8, RANTES, IL-4 and IL-13, indicating interference with NF-κB activity.[153] In a randomized controlled trial, although an unexpected increase in TNF-alpha was seen, bilberry juice resulted in significant decreases in plasma levels of C-reactive protein, IL-6, IL-15, and monokine induced by INF-γ.[154]

Regulation of Lipids

Though a number of reports point to the lipid-lowering effects of bilberry extracts, results from some studies report contradictory findings. A study in rabbits showed decreased levels of total and LDL cholesterol but no effect on triglyceride levels.[151] In a meta-analysis including 16 trials and a total of 1,109 patients, bilberry improved the lipid profile, showing a decrease in LDL cholesterol levels and increased levels of HDL.[155] In another meta-analysis, bilberry reduced LDL cholesterol levels and increased HDL cholesterol levels.[156] A recent clinical trial involving 36 patients showed a decrease in total cholesterol and LDL cholesterol and an increase in HDL cholesterol.[157] On the contrary, one study involving rabbits[148] and a clinical trial utilizing 40 g per day of *Vaccinium myrtillus* powder resulted in no improvements in total cholesterol and LDL cholesterol levels.[152]

Antiplatelet Activation

Anthocyanins demonstrate antiplatelet aggregation properties.[158] It is also suggested that metabolites of anthocyanins may possess antiplatelet aggregation properties.[159]

Safety, Toxicity, and Pharmacokinetics Data

Salvia Miltiorrhiza

Salvia miltiorrhiza is a perennial flowering herb of the family Labiatae and the gensus *Salvia*. The plant is found in China and Japan and grows at elevations of 90–1,200 m, reaching a height of between 30 and 60 cm. The plant has green leaves and blue-to-purple flowers, and the dried root or rhizome of the plant, known as *danshen*, is one of the oldest and well-known herbal medicines in traditional Chinese preparations; records of danshen can be found in

Shennong Bencao Jing (the first Chinese Materia Medica in China during the Eastern Han Dynasty, 25 AD–220 AD).[164][165] Danshen is now used extensively outside China due to its medicinal values and is mainly administered orally, with decoctions being the most common dosage forms. Tablets, capsules, granules, dripping pills, and parenteral preparations are also now available,[164] and the Fufang Danshen dripping pill for the treatment of cardiovascular diseases has passed FDA phase II trials.

Danshen is noted for its ability to promote blood circulation and remove blood stasis, but it has also been used for conditions including infections, palpitations, insomnia, pain in the chest and abdomen, numbness in the feet, stiffness in the spinal column, hepatocirrhosis, cancer, bone loss, Alzheimer's disease, and Parkinson's disease, among others.[164][165]

Over 200 compounds have been identified from danshen, and these can be grouped into three structural classes: diterpenoids, phenolic acids, and others. The most abundant compounds are the diterpenoids, which are known to have antibacterial, antioxidative, anti-inflammatory, and antineoplastic properties.[165][166] These compounds share a core structure of 20 carbons arranged in a ring and can further be grouped under tanshinones, which contain a common orthonaphtoquinone chromophore, and the abietane diterpenes, which have a common paranapthoquinone chromophore.[164] The total tanshinone content

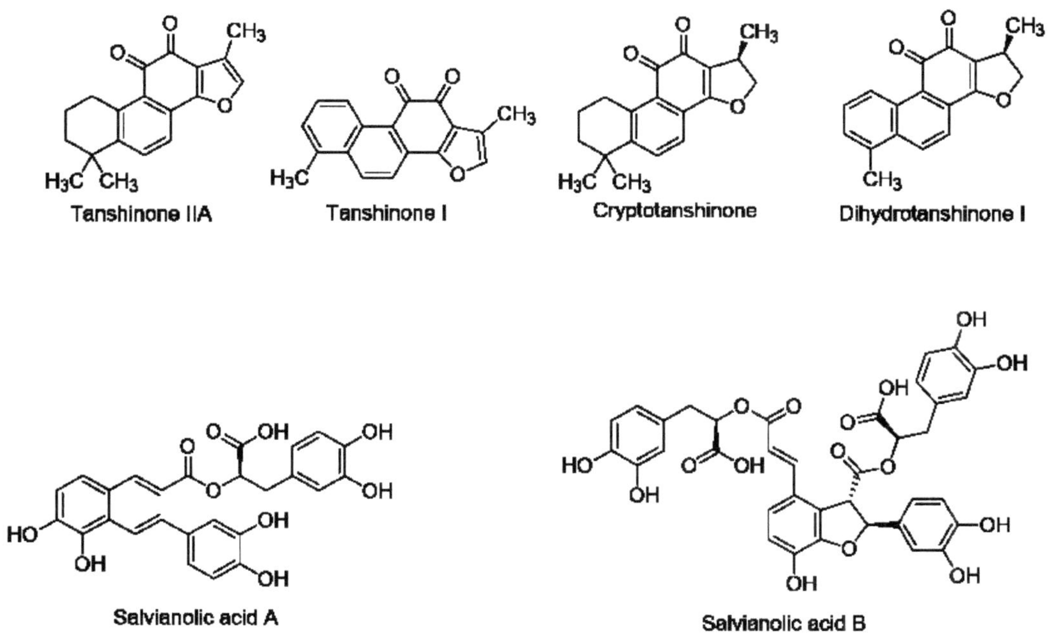

FIGURE 13.10 Structures of *Salvia miltiorrhiza* components.

of the root is about 1 percent,[167] with tanshinone IIA being the most abundant and most studied danshen compound. Along with tanshinone IIA, tanshinone I and cryptotanshinone are the most biologically active tanshinones.

More than 30 single- and polyphenolic compounds have also been isolated from *Salvia miltiorrhiza*, and these have antioxidative, anticoagulant, and anti-inflammatory properties.[164] The most abundant and pharmacologically active of these constituents are the salvianolic acids. In addition to these main classes of compounds, essential oils, flavones, amino acids, and metallic elements have been isolated.

The antiatherosclerotic and antithrombotic activity of danshen results from antioxidant, antiplatelet aggregation, hypolipidemic, and immunomodulatory properties.

Antiplatelet Aggregation

Salvianolic acid A has been shown to inhibit platelet secretion and aggregation and prevent thrombus formation in a mouse model,[168] while salvianolic acid B has also been demonstrated to inhibit human platelet aggregation.[169]

Anti-Inflammatory Effects

Studies have indicated that the tanshinones possess significant anti-inflammatory activity,[170] with tanshinone IIA treatment shown to reduce the expression of inflammatory mediators including TNF-α, CD40, IL-6, ICAM-1, VCAM-1, and MMP-2, -3, and -9 [171][172][173][174] These anti-inflammatory effects stem from the suppression of RAGE and interference with the activation of NF-κB.[172] Further, cryptotanshinone, dihydrotanshinone, and salvianolic acid B have all been shown to inhibit the activation of NF-κB.[169][175][176]

Antioxidative Effects

Using different models, the antioxidative effects of *S. miltiorrhiza* have been shown to contribute to its antiatherosclerotic effects. *S. miltiorrhiza* extracts and the compound tanshinone IIA have been shown to significantly decrease malondialdehyde content while increasing the activity of superoxide dismutase in rabbits.[171][177] Dihydrotanshinone I and cryptotanshinone have been shown to inhibit reactive oxygen species, resulting in a decrease in oxidative stress in mice.[175][176] The aqueous extracts of *S. miltiorrhiza* have also been shown to decrease oxidative stress,[178] with salvianolic acids A and B also demonstrated to have antioxidant activity.[164]

Hypolipidemic Effects

S. miltiorrhiza has also been shown to result in a reduction in total blood plasma cholesterol. Salvianolic acid A has been shown to decrease the levels of triglycerides, total cholesterol, and LDL while increasing HDL levels in rats.[179] Dihydrotanshinone also had a positive effect on the lipid profile of mice.[176]

Dosage and Toxicity

Danshen has been reported to be safe, with no severe adverse effects reported in humans when used within prescribed limits. According to the Chinese Pharmacopoeia, the recommended dose of danshen for the treatment of cardiovascular diseases is 9–15 g/day; however, doses of up to 60 g per day can be safely reached in other conditions.[167] The LD50 by injection is 40–80 g/kg.[167] Only minor side effects, such as stomach discomfort, itching, and pain, have been reported;[180] however, at higher doses, danshen could cause dry mouth, dizziness, shortness of breath, lassitude, and numbness.[167] In mice, high doses of IV-administered danshen (5.76 g/kg/day) resulted in peripheral vascular toxicity.[181] Being that it has potent anticoagulant activity, danshen should not be administered to patients who are prone to bleeding, and combination with other anticoagulants should be avoided or heavily monitored.[167]

Psyllium

Psyllium refers to the many species of the *Plantago* genus of the family Plantaginaceae. About 260 species have been identified, and these are found mostly in the tropical regions. Psyllium has, however, been used for medicinal purposes all over the world for thousands of years for constipation and diarrhea, hemorrhoids, high blood pressure, and skin irritation arising from insect bites and stings.[182] Currently, psyllium is available as seeds, seed husks, powders, flakes, granules, capsules, tablets, and oral preparations. Carbohydrates are the major phytochemical constituents of psyllium, with mucilage, dominated by D-xylose polysaccharides, accounting for up to 30 percent.[182] Other psyllium phytochemicals include carbohydrates, proteins, lipids, sterols, triterpenes, phenolic compounds, and glycosides, with the phenolic compounds thought to be the major bioactive constituents.[183][184]

Intake of psyllium is associated with cardiovascular benefits, including the prevention of atherosclerosis, and the main mechanism is via the regulation of the lipid profile. Several clinical trials show that psyllium significantly improves the lipid profile of both normal and patients with high risk for cardiovascular disease. These studies show significantly decreased total cholesterol, LDL cholesterol, triglycerides, and apolipoprotein levels.[185][186][187][188][189] A meta-analysis of three randomized controlled trials showed that coadministration of psyllium fiber with statins improved lipid profiles.[186]

Additionally, psyllium exerts anti-inflammatory and antioxidant activity.[184] Plantago extracts have been shown to prevent lipid peroxidation and also exert anti-inflammatory activity by interfering with NF-κB activity.[184] The specific phenolic compounds, acteoside and isoacteoside, are known to have both anti-inflammatory and antioxidant activity.[183]

Dosage, Side Effects, and Toxicity

The daily recommended dose of psyllium is determined by the particular preparation, and up to 30 g for seeds and 20 g for seed husk and seed husk powder can be used daily.[190] Common side effects of psyllium include gastrointestinal disturbances, and psyllium should be avoided in patients with intestinal obstruction and esophageal disease.[191] It is also not recommended for children younger than six years old. Psyllium is known to affect the absorption of drugs, including anticoagulant and antiplatelet drugs, carbamazepine, and minerals.[191][192]

Commiphora Mukul

Commiphora mukul, of the family Burseraceae, is a small, bushy thorn mainly found in India, Pakistan, and Bangladesh. This plant is usually bare and grows to a height of 1.2–1.8 m. At certain times of the year, however, its green leaves, red to brown flowers, and fruits, which ripen to a red color, can be seen.[193] The gum resin from the plant, also known as guggul, has been used for centuries for treating bone fractures, dyslipidemia, and inflammatory disorders. Guggul has also been used for its antimicrobial and anthelmintic properties.[193] A single plant can yield up to 500 g of guggul per year, and to obtain this, cuts are made in the bark of the tree, and the exudates are collected when they harden. Phytochemical constituents of

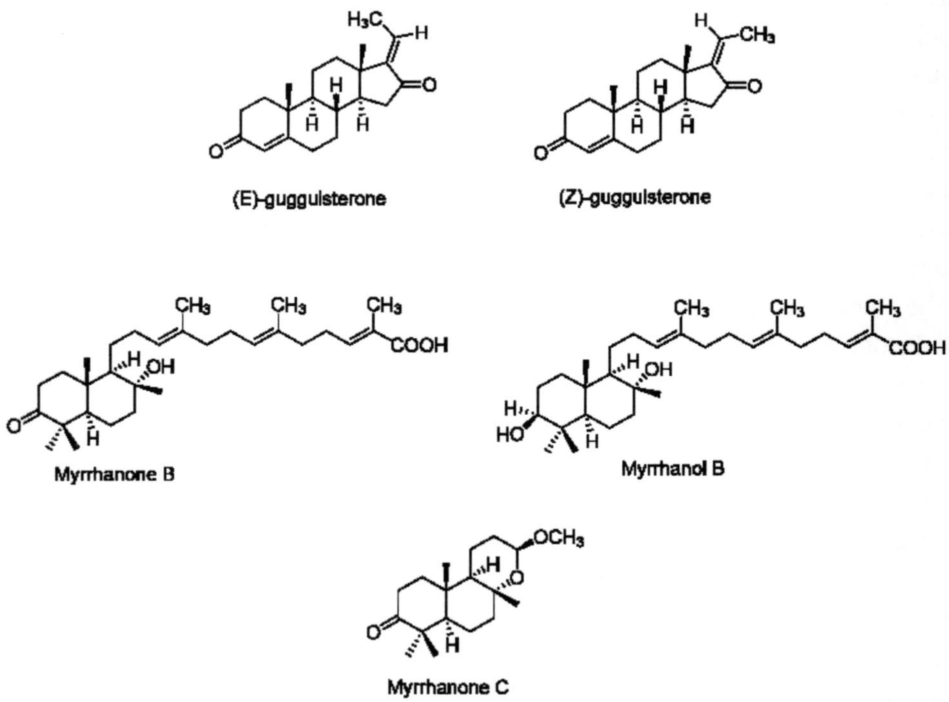

FIGURE 13.11 Structures of *Commiphora mukul* components.

Commiphora mukul include flavones, tannins, sterols, steroids, terpenes, essential oils, minerals, ferrulates and lignans. Guggulsterone (4,17(20)-pregnadiene-3,16-dione) is the most bioactive constituent of gum resin and has been shown to account for a lot of guggul's pharmacological activity.[194] Other bioactive compounds that have been identified are the myrrhanols and myrrhanones.[195]

Guggul has been shown to have anti-inflammatory, antiplatelet aggregation, and antioxidant properties, as well as the ability to improve the lipid profile. It is thought that these are the mechanisms by which antiatherosclerotic activity is achieved. Guggulsterone has also been shown to inhibit thrombus formation in mice.[196]

Anti-Inflammatory Activity

Guggulsterones have been shown to interfere with NF-κB activation and binding, leading to the decrease in expression of proinflammatory mediators, such as IL-6.[197][198][199] The ability of guggul to reduce the expression of proinflammatory markers in humans has also been demonstrated.[200]

Lipid Regulation

The lipid regulation activity of guggulsterones has been demonstrated in in vitro and in vivo assays.[201][202] Guggulsterone administration to rats resulted in decreased total cholesterol, triglycerides, VLDL, and LDL cholesterol levels and increased levels of HDL.[203][204] The hypolipidemic benefits of guggul extracts have also been observed in a number of clinical studies.[200] Guggulsterones have been shown to antagonize the bile acid receptor[205] and the farnesoid X receptor, a nuclear bile acid sensor,[206] and it is thought that these mechanisms contribute to its lipid-lowering properties.

Antioxidant Activity

In vitro studies have shown the ability of guggul to reduce the oxidation of LDL-cholesterol.[207] In rats, the administration of guggul extracts has been shown to decrease lipid and protein oxidation as well as increase the levels of enzymatic auto-oxidants, including superoxide dismutase, glutathione peroxidase, and glutathione reductase.[208]

Antiplatelet Activity

Guggul extracts have been reported to have antiplatelet aggregation properties.

Dosage, Toxicity, and Interactions

Preparations from *Commiphora mukul* typically contain 2.5–5 percent of guggulsterones and a daily dose of 1,000–3,000 mg of guggulipids, equivalent to 25–75 mg of guggulsterones, and have been used in cases of hyperlipidemia in adults.[201] There is, however, not sufficient data for dosing in children. Extracts from commiphora are thought to be generally safe, with gastrointestinal side effects, mainly diarrhea, being the most commonly reported. Other adverse reactions that have been reported include hypersensitivity skin reactions, headache, and rhabdomyolysis.[201] Guggul should be used with caution in patients with bleeding disorders, due to ability to potentiate bleeding, and in patients with thyroid disorders, as it has been found to stimulate thyroid function in animal studies.[201][209]

Allium Sativum

Allium sativum, of the family Amarylidaceae, is a perennial bulbous herb that is grown worldwide for culinary and medicinal purposes. Its use for medicinal purposes dates back thousands of years, and this includes uses for antimicrobial, antioxidant, anticancer, antiatherosclerotic, and antithrombotic purposes.[210][211] One of the most notable medicinal uses of garlic is for cardiovascular diseases, and epidemiological studies show that garlic use results in a decrease in progression of cardiovascular diseases.[212] In particular, garlic is known for its antiatherosclerotic properties.

Garlic contains several bioactive compounds and is thought to be one of the richest sources of total phenolic compounds among vegetables.[213] The compounds contained in garlic can be broadly grouped under sulfur-containing and non-sulfur-containing compounds, with the organosulfur compounds being responsible for the characteristic pungent smell of garlic.[213] Garlics cultivated from different parts of the world show wide variations in chemical

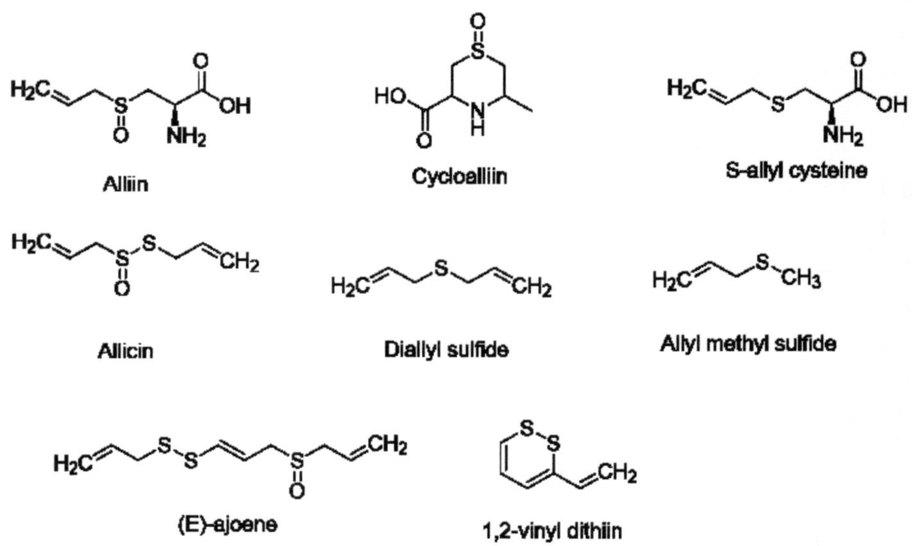

FIGURE 13.12 Structures of *Allium sativum* components.

constituents, and growing conditions have been shown to account for this.[213] The major sulfur-containing components of garlic are cysteine sulfoxides, including S-allyl-L-cysteine sulfoxide (alliin, and cycloallin, and the glutamylcysteines, such as gamma-glutamyl-S-allyl-L-cysteines).[214] The sulfoxide compounds are converted to thiosulfinates by the enzyme alliinase when garlic is cut or crushed. These thiosulfinate compounds, which include allicin, are very unstable and have relatively short half-lives, being decomposed to sulfide compounds such as diallyl, methyl, allyl, and dipropyl mono-, di-, tri-, and tetrasulfides.[213] Allicin, the major bioactive compound in aqueous garlic extract, has a half-life of less than 24 hours.[215] Non-sulfur-containing constituents of garlic include vitamins (especially C and B complex vitamins), flavonoids, saponins, sapogenins, phenolic compounds, nitrogen oxides, amides, and proteins and minerals. Due to the enzymatic activity and the instability of garlic's organosulfur compounds, several biochemical reactions take place during the processing of garlic that significantly alter the chemical constituents. Thus, garlic preparations vary significantly in type and amounts of sulfur compounds, with processed garlic containing a wider variety of organosulfur compounds than intact garlic. Analysis of processed garlic has identified over 20 sulfide compounds, the most abundant being diallyl sulfide (DAS) and allylmethyl sulfide (AMS). Others include the vinyldithiins, which are thermal-degradation products of allicin, and the ajoenes.[214] The common pharmaceutical preparations of garlic thus also have different chemical constituents. Garlic powder is rich in allicin. Aged garlic extract and aged black garlic, which are prepared by storing sliced garlic in 15–20 percent ethanol and heating fresh raw garlic at elevated temperatures under controlled humidity conditions for more than a month, respectively, do not contain allicin but are rich in S-allyl cysteine. Garlic oil, which is prepared by steam distillation, is rich in sulfide compounds.[215]

The antiatherosclerotic activity of *Allium sativum* has been demonstrated in a number of models. Aged garlic extract has been shown to suppress the development of atherosclerosis in mice.[216] It is thought that this is a result of the lipid-regulating, antioxidant, and anti-inflammatory properties.

Lipid Regulation

Garlic has been shown to significantly improve the lipid profile in both animal and human studies. In rabbits, it has been shown that garlic preparations decrease total serum lipid content about 1.5-fold and attenuate the accumulation of free and esterified cholesterol and triglycerides.[217] A clinical study in men with mild hypercholesterolemia reported an 11.8 percent decrease in LDL and about the same increase in HDL levels.[218] A meta-analysis that included 26 studies showed that garlic resulted in a significant reduction in total cholesterol and triglycerides.[219] Another meta-analysis including 39 trials showed that garlic preparations led to an 8 percent reduction in total cholesterol and a 9 percent reduction in

LDL in individuals with elevated cholesterol following use of garlic extract for longer than two months.[220]

Antioxidant Properties

Allium sativum is rich in antioxidants, and garlic extracts have been shown to result in a decrease in oxidative stress.[221] The organosulfur constituents, such as allicin, ajoenes, and 1,2-viniyldithiine, have potent antioxidant activity,[222] and studies indicate that aged garlic extracts may contain more antioxidant constituents than fresh extracts.[223] Enhanced levels of superoxide dismutase and glutathione peroxidase have been observed following treatment with garlic extracts in in vivo studies.[224]

Anti-Inflammatory Properties

The sulfur-containing compounds of garlic, including S-allyl-l-cysteine, diallyl sulfide, allicin, (Z, E)-ajoene, and their sulfonyl analogs, have been shown to play a role in the anti-inflammatory activity of garlic extract,[225] and in vivo studies show that aged garlic extracts suppressed the levels of c-reactive protein, TNF-α, and interleukin-1 receptor–associated kinase 4 (IRAK4), with a corresponding decrease in atherosclerotic lesions.[226] Other studies have also reported that garlic extracts reduce NF-κB activity and impact the expression of inflammatory mediators, including TNF-α, IL-1β and IL-6;[227] however, significant changes in these parameters have not been observed in clinical trials.[212]

Antiplatelet Adhesion

The antiplatelet aggregation properties of garlic are very important in its antiatherosclerotic properties. Aged garlic extracts have been shown to result in decreased thromboxane levels and decreased platelet aggregation.[228]

Dosage and Toxicity

Allium sativum and its constituents are relatively safe in humans, and toxicity and side effects are rare.[220] Bad breath and body odor are the most common complaints that accompany the use of garlic.[229] A daily dose of 1–7.2 g of aged garlic extract per day has been show to lower plasma cholesterol, with ingestion of large amounts having the possibility of causing burning sensations and diarrhea.[214] Allergic reactions to garlic, such as dermatitis, rhinitis, asthma, urticaria, photoallergy, and pemphigus, though rare, have been reported,[229] and anaphylaxis from garlic ingestion is also documented.[230] There are also rare cases of coagulation dysfunction. Garlic has no effect on CYP enzymes and can be administered safely with most drugs, with only a few herb-drug interactions having been observed.[229] Though potentiation of effects of anticoagulant drugs have been reported, garlic can be used with caution in these patients. There are also reports that garlic can reduce the efficacy of antiretrovirals.[229]

Fish Oil

Fish oil is the common name for oils derived from marine fish and is thought to have significant health benefit. It is commercially available as capsules and liquid preparations, with the main components being the ω-3 fatty acids, docosahexaenoic acid (DHA), and eicosapantaenoic acid (EPA), with concentrations of 18 and 12 percent w/w, respectively.[231] Omega-3 fatty acids are polyunsaturated fatty acids, and studies point to their beneficial roles in cardiovascular disease, cancer, diabetes, and inflammatory conditions, among others. In particular, their potential benefits to cardiovascular health have been highlighted.[232][233] Fish oil, and thus ω-3 fatty acids, are thought to help prevent the development of atherosclerotic and thrombotic disorders; however, the mechanisms underlying these are not very clear. Studies indicate that the anti-inflammatory and antiplatelet aggregation properties of the ω-3 fatty acids are the main contributors.[233][234][235] A few studies also point to the lipid regulation as a mechanism by which the ω-3 fatty acids prevent thrombosis and atherosclerosis.[232] It is, however, interesting to note that there are a number of studies that cast doubt on the veracity of these claims.[236][237][238]

Anti-Inflammatory Properties

The anti-inflammatory properties of ω-3 fatty acids are thought to significantly contribute to antiatherosclerotic activity. The anti-inflammatory effects of ω-3 fatty acids have been demonstrated in in vitro,[239] animal,[240] and clinical studies.[241] These studies show decreased expression of inflammatory mediators, including IL-6, C-reactive protein, TNF-alpha, ICAM-1, and IL-1β, among others.[234][240][241][242][243] The mechanisms by which ω-3 fatty acids attenuate inflammation are not well understood, but it has been shown that ω-3 fatty acid stimulation of the G protein-coupled receptor 120 (GPR120) plays a role.[239] Interestingly, other studies have not observed anti-inflammatory effects of ω-3 fatty acids.[244]

Antiplatelet Aggregation Effects

The ω-3 fatty acids demonstrate antithrombotic properties, and EPA in particular has been shown to inhibit the synthesis of thromboxane-A2, a prostaglandin

FIGURE 13.13 Structures of fish oil components.

involved in platelet aggregation and vasoconstriction.[233] A possible mechanism for the antiplatelet aggregation properties is competition of ω-3 fatty acids with arachidonic acid for esterification into platelets, resulting in platelets that have a decreased aggregation potential.[232] A clinical trial in men at risk of cardiovascular disease showed that ω-3 fatty acids led to reduced platelet aggregation.[245]

Lipid Regulation Properties

The lipid regulation properties of fish oil were shown in a clinical trial where patients receiving fish oil supplementation had significantly lowered VLDL-C, IDL-C and triglyceride levels.[232] A decrease in oxidized-LDL- β2 glycoprotein1 complex was also observed. It is thought that the regulation of the lipid profile is a result of modulation of VLDL-C and chylomicron metabolism.[246] A trial by Mori et al., however, found no improvements in the lipid profile with ω-3 fatty acid use.[247]

Dosage, Toxicity, and Interactions

According to the Food and Agricultural Administration, the combined daily recommended dose of EPA and DHA is 0.25 g. Doses of up to 2 g a day can be used, however.[234] No adverse effects or severe drug interactions have been reported with the use of fish oil preparations.

Avena Sativa

Avena sativa (oats), a whole grain plant of the family Poaceae, has been in use for over 4,000 years for food and medicinal purposes.[248] The plant, which grows to a height of about 1.5 m, is cultivated worldwide but has a preference for moderate climates and long day lengths.[249] Oats are a rich source of dietary fiber and a variety of phytochemicals, including carbohydrates, proteins, lipids, indole alkaloids, avenanthramides, tocols, flavonoids, organic acids, saponins, and minerals.[248][250][251] Climate and geographical location are known to affect the content and composition of oats.[249] Processing of oats, which helps improve the availability of nutrients, also alters the chemical constituents of oats.[251] Oats contain more soluble fiber than any other grain, and β-glucan, a mixed linkage of polysaccharide D-glucose units having primarily β1–3 linkages, is the most abundant component.[248] Beta-glucan is an important contributor to the health benefits associated with *Avena sativa*, and its structure and properties are also affected by growing conditions and processing.[252] *Avena sativa* also has the highest protein content of all cereals and is the only cereal to contain globulins, the major one being avenalin, which is also the most abundant protein. Avenanthramides are also an important constituent of *Avena sativa* and consist of anthranilic and hydroanthranilic acid linked to one of several hydroxycinnamic acids through an amide bond. Over 40 of these water-soluble low molecular weight compounds have been identified in oats.[253]

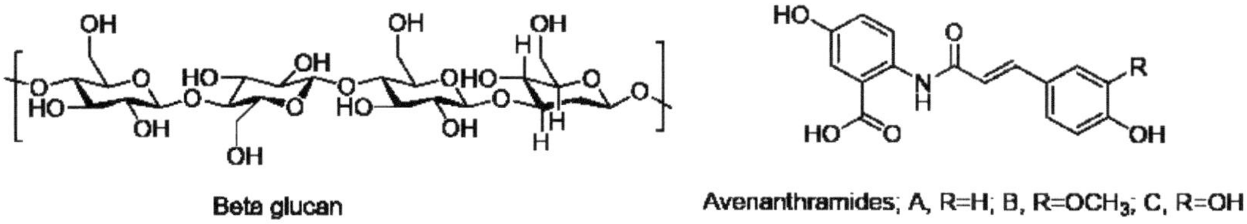

FIGURE 13.14 Structures of *Avena sativa* components.

Oats have antispasmodic, antitumor, cyanogenetic, demulscent, diuretic, neurotropic, stimulant, and tonic properties and have been used in traditional folklore medicine as teas, tinctures, and baths to treat conditions including insomnia, nerve weakness, nervous exhaustion, and anxiety.[248] Consumption of oats is also associated with reduced risk of cardiovascular diseases, including atherosclerosis,[250][254] and studies have shown that avenanthramides prevent the development of atherosclerosis in mice.[255] The antiatherosclerotic and antithrombotic activities of *Avena sativa* result from the lipid-regulation, antioxidant, anti-inflammatory, and antiplatelet aggregation properties of its phytochemical constituents.

Lipid Regulation

Avena sativa has long been thought of as having lipid-lowering properties. Thirty-seven and 34 out of 64 studies showed significant reduction in total cholesterol and LDL cholesterol, respectively.[254] Beta-glucan has been shown to be beneficial in improving the lipid profile by lowering total cholesterol and LDL cholesterol levels by 5–10 percent.[256] The physiochemical properties of β-glucan are important in its lipid lowering abilities, with a randomized clinical trial involving 345 patients showing that cereals containing higher molecular weight β-glucan had significantly better lipid-lowering effects.[257] Beta-glucan is thought to exert lipid-lowering effects by forming a viscous layer in the small intestine and preventing dietary cholesterol uptake and reabsorption of bile acids.[252][256]

Antioxidant Properties

The avenanthramides are potent antioxidant compounds and have up to 30 times higher antioxidant activity compared to other phenolic compounds.[253] Avenanthramide A, which is an ester of 5-hydroxyanthranilic acid with *p*-coumaric has the highest antioxidant activity.[253] An in vivo assay showed increased superoxide dismutase and glutathione peroxidase activity and decreased exercise-induced ROS and lipid peroxidation in rats following avenanthramide treatment.[258] In addition to the avenanthramides, *Avena sativa* contains tochopherols, tocotrienols, and flavonoids, which also possess antioxidant activity. Lunasin, a peptide found in oats, also exerts antioxidant activity.[259]

Anti-Inflammatory Activity

Some studies have pointed to the anti-inflammatory properties of oats, but other studies have cast doubt on this.[254] Avananthramides have been shown to decrease expression of inflammatory markers, including ICAM-1, VCAM-1, E-selectin, IL-8, IL-6, and MCP-1, and this is thought to be by interference with NF-κB activity.[253][260] Lunasin, a compound found in oats, also possesses anti-inflammatory activity.[259]

Antiplatelet Aggregation Activity

Enzymatic digestion of *Avena sativa* led to the release of peptides showing significant antiplatelet activity.[261] These peptides inhibited COX-1 activity, translating to decreased thromboxane A2 activity similar to acetyl salicylic acid.[261]

Toxicity and Safety

No toxicity has been reported, but some individuals may have hypersensitivity.

References

1. M. Naghavi et al., "Global, Regional, and National Age-Sex Specifc Mortality for 264 Causes of Death, 1980–2016: A Systematic Analysis for the Global Burden of Disease Study 2016," *Lancet* 390, no. 10100 (2017): 1151–210. https://doi.org/10.1016/S0140-6736(17)32152-9.
2. Ara Tachjian, Viqar Maria, and Arshad Jahangir, "Use of Herbal Products and Potential Interactions in Patients with Cardiovascular Diseases," *Journal of the American College of Cardiology* 55, no. 6 (2010): 515–25. https://doi.org/10.1016/j.jacc.2009.07.074.
3. Nick H. Mashour, George I. Lin, and William H. Frishman, "Herbal Medicine for the Treatment of Cardiovascular Disease," *Archives of Internal Medicine* 158, no. 20 (2003): 2225–34. https://doi.org/10.1001/archinte.158.20.2225.
4. Rosa Liperoti et al., "Herbal Medications in Cardiovascular Medicine," *Journal of the American College of Cardiology* 69, no. 9 (2017): 1188–99. https://doi.org/10.1016/j.jacc.2016.11.078.
5. Boback Ziaeian and Gregg C. Fonarow, "Epidemiology and Aetiology of Heart Failure Boback," *Nature Reviews Cardiology* 13, no. 6 (2016): 368–78. https://doi.org/10.1097/SLA.0000000000001177. Complications.
6. Arati A. Inamdar and Ajinkya C. Inamdar, "Heart Failure: Diagnosis, Management and Utilization," *Journal of Clinical Medicine* 5, no. 7 (2016): 62. https://doi.org/10.3390/jcm5070062.
7. Clyde W. Yancy et al., "2013 ACCF/AHA Guideline for the Management of Heart Failure," *Journal of the American College of Cardiology* 62, no. 16 (2013): e147–e239. https://doi.org/10.1016/j.jacc.2013.05.019.

8. G. Savarese and L. H. Lund, "Global Public Health Burden of Heart Failure," *Cardiac Failure Review* 3, no. 1 (2017): 7–11. https://doi.org/10.15420/cfr.2016.25.2
9. Michael C. Scott and Michael E. Winters, "Congestive Heart Failure," *Emergency Medicine Clinics of North America* 33, no. 3 (2015): 553–62. https://doi.org/10.1007/978-1-4471-4619-3_229.
10. Lars Køber et al., "Defibrillator Implantation in Patients with Nonischemic Systolic Heart Failure," *The New England Journal of Medicine* 375, no. 1 (2016): 1221–30. https://doi.org/10.1056/NEJMoa1608029.
11. Andrew P. Ambrosy et al., "The Use of Digoxin in Patients With Worsening Chronic Heart Failure," *Journal of the American College Cardiology* 63, no. 18 (2014): 1823–32. https://doi.org/10.1016/j.jacc.2014.01.051.
12. James J. DiNicolantonio et al., "Coenzyme Q10 for the Treatment of Heart Failure: A Review of the Literature," *Open Heart* 2, no. 1 (2015): e000326. https://doi.org/10.1136/openhrt-2015-000326.
13. Abhinav Sharma et al., "Coenzyme Q10 and Heart Failure. A State-of-the-Art-Review," *Circulation: Heart Failure* 9, no. 4 (2016): 1–8. https://doi.org/10.1161/CIRCHEARTFAILURE.115.002639.
14. Jerry Jankowski et al., "Coenzyme Q10—A New Player in the Treatment of Heart Failure?" *Pharmacological Reports* 68, no. 5 (2016): 1015–19. https://doi.org/10.1016/j.pharep.2016.05.012.
15. Anita Ayer, Peter Macdonald, and Roland Stocker, "CoQ 10 Function and Role in Heart Failure and Ischemic Heart Disease," *Annual Review of Nutrition* 35 (2015): 175–213. https://doi.org/10.1146/annurev-nutr-071714-034258.
16. Makoto Kawamukai, "Biosynthesis and Bioproduction of Coenzyme Q 10 by Yeasts and Other Organisms," *Biotechnology and Applied Biochemistry* 53, no. 4 (2009): 217–26. https://doi.org/10.1042/ba20090035.
17. Naoki Fukutomi et al., "Safety Assessment of Coenzyme Q 10 (CoQ 10)," *BioFactors* 32, no. 1–4 (2009): 199–208. https://doi.org/10.1002/biof.5520320124.
18. U. Singh, S. Devaraj, and I. Jialal, "Coenzyme Q10 Supplementation and Heart Failure," *Nutrition Reviews* 64, no. 6 (2007): 286–93. https://doi.org/10.1301/nr.2007.jun.286.
19. Adarsh Kumar et al., "Role of Coenzyme Q10 (CoQ10) in Cardiac Disease, Hypertension and Meniere-like Syndrome," *Pharmacology Therapeutics* 124, no. 3 (2009): 259–68. https://doi.org/10.1016/j.pharmthera.2009.07.003.
20. Barbara Sarter, "Coenzyme Q10 and Cardiovascular Disease: A Review," *Journal of Cardiovascular Nursing* 16, no. 4 (2013): 9–20. https://doi.org/10.1097/00005082-200207000-00003.
21. Catarina M. Quinzii, Michio Hirano, and Salvatore DiMauro, "CoQ10 Deficiency Diseases in Adults," *Mitochondrion* 7 (2007): S122–26. https://doi.org/10.1016/j.mito.2007.03.004.
22. Igor Pravst, Katja Žmitek, and Janko Žmitek, "Coenzyme Q10 Contents in Foods and Fortification Strategies," *Critical Reviews in Food Science and Nutrition* 50 (2010): 269–80. https://doi.org/10.1080/10408390902773037.

23. Leo Marcoff and Paul D. Thompson, "The Role of Coenzyme Q10 in Statin-Associated Myopathy: A Systematic Review," *Journal of the American College of Cardiology* 49, no. 23 (2007): 2231–37. https://doi.org/10.1016/j.jacc.2007.07.049.
24. Mehdi Jafari et al., "Coenzyme Q10 in the Treatment of Heart Failure: A Systematic Review of Systematic Reviews," *Indian Heart Journal* 70 (2018): S111–17. https://doi.org/10.1016/j.ihj.2018.01.031.
25. Li Lei and Yan Liu, "Efficacy of Coenzyme Q10 in Patients with Cardiac Failure: A Meta-Analysis of Clinical Trials," *BMC Cardiovascular Disorders*, 17, no. 1 (2017): 1–7. https://doi.org/10.1186/s12872-017-0628-9.
26. Rajiv Saini, "Coenzyme Q10: The Essential Nutrient," *Journal of Pharmacy and Bioallied Sciences* 3, no. 3 (2011): 466–67. https://doi.org/10.4103/0975-7406.84471.
27. H. W. Lack, "Floral Tributes," *Nature* 411 (2001): 137.
28. Thomas Courtney Lee, "Van Gogh's Vision Digitalis Intoxication?" *JAMA* 245, no. 7 (1981): 727–29.
29. Russell Collinson Davis, "ABC of Heart Failure. History and Epidemiology," *BMJ Clinical Research* 320 (2000): 39–42. https://doi.org/10.1016/S0001-6519(09)70311-5.
30. Seema Patel, "Plant-Derived Cardiac Glycosides: Role in Heart Ailments and Cancer Management," *Biomedicine and Pharmacotherapy* 84 (2016): 1036–41. https://doi.org/10.1016/j.biopha.2016.10.030.
31. Ionassis Prassas and Eleftherios P. Diamandis, "Novel Therapeutic Applications of Cardiac Glycosides," *Nature Reviews Drug Discovery* 7, no. 11 (2008): 926–35. https://doi.org/10.1038/nrd2682.
32. Ana Flavia Botelho et al., "A Review of Cardiac Glycosides: Structure, Toxicokinetics, Clinical Signs, Diagnosis and Antineoplastic Potential," *Toxicon* 158 (2019): 63–68. https://doi.org/10.1016/j.toxicon.2018.11.429.
33. Thomas W. Smith, "Digitalis—Mechanisms of Action and Clinical Use," *The New England Journal of Medicine* 318 (1988): 358–65. https://doi.org/10.1136/qshc.2004.010561.
34. Wolfgang Kreis, "The Foxgloves (Digitalis) Revisited," *Planta Medica* 83, no. 12–13 (2017): 962–76. https://doi.org/10.1055/s-0043-111240.
35. Thomas F. Whayne, Jr., "Clinical Use of Digitalis: A State of the Art Review," *American Journal of Cardiovascular Drugs* 18, no. 6 (2018): 427–40. https://doi.org/10.1007/s40256-018-0292-1.
36. Parminder S. Chaggar, Steven M. Shaw, and Simon G. Williams, "Is Foxglove Effective in Heart Failure?" *Cardiovascular Therapeutics* 33, no. 4 (2015): 236–41. https://doi.org/10.1111/1755-5922.12130.
37. Paul J. Hauptman and R. A. Kelly, "Digitalis," *Circulation* 99 (1999): 1265–70. https://doi.org/10.1161/01.cir.99.9.1265.

38. Darren M. Roberts et al., "Pharmacological Treatment of Cardiac Glycoside Poisoning," *British Journal of Clinical Pharmacology* 81, no. 3 (2015): 488–95. https://doi.org/10.1111/bcp.12814.
39. S. H. Rahimtoola and T. Tak, "The Use of Digitalis in Heart Failure," *Current Problems in Cardiology* 21, no. 12 (1996): 783–845.
40. Oliver J. Ziff and Dipak Kotecha, "Digoxin: The Good and the Bad," *Trends in Cardiovascular Medicine* 26, no. 7 (2016): 585–95. https://doi.org/http://dx.doi.org/10.1016/j.tcm.2016.03.011.
41. Ana Martin-Suarez et al., "Pharmacokinetics and Dosing Requirements of Digoxin in Pregnant Women Treated for Fetal Supraventricular Tachycardia," *Expert Review of Clinical Pharmacology* 10, no. 8 (2017), 911–17. https://doi.org/10.1080/17512433.2017.1344096.
42. Monica Ahluwalia and Sripal Bangalore, "Management of Hypertension in 2017: Targets and Therapies," *Current Opinion in Cardiology* 32, no. 4 (2017): 413–21. https://doi.org/10.1097/HCO.0000000000000408.
43. Euan Ashley and Josef Niebauer, "Hypertension," in *Cardiology Explained* (London: Remedica, 2004), 77–92.
44. Feng J. He, Jiafu Li, and Graham A. MacGregor, "Effect of Longer Term Modest Salt Reduction on Blood Pressure: Cochrane Systematic Review and Meta-Analysis of Randomised Trials," *British Medical Journal* 346 (2013): 1–15. https://doi.org/10.1136/bmj.f1325.
45. Stéphane Laurent, "Antihypertensive Drugs," *Pharmacological Research* 124 (2017): 116–25. https://doi.org/10.1016/j.phrs.2017.07.026.
46. Mary E. Endress and Peter V. Bruyns, "A Revised Classification of the Apocynaceae s.L.," *The Botanical Review* 66, no. 1 (2000): 1–56. https://doi.org/10.1007/BF02857781.
47. Eric Yarnell and Kathy Abascal, "Treating Hypertension Botanically," *Alternative and Complementary Therapies* 7, no. 5 (2001): 284–90. https://doi.org/10.1089/107628001753312121.
48. Rustom Jal Vakil, "A Clinical Trail of Rauwolfia Serpentina in Essential Hypertension," *British Heart Journal* 11, no. 4 (1949): 350–55. https://doi.org/10.1136/hrt.11.4.350.
49. Robert E. Woodson, Jr., et al., "Rauwolfia: Botany, Pharmacognosy, Chemistry and Pharmacology," *Journal of the American Pharmaceutical Association* 46, no. 6 (1957): 390.
50. Kuldip C. Verma and S. K. Verma, "Alkaloids Analysis in Root and Leaf Fractions of Sarpaghanda (*Rauwolfia serpentina*)," *Agricultural Science Digest* 30, no. 2 (2010): 133–35.
51. Satyanarayanaraju Sagi et al., "Quantification and Characterization of Alkaloids from Roots of Rauwolfia Serpentina Using Ultra-High Performance Liquid Chromatography-Photo Diode Array-Mass Spectrometry," *Analytical and Bioanalytical Chemistry* 408, no. 1 (2016): 177–90. https://doi.org/10.1007/s00216-015-9093-4.
52. Douglas Lobay, "Rauwolfia in the Treatment of Hypertension," *Integrative Medicine* 14, no. 3 (2015): 40–46.

53. S. Schuldiner, Y. Liu, and R. H. Edwards, "Reserpine Binding to a Vesicular Amine Transporter Expressed in Chinese Hamster Ovary Fibroblasts," *Journal of Biological Chemistry* 268, no. 1 (1993): 29–34.
54. S. D. Shamon and M. I. Perez, "Blood Pressure Lowering Efficacy of Reserpine for Primary Hypertension," *Cochrane Database of Systematic Reviews* 4 (2009, Oct. 7): CD007655. https://doi.org/10.1002/14651858.CD007655.pub2.
55. R. Harisaranraj, K. Suresh, and S. Saravanababu, "Evaluation of the Chemical Composition Rauwolfia Serpentina and Ephedra Vulgaris," *Advances in Biological Regulations (Rennes)* 3, no. 56 (2009): 174–78.
56. David Healy and Marie Savage, "Reserpine Exhumed," *British Journal of Psychiatry* 172, no. 1958 (1998): 376–78.
57. Guy Lemieux, Andre Davignon, and Jacques Genest, "Depressive States during Rauwolfia Therapy for Arterial Hypertension; a Report of 30 Cases," *Canadian Medical Association Journal* 74, no. 7 (1956): 522–26.
58. Jennifer Joan Ryan et al., "Prospective Safety Evaluation of a Cardiovascular Health Dietary Supplement in Adults with Prehypertension and Stage I Hypertension," *Journal of Alternative and Complementary Medicine* 25, no. 2 (2018): 249–56. https://doi.org/10.1089/acm.2018.0311.
59. Yi-Tsau Huang and Chuang Ye Hongt, "Tetrandrine," *Cardiovascular Drug Reviews* 16, no. 1 (1998): 1–15.
60. K. K. Chen and A. L. Chen, "The Alkaloids of Han-Fang-Chi," *Journal of Biological Chemistry* 109 (1935): 681–85.
61. X.-C. Yu et al., "Antihypertensive and Anti-Arrhythmic Effects of an Extract of Radix Stephaniae Tetrandrae in the Rat," *Journal of Pharmacy and Pharmacology* 56, no. 1 (2004): 115–22. https://doi.org/10.1211/0022357022458.
62. M. Catret et al., "α-Adrenoceptor Interaction of Tetrandrine and Isotetrandrine in the Rat: Functional and Binding Assays," *Journal of Pharmacy and Pharmacology* 50, no. 11 (1998): 1267–73. https://doi.org/10.1111/j.2042-7158.1998.tb03344.x.
63. V. Frank King et al., "Interaction of Tetrandrine with Slowly Inactivating Calcium Channels. Characterization of Calcium Channel Modulation by an Alkaloid of Chinese Medicinal Herb Origin," *Journal of Biological Chemistry* 263, no. 5 (1988): 2238–44.
64. Y. I. T. Huang et al., "Haemodynamic Effects of Chronic Tetrandrine Treatment in Portal Hypertensive Rats," *Journal of Gastroenterology and Hepatology* 12, no. 8 (1997): 585–89. https://doi.org/10.1111/j.1440-1746.1997.tb00490.x.
65. Huai-Liang Wang et al., "Tetrandrine Prevents Monocrotaline-Induced Pulmonary Hypertension in Rats," *Drug Development Research* 160, no. 931 (1997): 158–60.
66. Qiang-Min Xie et al., "Pharmacological Actions of Tetrandrine in Inflammatory Pulmonary Diseases," *Acta Pharmacological Sinica* 23, no. 12 (2002): 1107–13.

67. Wenchao Liu et al., "Tetrandrine Combined with Gemcitabine and Cisplatin for Patients with Advanced Non-Small Cell Lung Cancer Improve Efficacy," *International Journal of Biomedical Science* 8, no. 1 (2012): 28–35.
68. N. Bhagya and K. R. Chandrashekar, "Tetrandrine - A Molecule of Wide Bioactivity," *Phytochemistry* 125 (2016): 5–13. https://doi.org/10.1016/j.phytochem.2016.02.005.
69. Chunhul Song et al., "Tetrandrine Down-Regulates Expression of MiRNA-155 to Inhibit Signal-Induced NF-κB Activation in a Rat Model of Diabetes Mellitus," *International Journal of Clinical and Experimental Medicine* 8, no. 3 (2015): 4024–30.
70. Zhe Zhang et al., "Tetrandrine Reverses Drug Resistance in Isoniazid and Ethambutol Dual Drug-Resistant Mycobacterium Tuberculosis Clinical Isolates," *BMC Infectious Diseases* 15, no. 1 (2015): 1–7. https://doi.org/10.1186/s12879-015-0905-0.
71. Yuan-Li Huang et al., "Tetrandrine, an Alkaloid from S. Tetrandra Exhibits Anti-Hypertensive and Sleep-Enhancing Effects in SHR via Different Mechanisms," *Phytomedicine* 23, no. 14 (2016): 1821–29. https://doi.org/10.1016/j.phymed.2016.10.021.
72. Xia Ran et al., "Ligusticum Chuanxiong Hort: A Review of Chemistry and Pharmacology," *Pharmaceutical Biology* 49, no. 11 (2011): 1180–89. https://doi.org/10.3109/13880209.2011.576346.
73. Eun-Young Kim and Mee-Ra Rhyu, "Synergistic Vasorelaxant and Antihypertensive Effects of Ligusticum Wallichii and Angelica Gigas," *Journal of Ethnopharmacology* 130, no. 3 (2010): 545–51. https://doi.org/10.1016/j.jep.2010.05.048.
74. Fang-Chi Chang et al., "Effects of Tetramethylpyrazine on Portal Hypertensive Rats," *Journal of Pharmacy and Pharmacology* 50, no. 8 (1998): 881–84. https://doi.org/10.1111/j.2042-7158.1998.tb04003.x.
75. Chin-Chuan Tsai et al., "Inhibitory Effects of Potassium Channel Blockers on Tetramethylpyrazine-Induced Relaxation of Rat Aortic Strip in Vitro," *Life Sciences* 71, no. 11 (2002): 1321–30. https://doi.org/10.1016/S0024-3205(02)01852-0.
76. Atsushi Suzuki et al., "Short- and Long-Term Effects of Ferulic Acid on Blood Pressure in Spontaneously Hypertensive Rats," *American Journal of Hypertension* 15, no. 4 (2002): 351–57.
77. C. E. Ridsdale, "A Revision of Mitragyna and Uncaria (Rubiaceae)," *Blumea* 24 (1978): 43–100.
78. Arturo Alejandro Dreifussa et al., "Antitumoral and Antioxidant Effects of a Hydroalcoholic Extract of Cat's Claw (Uncaria Tomentosa) (Willd. Ex Roem. & Schult) in an in Vivo Carcinosarcoma Model," *Journal of Ethnopharmacology* 130, no. 1 (2010): 127–33. https://doi.org/10.1016/j.jep.2010.04.029.
79. Zhi-Wei Wang et al., "α-Glucosidase Inhibitory Triterpenoids from the Stem Barks of Uncaria Laevigata," *Fitoterapia* 90 (2013): 30–37. https://doi.org/10.1016/j.fitote.2013.07.005.
80. Daniel R. Herrera et al., "In Vitro Antimicrobial Activity of Phytotherapic Uncaria Tomentosa against Endodontic Pathogens," *Journal of Oral Science* 52, no. 3 (2010): 473–76. https://doi.org/10.2334/josnusd.52.473.

81. Ji-Hee Kim et al., "Uncaria Rhynchophylla Inhibits the Production of Nitric Oxide and Interleukin-1β through Blocking Nuclear Factor KB, Akt, and Mitogen-Activated Protein Kinase Activation in Macrophages," *Journal of Medicinal Food* 13, no. 5 (2010): 1133–40.
82. Jeff Holderness et al., "Select Plant Tannins Induce IL-2R Up-Regulation and Augment Cell Division in Γδ T Cells," *The Journal of Immunology* 179, no. 10 (2007): 6468–78. https://doi.org/10.4049/jimmunol.179.10.6468.
83. Arturo Alejandro Dreifuss et al., "Uncaria Tomentosa Exerts Extensive Anti-Neoplastic Effects Against the Walker-256 Tumour by Modulating Oxidative Stress and Not by Alkaloid Activity," *PLoS One* 8, no. 2 (2013): e54618. https://doi.org/10.1371/journal.pone.0054618.
84. Lieh-Ching Hsu et al., "Antidepressant-like Activity of the Ethanolic Extract from Uncaria Lanosa Wallich Var. Appendiculata Ridsd in the Forced Swimming Test and in the Tail Suspension Test in Mice," *Evidence-Based Complementary and Alternative Medicine* 2012 (2012): 497302. https://doi.org/10.1155/2012/497302.
85. Haipeng Guo et al., "Isorhynchophylline Protects Against Pulmonary Arterial Hypertension and Suppresses PASMCs Proliferation," *Biochemical and Biophysical Research Communications* 450, no. 1 (2014): 729–34. https://doi.org/10.1016/j.bbrc.2014.06.044.
86. Yutaka Shimada et al., "Choto-San Prevents Occurrence of Stroke and Prolongs Life Span in Stroke-Prone Spontaneously Hypertensive Rats," *American Journal of Chinese Medicine* 31, no. 1 (2003): 79–85. https://doi.org/10.1142/s0192415x03000837.
87. Ana Liu et al., "Serum Metabolomics Study Based on LC-MS and Antihypertensive Effect of Uncaria on Spontaneously Hypertensive Rats," *Evidence-Based Complementary and Alternative Medicine* 2018 (2018): 1–11. https://doi.org/10.1155/2018/9281946.
88. Wen-Bo Zhang et al., "In Vitro Vasodilator Mechanisms of the Indole Alkaloids Rhynchophylline and Isorhynchophylline, Isolated from the Hook of Uncaria Rhynchophylla (Miquel)," *Naunyn-Schmiedeberg's Archives of Pharmacology* 369, no. 2 (2004): 232–38. https://doi.org/10.1007/s00210-003-0854-9.
89. Yean Chun Loh et al., "Mechanisms of Action of Uncaria Rhynchophylla Ethanolic Extract for Its Vasodilatory Effects," *Journal of Medicinal Food* 20, no. 9 (2017): 895–911. https://doi.org/10.1089/jmf.2016.3804.
90. Wendy B. Zomlefer, et al., "An Overview of Veratrum s. l. (Liliales : Melanthiaceae) and an Infrageneric Phylogeny Based on ITS Sequence Data," *Systematic Botany* 28, no. 2 (2003): 250–69.
91. Hui-Jun Li, Yan Jiang, and Ping Li, "Chemistry, Bioactivity and Geographical Diversity of Steroidal Alkaloids from the Liliaceae Family," *Natural Product Reports* 23, no. 5 (2006): 735–52. https://doi.org/10.1039/b609306j.
92. Ralph Hirschmann et al., "The Rearrangement of the Steroid C/D Rings," *Journal of the American Chemical Society* 76, no. 15 (1954): 4013–25. https://doi.org/10.1021/ja01644a046.

93. K. S. Grimson, "Drugs Recently Introduced for Hypertension," *Journal of the American Medical Association* 158, no. 5 (1955): 359–67.
94. Peter Nánási et al., "Different Actions of Aconitine and Veratrum Alkaloids on Frog Skeletal Muscle," *General Pharmacology* 21, no. 6 (1990): 863–68. https://doi.org/10.1016/0306-3623(90)90446-S.
95. T. Grobosch et al., "Accidental Intoxication with Veratrum Album," *Journal of Analytical Toxicology* 32, no. 9 (2008): 768–73. https://doi.org/10.1093/jat/32.9.768.
96. L. B. Page and J. J. Sidd, "Medical Management of Primary Hypertension (Third of Three Parts)," *New England Journal of Medicine* 287 (1972): 1074–79. https://doi.org/10.1056/NEJM197211232872106.
97. Mohammed S. Ellulu et al., "Atherosclerotic Cardiovascular Disease: A Review of Initiators and Protective Factors," *Inflammopharmacology* 24, no. 1 (2016): 1–10. https://doi.org/10.1007/s10787-015-0255-y.
98. R. Ross and L. Harker, "Hyperlipidemia and Atherosclerosis," *Science* 193, no. 4258 (1976): 1094–1100.
99. Dennis Wolf and Klaus Ley, "Immunity and Inflammation in Atherosclerosis," *Circulation Research* 124, no. 2 (2019): 315–27. https://doi.org/10.1161/CIRCRESAHA.118.313591.
100. Peter Libby, "Inflammation in Atherosclerosis," *Nature* 420, no. 6917 (2002): 868–74. https://doi.org/10.1161/ATVBAHA.108.179705.
101. Paul M. Ridker et al., "Antiinflammatory Therapy with Canakinumab for Atherosclerotic Disease," *New England Journal of Medicine* 377, no. 12 (2017): 1119–31. https://doi.org/10.1056/nejmoa1707914.
102. Judith A. Berliner et al., "Atherosclerosis: Basic Mechanisms Oxidation, Inflammation and Genetics," *Circulation* 91,, no. 9 (1995): 2488–96.
103. D. Collen, "Oxidized Lipoproteins in Atherosclerosis and Thrombosis," *FASEB Journal* 980582 (2019): 1279–84.
104. Ulrich Förstermann, Ning Xia, and Huige Li, "Roles of Vascular Oxidative Stress and Nitric Oxide in the Pathogenesis of Atherosclerosis," *Circulation Research* 120, no. 4 (2017): 713–35. https://doi.org/10.1161/CIRCRESAHA.116.309326.
105. Caroline S. Bruikman et al., "New Drugs for Atherosclerosis," *Canadian Journal of Cardiology* 33, no. 3 (2017): 350–57. https://doi.org/10.1016/j.cjca.2016.09.010.
106. Chuan Wang et al., "Treatment of Atherosclerosis by Traditional Chinese Medicine: Questions and Quandaries," *Atherosclerosis* 277 (2018): 136–44. https://doi.org/10.1016/j.atherosclerosis.2018.08.039.
107. Cui-Qing Liu and Yu Huang, "Chinese Herbal Medicine on Cardiovascular Diseases and the Mechanisms of Action," *Frontiers in Pharmacology* 7 (2016): 1–21. https://doi.org/10.3389/fphar.2016.00469.

108. Adolf Nahrstedt et al., "Willow Bark Extract: The Contribution of Polyphenols to the Overall Effect," *Wiener Medizinische Wochenschrift* 157, no. 13–14 (2007): 348–51. https://doi.org/10.1007/s10354-007-0437-3.
109. Maria Rosa Montinari, Sergio Minelli, Raffaele De Caterina, "The First 3500 years of Aspirin History from Its Roots—A Concise Summary," *Vascular Pharmacology* 113 (2018): 1–8. https://doi.org/10.1016/j.vph.2018.10.008.
110. Sarah E. Edwards et al., "Willow (Bark)," in *Phyopharmacy: An Evidence-Based Guide to Herbal Medical Products* (Chichester, UK: John Wiley & Sons, Ltd, 2015).
111. Mohd Shara and Sidney J. Stohs, "Efficacy and Safety of White Willow Bark (Salix Alba) Extracts," *Phytherapery Research* 29, no. 8 (2015): 1112–16. https://doi.org/10.1002/ptr.5377.
112. Shabnam Enayat and Sreeparna Banerjee, "Comparative Antioxidant Activity of Extracts from Leaves, Bark and Catkins of *Salix aegyptiaca* Sp," *Food Chemistry* 116, no. 1 (2009): 23–28. https://doi.org/10.1016/j.foodchem.2009.01.092.
113. Sara Agnolet et al., "Comprehensive Analysis of Commercial Willow Bark Extracts by New Technology Platform: Combined Use of Metabolomics, High-Performance Liquid Chromatography-Solid-Phase Extraction-Nuclear Magnetic Resonance Spectroscopy and High-Resolution Radical Scavenging Assay," *Journal of Chromatography A* 1262 (2012): 130–37. https://doi.org/10.1016/j.chroma.2012.09.013.
114. Nadja Förster et al., "Factors Influencing the Variability of Antioxidative Phenolic Glycosides in Salix Species," *Journal of Agricultural and Food Chemistry* 58, no. 14 (2010): 8205–10. https://doi.org/10.1021/jf100887v.
115. Mehdi Shakibaei et al., "Botanical Extracts from Rosehip (Rosa Canina), Willow Bark (Salix Alba), and Nettle Leaf (Urtica Dioica) Suppress IL-1 β -Induced NF-κB Activation in Canine Articular Chondrocytes," *Evidence-Based Complementary and Alternative Medicine* 2012 (2012): 509383. https://doi.org/10.1155/2012/509383.
116. G. A. Bonaterra et al., "Anti-Inflammatory Effects of the Willow Bark Extract STW 33-I (Proaktiv®) in LPS-Activated Human Monocytes and Differentiated Macrophages," *Phytomedicine* 17, no. 14 (2010): 1106–13. https://doi.org/10.1016/j.phymed.2010.03.022.
117. Mohamed T. Khayyal et al., "Mechanisms Involved in the Anti-Inflammatory Effect of a Standardized Willow Bark Extract," *Arzneimittelforschung* 55, no. 11 (2012): 677–87. https://doi.org/10.1055/s-0031-1296917.
118. A. Freischmidt et al., "Contribution of Flavonoids and Catechol to the Reduction of ICAM-1 Expression in Endothelial Cells by a Standardised Willow Bark Extract," *Phytomedicine* 19, no. 3–4 (2011): 245–52. https://doi.org/10.1016/j.phymed.2011.08.065.
119. Urszula Gawlik-Dziki, et al., "Bioaccessibility In Vitro of Nutraceuticals from Bark of Selected Salix Species," *Scientific World Journal* 14 (2014). https://doi.org/10.1155/2014/782763.

120. Narges Amel Zabihi et al., "Salix Alba Attenuated Oxidative Stress in the Heart and Kidney of Hypercholesterolemic Rabbits," *Avicenna Journal of Phytomedicine* 8, no. 1 (2018): 63–72.
121. Norberto Krivoy et al., "Effect of Salicis Cortex Extract on Human Platelet Aggregation," *Planta Medica* 67, no. 3 (2001): 209–12. https://doi.org/10.1055/s-2001-12000.
122. Baoru Yang and Pengzhan Liu, "Composition and Health Effects of Phenolic Compounds in Hawthorn (Crataegus Spp.) of Different Origins," *Journal of the Science of Food and Agriculture* 92, no. 8 (2012): 1578–90. https://doi.org/10.1002/jsfa.5671.
123. Qi Chang et al., "Hawthorn," *Journal of Clinical Pharmacology* 42, no. 6 (2002): 605–12.
124. Janene M. Rigelsky and Burgunda V. Sweet, "Hawthorn: Pharmacology and Therapeutic Uses," *American Journal of Health-System Pharmacy* 59, no. 5 (2002): 417–22.
125. Seyed Fazel Nabavi et al., "Polyphenolic Composition of Crataegus Monogyna Jacq.: From Chemistry to Medical Applications," *Nutrients* 7, no. 9 (2015): 7708–28. https://doi.org/10.3390/nu7095361.
126. Mary C. Tassell et al., "Hawthorn (Crataegus Spp.) in the Treatment of Cardiovascular Disease," *Pharmacognosy Review* 4, no. 7 (2010): 32–41. https://doi.org/10.4103/0973-7847.65324.
127. N. Hellenbrand et al., "Isolation and Quantification of Oligomeric and Polymeric Procyanidins in Leaves and Flowers of Hawthorn (Crataegus Spp.)," *Fitoterapia* 104 (2015): 14–22. https://doi.org/10.1016/j.fitote.2015.04.010.
128. Jiaqi Wu et al., "Crataegus Pinnatifida: Chemical Constituents, Pharmacology, and Potential Applications," *Molecules* 19, no. 2 (2014): 1685–712. https://doi.org/10.3390/molecules19021685.
129. Pengzhi Dong et al., "Hawthorn (*Crataegus pinnatifida* Bunge) Leave Flavonoids Attenuate Atherosclerosis Development in ApoE Knock-out Mice," *Journal of Ethnopharmacology* 198 (2017): 479–88. https://doi.org/10.1016/j.jep.2017.01.040.
130. Sarah E. Edwards et al., "Hawthorn," in *Phytopharmacy: An Evidence-Based Guide to Herbal Medicinal Products, First* (Chichester, UK: Wiley Blackwell, 2015), 195–97.
131. Shanthi Rajendran et al., "Effect of Tincture of Crataegus on the LDL-Receptor Activity of Hepatic Plasma Membrane of Rats Fed an Atherogenic Diet," *Atherosclerosis* 123, no. 1–2 (1996): 235–41. https://doi.org/10.1016/0021-9150(96)05813-3.
132. Lingrong Wen et al., "Phenolic Contents and Cellular Antioxidant Activity of Chinese Hawthorn '*Crataegus pinnatifida*,'" *Food Chemistry* 186 (2015): 54–62. https://doi.org/10.1016/j.foodchem.2015.03.017.
133. Raiendran Shanthi et al., "Protective Effect of Tincture of Crataegus on Oxidative Stress in Experimental Atherosclerosis in Rats," *Journal of Clinical Biochemistry and Nutrition* 20, no. 3 (1996): 211–23.
134. Pinyi Gao et al., "Antiplatelet Aggregation and Antithrombotic Benefits of Terpenes and Flavones from Hawthorn Leaf Extract Isolated Using the Activity-Guided Method," *Food and Function* 2019, no. 2 (2019). https://doi.org/10.1039/C8FO01862F.

135. Ling-zhi Li et al., "Monoterpenes and Flavones from the Leaves of Crataegus Pinnatifida with Anticoagulant Activities," *Journal of Functional Foods* 12 (2015): 237–45. https://doi.org/10.1016/j.jff.2014.11.012.
136. Pin-Yi Gao et al., "Natural Terpenoid Glycosides with: In Vitro / Vivo Antithrombotic Profiles from the Leaves of Crataegus Pinnatifida," *RSC Advances* 76 (2017): 48466–74. https://doi.org/10.1039/c7ra10768d.
137. Claudia Daniele et al., "Adverse-Event Profile of Crataegus Spp," *Drug Safety* 29, no. 6 (2006): 523–35.
138. W. Chu, S. Cheung, R. Lau, I. Benzie, "Bilberry (Vaccinium Myrtillus L.)," In *Herbal Medicine: Biomolecular and Clinicial Aspects* (eds. Iris F. F. Benzie and Sissi Wachtel-Galor) (Boca Raton, FL: CRC Press, 2011), 55–72.
139. Oana-Crina Bujor et al., "Seasonal Variations of the Phenolic Constituents in Bilberry (Vaccinium Myrtillus L.) Leaves, Stems and Fruits, and Their Antioxidant Activity," *Food Chemistry* 213 (2016): 58–68. https://doi.org/10.1016/j.foodchem.2016.06.042.
140. Mirosława Teleszko and Aneta Wojdyło, "Comparison of Phenolic Compounds and Antioxidant Potential between Selected Edible Fruits and Their Leaves," *Journal of Functional Foods* 14 (2015): 736–46. https://doi.org/10.1016/j.jff.2015.02.041.
141. Sonia de Pascual-Teresa and Maria Teresa Sanchez-Ballesta, "Anthocyanins: From Plant to Health," *Phytochemistry Reviews* 7 (2008): 281–99. https://doi.org/10.1007/s11101-007-9074-0.
142. Michael N. Clifford, "Anthocyanins – Nature, Occurrence and Dietary Burden," *Journal of the Science of Food and Agriculture* 1072 (2000): 1063–72.
143. Andreas Juadjur and Peter Winterhalter, "Development of a Novel Adsorptive Membrane Chromatographic Method for the Fractionation of Polyphenols from Bilberry," *Journal of Agricultural and Food Chemistry* 60, no. 10 (2012): 2427–33. https://doi.org/10.1021/jf2047724.
144. Peter Heffels et al., "Influence of Common and Excessive Enzymatic Treatment on Juice Yield and Anthocyanin Content and Profile during Bilberry (Vaccinium Myrtillus L.) Juice Production," *European Food Research and Technology* 243, no. 1 (2017): 59–68. https://doi.org/10.1007/s00217-016-2722-0.
145. Dolores Müller, Markus Schantz, and Elke Richling, "High Performance Liquid Chromatography Analysis of Anthocyanins in Bilberries (Vaccinium Myrtillus L.), Blueberries (Vaccinium Corymbosum L.), and Corresponding Juices," *Journal of Food Science* 77, no. 4 (2012): 340–45. https://doi.org/10.1111/j.1750-3841.2011.02605.x.
146. Spela Mose Bornsek et al., "Bilberry and Blueberry Anthocyanins Act as Powerful Intracellular Antioxidants in Mammalian Cells," *Food Chemistry* 134, no. 4 (2012): 1878–84. https://doi.org/10.1016/j.foodchem.2012.03.092.

147. Aurelie Mauray et al., "Bilberry Anthocyanin-Rich Extract Alters Expression of Genes Related to Atherosclerosis Development in Aorta of Apo E-Deficient Mice," *Nutrition, Metabolism, and Cardiovascular Diseases* 22, no. 1 (2012): 72–80. https://doi.org/10.1016/j.numecd.2010.04.011.
148. Jean-Max Rouanet et al., "Berry Juices, Teas, Antioxidants and the Prevention of Atherosclerosis in Hamsters," *Food Chemistry* 118, no. 2 (2009): 266–71. https://doi.org/10.1016/j.foodchem.2009.04.116.
149. Ana Faria et al., "Antioxidant Properties of Prepared Blueberry (Vaccinium Myrtillus) Extracts," *Journal of Agricultural and Food Chemistry* 53, no. 17 (2005): 6896–902. https://doi.org/10.1021/jf0511300.
150. A. Juadjur et al., "Fractionation of an Anthocyanin-Rich Bilberry Extract and in Vitro Antioxidative Activity Testing," *Food Chemistry* 167 (2014): 418–24. https://doi.org/10.1016/j.foodchem.2014.07.004.
151. Yahya Madihi et al., "Bioactive Components and the Effect of Hydroalcoholic Extract of Vaccinium Myrtillus on Postprandial Atherosclerosis Risk Factors in Rabbits," *Pakistan Journal of Medical Sciences* 29, no. 1 (2013): 384–89. https://doi.org/10.12669/pjms.291(Suppl).3539.
152. Lilith Arevström et al., "Freeze-Dried Bilberry (Vaccinium Myrtillus) Dietary Supplement Improves Walking Distance and Lipids after Myocardial Infarction: An Open-Label Randomized Clinical Trial," *Nutrition Research* 62 (2018): 13–22. https://doi.org/10.1016/j.nutres.2018.11.008.
153. Anette Karlsen et al., "Anthocyanins Inhibit Nuclear Factor-KB Activation in Monocytes and Reduce Plasma Concentrations of Pro-Inflammatory Mediators in Healthy Adults," *Journal of Nutrition* 137, no. 8 (2018): 1951–54. https://doi.org/10.1093/jn/137.8.1951.
154. Anette Karlsen et al., "Bilberry Juice Modulates Plasma Concentration of NF-κB Related Inflammatory Markers in Subjects at Increased Risk of CVD," *European Journal of Nutrition* 49, no. 6 (2010): 345–55. https://doi.org/10.1007/s00394-010-0092-0.
155. Yitong Zhu et al., "Effects of Vaccinium Berries on Serum Lipids: A Meta-Analysis of Randomized Controlled Trials," *Evidence-Based Complementary and Alternative Medicine* 2015 (2015): 790329. https://doi.org/10.1155/2015/790329.
156. Hoahai Huang et al., "Effects of Berries Consumption on Cardiovascular Risk Factors: A Meta-Analysis with Trial Sequential Analysis of Randomized Controlled Trials," *Scientific Reports* 6 (2016). https://doi.org/10.1038/srep23625.
157. Marta Habanova et al., "Intake of Bilberries (Vaccinium Myrtillus L.) Reduced Risk Factors for Cardiovascular Disease by Inducing Favorable Changes in Lipoprotein Profiles," *Nutrition Research* 36, no. 12 (2016): 1415–22. https://doi.org/10.1016/j.nutres.2016.11.010.
158. Almottesembellah Abdalruhman Gaiz et al., "Potential of Anthocyanin to Prevent Cardiovascular Disease in Diabetes," *Alternative Therapies in Health and Medicine* 24, no. 3 (2018): 40–47.

159. Kiara Thompson, Wayne Pederick, and Abishek Bommanna Santhakumar, "Anthocyanins in Obesity-Associated Thrombogenesis: A Review of the Potential Mechanism of Action," *Food and Function* 7, no. 5 (2016): 2169–78. https://doi.org/10.1039/c6fo00154h.
160. Dolores Mueller et al., "Encapsulation of Anthocyanins from Bilberries – Effects on Bioavailability and Intestinal Accessibility in Humans," *Food Chemistry* 248 (2017): 217–24. https://doi.org/10.1016/j.foodchem.2017.12.058.
161. Dolores Mueller et al., "Human Intervention Study to Investigate the Intestinal Accessibility and Bioavailability of Anthocyanins from Bilberries," *Food Chemistry* 231 (2017): 275–86. https://doi.org/10.1016/j.foodchem.2017.03.130.
162. Taylor C. Wallace, "Anthocyanins," *Advances in Nutrition* 6, no. 5 (2015): 620–22. https://doi.org/10.3945/an.115.009233.
163. Hamid Rouhi-Boroujeni et al., "A Systematic Review on Safety and Drug Interaction of Herbal Therapy in Hyperlipidemia: A Guide for Internist," *Acta Biomedica: Atenei Parmensis* 86, no. 2 (2015): 130–36.
164. Xiao-Dan Mei et al., "Danshen: A Phytochemical and Pharmacological Overview," *Chinese Journal of Natural Medicines* 17, no. 1 (2019): 59–80. https://doi.org/10.1016/S1875-5364(19)30010-X.
165. Chun-Yan Su et al., "Salvia Miltiorrhiza: Traditional Medicinal Uses, Chemistry, and Pharmacology," *Chinese Journal of Natural Medicines* 13, no. 3 (2015): 163–82. https://doi.org/10.1016/S1875-5364(15)30002-9.
166. Wen-JunWei et al., "Diterpenoids from Salvia Miltiorrhiza and Their Immune-Modulating Activity," *Journal of Agricultural and Food Chemistry* 65, no. 29 (2017): 5985–93. https://doi.org/10.1021/acs.jafc.7b02384.
167. Bao-Qing Wang, "Salvia Miltiorrhiza: Chemical and Pharmacological Review of a Medicinal Plant," *Journal of Medicinal Plants Research* 4, no. 25 (2010): 2813–20.
168. Zhangsen S. Huang et al., "Salvianolic Acid A Inhibits Platelet Activation and Arterial Thrombosis via Inhibition of Phosphoinositide 3-Kinase," *Journal of Thrombosis and Haemostasis* 8, no. 6 (2010): 1383–93. https://doi.org/10.1111/j.1538-7836.2010.03859.x.
169. Shixin Xu et al., "Salvianolic Acid B Inhibits Platelets-Mediated Inflammatory Response in Vascular Endothelial Cells," *Thrombosis Research* 135, no. 1 (2015): 137–45. https://doi.org/10.1016/j.thromres.2014.10.034.
170. Shuli Ma et al., "Evaluation of the Anti-Inflammatory Activities of Tanshinones Isolated from Salvia Miltiorrhiza Var. Alba Roots in THP-1 Macrophages," *Journal of Ethnopharmacology* 188 (2016): 193–99. https://doi.org/10.1016/j.jep.2016.05.018.
171. Jun Feng, Shusheng Li, and Huawen Chen, "Tanshinone IIA Inhibits Myocardial Remodeling Induced by Pressure Overload via Suppressing Oxidative Stress and Inflammation: Possible Role of Silent Information Regulator 1," *European Journal of Pharmacology* 791 (2016): 632–39. https://doi.org/10.1016/j.ejphar.2016.09.041.

172. Jin-Xiu Yang et al., "Tanshinone II A Attenuates TNF-α-Induced Expression of VCAM-1 and ICAM-1 in Endothelial Progenitor Cells by Blocking Activation of NF-κB," *Cellular Physiology and Biochemistry* 41, no. 1 (2016): 195–206. https://doi.org/10.1159/000452537.
173. Dong Zhao et al., "Tanshinone II A Stabilizes Vulnerable Plaques by Suppressing RAGE Signaling and NF-κB Activation in Apolipoprotein-E-Deficient Mice," *Molecular Medicine Reports* 14, no. 6 (2016): 4983–90. https://doi.org/10.3892/mmr.2016.5916.
174. Zhi-yuan Fang et al., "Tanshinone IIA Downregulates the CD40 Expression and Decreases MMP-2 Activity on Atherosclerosis Induced by High Fatty Diet in Rabbit," *Journal of Ethnopharmacology* 115, no. 2 (2008): 217–22. https://doi.org/10.1016/j.jep.2007.09.025.
175. Zhiping Liu et al., "Cryptotanshinone, an Orally Bioactive Herbal Compound from Danshen, Attenuates Atherosclerosis in Apolipoprotein E-Deficient Mice: Role of Lectin-like Oxidized LDL Receptor-1 (LOX-1)," *British Journal of Pharmacology* 172, no. 23 (2015): 5661–75. https://doi.org/10.1111/bph.13068.
176. Wenwen Zhao et al., "Dihydrotanshinone I Attenuates Atherosclerosis in ApoE-Deficient Mice: Role of NOX4/NF-κB Mediated Lectin-like Oxidized LDL Receptor-1 (LOX-1) of the Endothelium," *Frontiers in Pharmacology* 7 (2016): 1–13. https://doi.org/10.3389/fphar.2016.00418.
177. Fei Cao et al., "Antiviral C-25 Epimers of 26-Acetoxy Steroids from the South China Sea Gorgonian Echinogorgia Rebekka," *Journal of Natural Products* 77, no. 6 (2014): 1488–93. https://doi.org/10.1021/np500252q.
178. Yu-Chiang Hung, Pei-Wen Wang, and Tai-Long Pan, "Functional Proteomics Reveal the Effect of Salvia Miltiorrhiza Aqueous Extract Against Vascular Atherosclerotic Lesions," *Biochemica et Biophysica Acta (BBA) - Proteins and Proteomics* 1804, no. 6 (2010): 1310–21. https://doi.org/10.1016/j.bbapap.2010.02.001.
179. Qiongtao Song et al., "Potential Mechanisms Underlying the Protective Effects of Salvianic Acid A against Atherosclerosis in Vivo and Vitro," *Biomedicine and Pharmacotherapy* 109 (2019): 945–56. https://doi.org/10.1016/j.biopha.2018.10.147.
180. Yu Liu et al., "Salvia Miltiorrhiza Injection on Pulmonary Heart Disease: A Systematic Review and Meta-Analysis," *Amerian Journal of Chinese Medicine* 42, no. 6 (2014): 1315–31. https://doi.org/10.1142/S0192415X14500827.
181. C. Wang et al., "An in Vivo and in Vitro Study: High-Dosage Danshen Injection Induces Peripheral Vascular Endothelial Cells Injury," *Human and Experimental Toxicology* 35, no. 4 (2016): 404–17. https://doi.org/10.1177/0960327115591374.
182. Ashwini R. Madgulkar, Monica R. P. Rao, and Deepa Warrier, "Characterization of Psyllium (Plantago Ovata) Polysaccharide and Its Uses," *Polysaccharides*, edited by Kishan Gopal Ramawat and Jean-Michel Mérillon (Cham: Springer, 2015), 872–90. https://doi.org/10.1007/978-3-319-16398-0_49.

183. Li Li et al., "Isolation and Purification of Acteoside and Isoacteoside from Plantago Psyllium L. by High-Speed Counter-Current Chromatography," *Journal of Chromatography A* 1063, no. 1–2 (2005): 161–69. https://doi.org/10.1016/j.chroma.2004.11.024.
184. Sandra Gonçalves and Anabela Romano, "The Medicinal Potential of Plants from the Genus Plantago (Plantaginaceae)," *Industrial Crops and Products* 83 (2016): 213–26. https://doi.org/10.1016/j.indcrop.2015.12.038.
185. Rosa Solà et al., "Soluble Fibre (Plantago Ovata Husk) Reduces Plasma Low-Density Lipoprotein (LDL) Cholesterol, Triglycerides, Insulin, Oxidised LDL and Systolic Blood Pressure in Hypercholesterolaemic Patients: A Randomised Trial," *Atherosclerosis* 211, no. 2 (2010): 630–37. https://doi.org/10.1016/j.atherosclerosis.2010.03.010.
186. Elena Jovanovski et al., "Effect of Psyllium (Plantago Ovata) Fiber on LDL Cholesterol and Alternative Lipid Targets, Non-HDL Cholesterol and Apolipoprotein B: A Systematic Review and Meta-Analysis of Randomized Controlled Trials," *American Journal of Clinical Nutrition* 108, no. 5 (2018): 922–32. https://doi.org/10.1093/ajcn/nqy115.
187. Z. H. Wei et al., "Time- and Dose-Dependent Effect of Psyllium on Serum Lipids in Mild-to-Moderate Hypercholesterolemia: A Meta-Analysis of Controlled Clinical Trials," *European Journal of Clinical Nutrition* 63, no. 7 (2009): 821–27. https://doi.org/10.1038/ejcn.2008.49.
188. Rosa Solà et al., "Effects of Soluble Fiber (Plantago Ovata Husk) on Plasma Lipids, Lipoproteins, and Apolipoproteins in Men with Ischemic Heart Disease," *American Journal of Clinical Nutrition* 85, no. 4 (2007): 1157–63. https://doi.org/10.1093/ajcn/85.4.1157.
189. Simone Augusta Ribas et al., "Effects of Psyllium on LDL-Cholesterol Concentrations in Brazilian Children and Adolescents: A Randomised, Placebo-Controlled, Parallel Clinical Trial," *British Journal of Nutrition* 113, no. 1 (2015): 134–41. https://doi.org/10.1017/S0007114514003419.
190. K. Haddadian, K. Haddadian, and M. A. Zahmatkash, "A Review of Plantago Plant," *Indian Journal Traditional Knowledge* 13, no. 4 (2014): 681–85. http://nopr.niscair.res.in/handle/123456789/29518.
191. Catherine Ulbricht et al., "Clinical Evidence of Herb-Drug Interactions: A Systematic Review by the Natural Standard Research Collaboration," *Current Drug Metabolism* 9, no. 10 (2008): 1063–1120. https://doi.org/10.2174/138920008786927785.
192. A. Fugh-Berman, "Herb-Drug Interactions," *Lancet* 355, no. 9198 (2000): 134–38.
193. Rohan Shah, Vandana Gulati, and Enzo Palomno, "Pharmacological Properties of Guggulsterones, the Major Active Components of Gum Guggul," *Phytotherapy Research* 26, no. 11 (2012): 1594–605. https://doi.org/10.1002/ptr.4647.
194. Shishir Shishodia et al., "The Guggul for Chronic Diseases: Ancient Medicine, Modern Targets," *Anticancer Research* 28, no. 6A (2008): 3647–64.

195. Najeeb Ur Rehman et al., "A Norterpenoid and Tripenoids from Commiphora Mukul: Isolation and Biological Activity," *Zeitschrift fur Naturforsch. - Sect. B* 72, no. 1 (2017): 11–15. https://doi.org/10.1515/znb-2016-0062.
196. Catherine Gebhard et al., "Guggulsterone, an Anti-Inflammatory Phytosterol, Inhibits Tissue Factor and Arterial Thrombosis," *Basic Research in Cardiology* 104, no. 3 (2009): 285–94. https://doi.org/10.1007/s00395-008-0757-5.
197. Shishir Shishodia and Bharat B. Aggarwal, "Guggulsterone Inhibits NF-κB and IκBα Kinase Activation, Suppresses Expression of Anti-Apoptotic Gene Products, and Enhances Apoptosis," *Journal of Biological Chemistry* 279, no. 45 (2004): 47148–58. https://doi.org/10.1074/jbc.M408093200.
198. Young-Rae Lee et al., "Guggulsterone Blocks IL-1β-Mediated Inflammatory Responses by Suppressing NF-κB Activation in Fibroblast-like Synoviocytes," *Life Sciences* 82, no. 23–24 (2008): 1203–09. https://doi.org/10.1016/j.lfs.2008.04.006.
199. Dong-Goo Kim et al., "Guggulsterone Attenuated Lipopolysaccharide-Induced Inflammatory Responses in Mouse Inner Medullary Collecting Duct-3 Cells," *Inflammation* 39, no. 1 (2016): 87–95. https://doi.org/10.1007/s10753-015-0226-x.
200. Ruitang Deng "Therapeutic Effects of Guggul and Its Constituent Guggulsterone: Cardiovascular Benefits," *Cardiovascular Drug Reviews* 25, no. 4 (2007): 375–90. https://doi.org/10.1111/j.1527-3466.2007.00023.x.
201. Catherine Ulbricht et al., "Guggul for Hyperlipidemia: A Review by the Natural Standard Research Collaboration," *Complementary Therapies in Medicine* 13, no. 4 (2005): 279–90. https://doi.org/10.1016/j.ctim.2005.08.003.
202. Saibal Das et al., "A Comparative Study of Lipid-Lowering Effects of Guggul and Atorvastatin Monotherapy in Comparison to Their Combination in High Cholesterol Diet-Induced Hyperlipidemia in Rabbits," *Journal of Dietary Supplements* 13, no. 5 (2016): 495–504. https://doi.org/10.3109/19390211.2015.1118654.
203. Ramesh Chander, A. K. Khanna, and N. K. Kapoor, "Lipid Lowering Activity of Guggulsterone from Commiphora Mukul in Hyperlipaemic Rats," *Phytotherapy Research* 10, no. 6 (1996): 508–11. https://doi.org/10.1002/(SICI)1099-1573(199609)10:6<508::AID-PTR895>3.0.CO;2-P.
204. Bhavna Sharma et al., "Effects of Guggulsterone Isolated from Commiphora Mukul in High Fat Diet Induced Diabetic Rats," *Food and Chemical Toxicology* 47, no. 10 (2009): 2631–39. https://doi.org/10.1016/j.fct.2009.07.021.
205. Jun Wu et al., "The Hypolipidemic Natural Product Guggulsterone Acts as an Antagonist of the Bile Acid Receptor," *Molecular Endocrinology* 16, no. 7 (2002): 1590–97. https://doi.org/10.1210/mend.16.7.0894.

206. Hamid Mollazadeh, Davood Mahdian, and Hossein Hosseinzadeh, "Medicinal Plants in Treatment of Hypertriglyceridemia: A Review Based on Their Mechanisms and Effectiveness," *Phytomedicine* 53 (2019): 43–52. https://doi.org/10.1016/j.phymed.2018.09.024.
207. Xiaosong Wang et al., "The Hypolipidemic Natural Product Commiphora Mukul and Its Component Guggulsterone Inhibit Oxidative Modification of LDL," *Atherosclerosis* 172, no. 2 (2004): 239–46. https://doi.org/10.1016/j.atherosclerosis.2003.10.008.
208. Bellamkonda Ramesh and Dessireddy Saralakumari, "Antihyperglycemic, Hypolipidemic and Antioxidant Activities of Ethanolic Extract of Commiphora Mukul Gum Resin in Fructose-Fed Male Wistar Rats," *Journal of Physiology and Biochemistry* 68, no. 4 (2012): 573–82. https://doi.org/10.1007/s13105-012-0175-x.
209. Brock McGregor, "Extra-Thyroidal Factors Impacting Thyroid Hormone Homeostasis: A Review," *Journal of Restorative Medicine* 4, no. 1 (2016): 40–49. https://doi.org/10.14200/jrm.2015.4.0110.
210. Peyman Mikaili et al., "Therapeutic Uses and Pharmacological Properties of Garlic, Shallot, and Their Biologically Active Compounds," *Iranian Journal of Basic Medical Science* 16, no. 10 (2013): 1031–48.
211. Michal Majewski, "*Allium sativum*: Facts and Myths Regarding Human Health," *Roczniki Panstwowego Zakladu Higieny* 65, no. 1 (2014): 1–8.
212. Yequan Zhu et al., "A Mini Review: Garlic Extract and Vascular Diseases," *Neurological Research* 40, no. 6 (2018): 421–25. https://doi.org/10.1080/01616412.2018.1451269.
213. Natália Martins, Spyridon Petropoulos, and Isabel C. F. R. Ferreira, "Chemical Composition and Bioactive Compounds of Garlic (Allium Sativum L.) as Affected by Pre- and Post-Harvest Conditions: A Review," *Food Chemistry* 211 (2016): 41–50. https://doi.org/10.1016/j.foodchem.2016.05.029.
214. Richard S. Rivlin, Matthew Budoff, and Harunobu Amagase, "Clarifying the Real Bioactive Constituents of Garlic," *Journal of Nutrition* 136, no. 3 (2006): S716–25. https://doi.org/10.1093/jn/136.3.v.
215. Feras Q. Alali et al., "Garlic for Cardiovascular Disease: Prevention or Treatment?" *Current Pharmaceutical Design* 23, no. 7 (2017): 1028–41. https://doi.org/10.2174/1381612822666161010124530.
216. Naoaki Morihara et al., "Aged Garlic Extract Suppresses the Development of Atherosclerosis in Apolipoprotein E–Knockout Mice," *Journal of Nutrition* 146, no. 2 (2016): S460–63. https://doi.org/10.3945/jn.114.206953.
217. Igor A. Sobenin et al., "Anti-Atherosclerotic Effects of Garlic Preparation in Freeze Injury Model of Atherosclerosis in Cholesterol-Fed Rabbits," *Phytomedicine* 23, no. 11 (2016): 1235–39. https://doi.org/10.1016/j.phymed.2015.10.014.

218. Vasily P. Karagodin, Igor A. Sobenin, and Alexander N. Orekhov, "Antiatherosclerotic and Cardioprotective Effects of Time-Released Garlic Powder Pills," *Current Pharmaceutical Design* 22, no. 2 (2015): 196–213. https://doi.org/10.2174/1381612822666151112153351.
219. Tao Zeng et al., "A Meta-Analysis of Randomized, Double-Blind, Placebo-Controlled Trials for the Effects of Garlic on Serum Lipid Profiles," *Journal of the Science of Food and Agriculture* 92, no. 9 (2012): 1892–1902. https://doi.org/10.1002/jsfa.5557.
220. Karin Ried, Catherine Toben, and Peter Fakler, "Effect of Garlic on Serum Lipids: An Updated Meta-Analysis," *Nutrition Reviews* 71, no. 5 (2013): 282–99. https://doi.org/10.1111/nure.12012.
221. Anna Capasso, "Antioxidant Action and Therapeutic Efficacy of Allium Sativum L.," *Molecules* 18, no. 1 (2013): 690–700. https://doi.org/10.3390/molecules18010690.
222. Daniela A. Locatelli et al., "Cooked Garlic and Antioxidant Activity: Correlation with Organosulfur Compound Composition," *Food Chemistry* 220 (2017): 219–24. https://doi.org/10.1016/j.foodchem.2016.10.001.
223. Abdulhakim Elosta et al., "Aged Garlic Has More Potent Antiglycation and Antioxidant Properties Compared to Fresh Garlic Extract in Vitro," *Scientific Reports* 7 (2017). https://doi.org/10.1038/srep39613.
224. Roya Naderi et al., "Preventive Effects of Garlic (*Allium sativum*) on Oxidative Stress and Histopathology of Cardiac Tissue in Streptozotocin-Induced Diabetic Rats," *Acta Physiologica Hungarica* 102, no. 4 (2015): 380–90. https://doi.org/10.1556/036.102.2015.4.5.
225. Da Yeon Lee et al., "Anti-Inflammatory Activity of Sulfur-Containing Compounds from Garlic," *Journal of Medicinal Food* 15, no. 11 (2012): 992–99. https://doi.org/10.1089/jmf.2012.2275.
226. Naoaki Morihara et al., "Aged Garlic Extract Suppresses Inflammation in Apolipoprotein E-Knockout Mice," *Molecular Nutrition and Food Research* 61, no. 10 (2017): 1–7. https://doi.org/10.1002/mnfr.201700308.
227. Hans-Peter Keiss et al., "Biochemical and Molecular Actions of Nutrients Garlic (*Allium sativum* L.) Modulates Cytokine Expression in Lipopolysaccharide-Activated Human Blood Thereby Inhibiting," *Journal of Nutrition* 133, no. 7 (2003): 2171–75.
228. Naoaki Morihara and Atsuko Hino, "Aged Garlic Extract Suppresses Platelet Aggregation by Changing the Functional Property of Platelets," *Journal of Natural Medicines* 71, no. 1 (2017): 249–56. https://doi.org/10.1007/s11418-016-1055-4.
229. Francesca Borrelli, Rafaelle Capasso, and Angelo A. Izzo, "Garlic (*Allium sativum* L.): Adverse Effects and Drug Interactions in Humans," *Molecular Nutrition and Food Research* 51, no. 11 (2007): 1386–97. https://doi.org/10.1002/mnfr.200700072.
230. Ravi Varshney and Matthew J. Budoff, "Garlic and Heart Disease," *Journal of Nutrition* 146, no. 2 (2016): S416–21. https://doi.org/10.3945/jn.114.202333.

231. Leslie G. Cleland, Michael J. James, and Susanna M. Proudman, "Fish Oil: What the Prescriber Needs to Know," *Arthritis Research and Therapy* 8, no. 1 (2006): 202. https://doi.org/10.1186/ar1876.
232. Christopher J. Franzese et al., "Relation of Fish Oil Supplementation to Markers of Atherothrombotic Risk in Patients with Cardiovascular Disease Not Receiving Lipid-Lowering Therapy," *American Journal of Cardiology* 115, no. 9 (2015): 1204–11. https://doi.org/10.1016/j.amjcard.2015.02.002.
233. A. P. Jain, K. K. Aggarwal, and P. Y. Zhang, "Omega-3 Fatty Acids and Cardiovascular Disease," *European Review for Medical and Pharmacological Sciences* 19, no. 3 (2015): 441–45.
234. Mohammed S. Ellulu et al., "Role of Fish Oil in Human Health and Possible Mechanism to Reduce the Inflammation," *Inflammopharmacology* 23 (2015): 79–89. https://doi.org/10.1007/s10787-015-0228-1.
235. Stein Harald Johnson et al., "Fish Consumption, Fish Oil Supplements and Risk of Atherosclerosis in the Tromsø Study," *Nutrition Journal* 17, no. 56 (2018): 79–89. https://doi.org/10.1186/s12937-018-0364-8.
236. Theingi Aung et al., "Associations of Omega-3 Fatty Acid Supplement Use with Cardiovascular Disease Risks Meta-Analysis of 10 Trials Involving 77 917 Individuals," *JAMA Cardiology* 3, no. 3 (2018): 225–34. https://doi.org/10.1001/jamacardio.2017.5205.
237. Akshay Goel et al., "Fish, Fish Oils and Cardioprotection: Promise or Fish Tale?" *International Journal of Molecular Sciences* 1, no. 12 (2018): 3703. https://doi.org/10.3390/ijms19123703.
238. JoAnn E. Manson et al., "Marine N–3 Fatty Acids and Prevention of Cardiovascular Disease and Cancer," *New England Journal of Medicine* 380, no. 1 (2018): 23–32. https://doi.org/10.1056/nejmoa1811403.
239. Da Young Oh et al., "GPR120 Is an Omega-3 Fatty Acid Receptor Mediating Potent Anti-Inflammatory and Insulin-Sensitizing Effects," *Cell* 142, no. 5 (2010): 687–98. https://doi.org/10.1016/j.cell.2010.07.041.
240. Robert K. McNamara et al., "Omega-3 Fatty Acid Deficiency Increases Constitutive pro-Inflammatory Cytokine Production in Rats: Relationship with Central Serotonin Turnover," *Prostaglandins Leukotrienes and Essential Fatty Acids* 83, no. 4–6 (2010): 185–91. https://doi.org/10.1016/j.plefa.2010.08.004.
241. Y. T. Zhao et al., "Effects of n -3 Polyunsaturated Fatty Acid Therapy on Plasma Inflammatory Markers and N-Terminal Pro-Brain Natriuretic Peptide in Elderly Patients with Chronic Heart Failure," *Journal of International Medical Research* 37, no. 6 (2009): 1831–41. https://doi.org/10.1177/147323000903700619.
242. Clara M. Yates, Philip C. Calder, and G. Ed Rainger, "Pharmacology and Therapeutics of Omega-3 Polyunsaturated Fatty Acids in Chronic Inflammatory Disease," *Pharmacology and Therapeutics* 141, no. 3 (2014): 272–82. https://doi.org/10.1016/j.pharmthera.2013.10.010.

243. Hanne K. Maehre et al., "ω-3 Fatty Acids and Cardiovascular Diseases: Effects, Mechanisms and Dietary Relevance," *International Journal of Molecular Sciences* 16, no. 9 (2015): 22636–61. https://doi.org/10.3390/ijms160922636.
244. M. F. Muldoon et al., "Fish Oil Supplementation Does Not Lower C-Reactive Protein or Interleukin-6 Levels in Healthy Adults," *Journal of Internal Medicine* 279, no. 1 (2016): 98–109. https://doi.org/10.1111/joim.12442.
245. Trevor A. Mori et al., "Interactions between Dietary Fat, Fish, and Fish Oils and Their Effects on Platelet Function in Men at Risk of Cardiovascular Disease," *Arteriosclerosis, Thrombosis, and Vascular Biology* 17, no. 2 (1997): 279–86. https://doi.org/10.1161/01.ATV.17.2.279.
246. Daniel Weitz et al., "Fish Oil for the Treatment of Cardiovascular Disease," *Cardiology in Review* 18, no. 5 (2010): 258–63. https://doi.org/10.1097/CRD.0b013e3181ea0de0.
247. Trevor A. Mori et al., "Dietary Fish as a Major Component of a Weight-Loss Diet: Effect on Serum Lipids, Glucose, and Insulin Metabolism in Overweight Hypertensive Subjects," *American Journal of Clinical Nutrition* 70, no. 5 (1999): 817–25. https://doi.org/10.1093/ajcn/70.5.817.
248. Rajinder Singh, Subrata De, and Asma Belkheir, "*Avena sativa* (Oat), A Potential Neutraceutical and Therapeutic Agent: An Overview," *Critical Reviews in Food Science and Nutrition* 53, no. 2 (2013): 126–44. https://doi.org/10.1080/10408398.2010.526725.
249. Derek Stewart and Gordon McDougall, "Oat Agriculture, Cultivation and Breeding Targets: Implications for Human Nutrition and Health," *British Journal of Nutrition* 112, no. S2 (2014): S50–57. https://doi.org/10.1017/S0007114514002736.
250. Roger Clemens and B. Jan-Willem van Klinken, "Oats, More than Just a Whole Grain: An Introduction," *British Journal of Nutrition* 112, no. S2 (2014): S1–S3. https://doi.org/10.1017/S0007114514002712.
251. Eric A. Decker, Devin J. Rose, and Derek Stewart, "Processing of Oats and the Impact of Processing Operations on Nutrition and Health Benefits," *British Journal of Nutrition* 112, no. S2 (2014): S58–64. https://doi.org/10.1017/S000711451400227X.
252. Qi Wang and Peter R. Ellis, "Oat β-Glucan: Physico-Chemical Characteristics in Relation to Its Blood-Glucose and Cholesterol-Lowering Properties," *Brirish Journal of Nutrition* 112, no. S2 (2014): S4–13. https://doi.org/10.1017/S0007114514002256.
253. Hüseyin Boz, "Phenolic Amides (Avenanthramides) in Oats—A Review," *Czech Journal of Food Sciences* 33, no. 5 (2015): 399–404. https://doi.org/10.17221/696/2014-CJFS.
254. Frank Thies et al., "Oats and CVD Risk Markers: A Systematic Literature Review," *British Journal of Nutrition* 112, no. S2 (2014): S19–30. https://doi.org/10.1017/S0007114514002281.
255. Michael Thomas et al., "High Levels of Avenanthramides in Oat-Based Diet Further Suppress High Fat Diet-Induced Atherosclerosis in Ldlr -/- Mice," *Journal of Agricultural and Food Chemistry* 66, no. 2 (2018): 498–504. https://doi.org/10.1021/acs.jafc.7b04860.

256. Rgia A. Othman, Mohammed H. Moghadasian, and Peter J. H. Jones, "Cholesterol-Lowering Effects of Oat β-Glucan," *Nutrition Reviews* 69, no. 6 (2011): 299–309. https://doi.org/10.1111/j.1753-4887.2011.00401.x.
257. Thomas M. S. Wolever et al., "Physicochemical Properties of Oat B-Glucan Influence Its Ability to Reduce Serum LDL Cholesterol in Humans: A Randomized Clinical Trial," *American Journal of Clinical Nutrition* 92, no. 4 (2010): 723–32. https://doi.org/10.3945/ajcn.2010.29174.
258. Li Li Ji et al., "Effects of Avenanthramides on Oxidant Generation and Antioxidant Enzyme Activity in Exercised Rats," *Nutrition Research* 23, no. 11 (2003): 1579–90. https://doi.org/10.1016/S0271-5317(03)00165-9.
259. Ilva Nakurte et al., "Detection of the Lunasin Peptide in Oats (Avena Sativa L)," *Journal of Cereal Science* 57, no. 3 (2013): 319–24. https://doi.org/10.1016/j.jcs.2012.12.008.
260. Liping Liu et al., "The Antiatherogenic Potential of Oat Phenolic Compounds," *Atherosclerosis* 175, no. 1 (2004): 39–49. https://doi.org/10.1016/j.atherosclerosis.2004.01.044.
261. Guoyong Yu et al., "In Vitro Inhibition of Platelet Aggregation by Peptides Derived from Oat (Avena Sativa L.), Highland Barley (Hordeum Vulgare Linn. Var. Nudum Hook. f.), and Buckwheat (Fagopyrum Esculentum Moench) Proteins," *Food Chemistry* 194 (2016): 577–86. https://doi.org/10.1016/j.foodchem.2015.08.058.

Chapter 14

Natural Products in Endocrine System Diseases Treatment

Anfal S. Aljahdali, James Burnett, and Martin Safo

Introduction

The endocrine system is a collection of glands that secrete hormones into the circulatory system to regulate the function and/or activity of organs throughout the body.[1][2] The hormones bind to specific receptor sites in the various organs to regulate physiological and behavioral activities, such as development, digestion, metabolism, respiration, sleep, stress, growth, mood, reproduction, and so on.[1][2] Very low hormone concentrations have profound effects on organs, with each organ requiring precise amounts that change throughout the life cycle or in response to the environment.[3] Examples of hormones, their secreting glands, and functions are shown in Table 14.1.

TABLE 14.1 Major Endocrine Glands and Hormones

Endocrine Gland	Major Hormone(s)	General Effect/Function
Pituitary	1. Growth hormone	1. Growth
	2. Thyroid stimulating hormone (TSH)	2. Metabolism
	3. Oxytocin	3. Reproduction, childbirth, nursing
	4. Prolactin	4. Milk production
	5. Vasopressin	5. Electrolyte/water balance
	6. Adrenocorticotropic hormone (ACTH)	6. Regulate levels of cortisol
	7. Luteinizing hormone (LH)	7. Female and male reproduction
	8. Follicle stimulating hormone (FSH)	8. Female and male reproduction
Adrenal	1. Glucocorticoids (cortisol)	1. Stress, metabolism, immune system
	2. Mineralocorticoids (aldosterone)	2. Electrolyte/water balance
	3. Androgen (sex steroids)	3. Sex development

(Continued)

TABLE 14.1 *(Continued)*

Endocrine Gland	Major Hormone(s)	General Effect/Function
Pancreas	1. Insulin 2. Glucagon	1. Blood sugar regulation 2. Blood sugar regulation
Thyroid	1. Thyroid hormone 2. Calcitonin	1. Metabolism 2. Calcium homeostasis
Parathyroid	1. Parathyroid hormone	1. Calcium balance
Pineal	1. Melatonin	1. Circadian rhythm, reproductive hormones regulation
Ovary	1. Sex steroids (estrogens, progesterone)	1. Female reproduction
Testes	2. Sex steroids (androgens, e.g., testosterone)	1. Male reproduction
Hypothalamus	1. Corticotropin-releasing hormone (CRH) 2. Thyrotropin-releasing hormone (TRH) 3. Gonadotropin-releasing hormone (GnRH) 4. Oxytocin 5. Prolactin	1. Stress and immune response 2. Metabolism 3. Reproduction 4. Reproduction, childbirth, nursing 5. Breast milk

Endocrine Modulators

Every hormone binds to a receptor(s) on the target organ it regulates. Shown in Figure 14.1 are examples of chemical or crystal structures of hormones and/or complexes with their respective endocrine receptors. The ability of a hormone to activate its receptor depends on several factors, including the concentration of the hormone in circulation, the amount that reaches the target organ, potency, and the duration of hormonal activation. Natural products, environmental compounds, manufactured chemicals, and pollutants can interfere with any or some of these steps, thereby modulating or disrupting the endocrine system and potentially affecting many body functions or biological processes.[4][5] These compounds activate hormone receptors and trigger processes that are normally activated only by natural hormones, while others may prevent activation of the endocrine system by blocking a natural hormone from binding to its receptor.[4][5]

Endocrine Disorders and Natural Products

Because of its critical role in many important biological and physiological functions, impairments in any part of the endocrine system can lead to poor quality of life, disease, and death.[6]

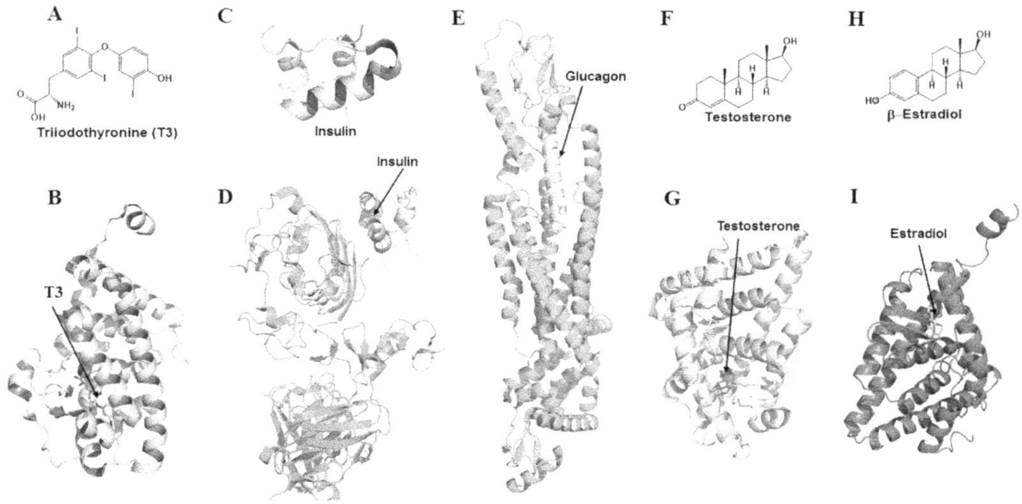

FIGURE 14.1 The endocrine system. (A) Chemical structure of the thyroid hormone, triiodothyronine (T3). (B) Crystal structure of human thyroid hormone receptor in complex with T3 (PDB code 3GWS). (C) Crystal structure of human insulin (PDB code 3I40). (D) Crystal structure of human insulin receptor in complex with insulin (PDB code 4OGA). (E) Crystal structure of human glucagon receptor in complex with glucagon analog (PDB code 5YQZ). (F) Chemical structure of testosterone. (G) Crystal structure of human androgen receptor ligand binding domain in complex with testosterone (PDB code 2AM9). (H) Chemical structure of β-estradiol (estrogen). (I) Crystal structure of human estrogen receptor ligand binding domain in complex with β-estradiol (PDB code 1A52).

The disturbance may take the form of excessive or attenuated activity, and to varying degrees. These include but are not limited to blood sugar/metabolism imbalance, heart disease, gut issues, stress, premenstrual syndrome, fatigue, inflammation, mood issues, fibromyalgia, hormone imbalance, infertility, benign prostatic hyperplasia, thyroid disease, autoimmune disease, and sleep disorder.[6] One of the most common endocrine diseases is diabetes mellitus, which is characterized by an inability to properly process glucose. Another common endocrine disorder is hypothyroidism, which occurs when the thyroid gland does not produce enough thyroid hormone. Hormone imbalances can also have a significant impact on the reproductive system.

Natural products from plants and other sources, as well as major drugs that have their origin from natural products, have been used for centuries to treat a number of diseases arising from dysfunction of the endocrine system.[6][7] These natural products, derived from plant root, seed, fruit, or bark, contain several phytochemicals and are suggested to inhibit the binding of hormones at receptor sites, improve hormone metabolism, or synergize with the effects of naturally occurring hormones. While there is a scientific basis for the use of some of these phytochemicals, others are based on anecdotal or inconclusive scientific/clinical data or poorly conducted studies. Regardless, the use of natural products and/or screening for new compounds from natural products is very attractive, as they contain substances that have relatively less toxic side effects.[7] Nonetheless, serious side effects from natural product therapy are known to occur but can be minimized if care is taken to balance the body's need and the administered dose. This chapter focuses on natural products that are used to treat diabetes mellitus, sex hormone (estrogen) imbalance disorders, and benign prostatic hyperplasia. The therapeutic actions of select plants, highlighting possible phytochemicals and their mechanism-based activities, and examples of reported preclinical and/or clinical studies are discussed.

Diabetes Mellitus and Medicinal Plants

Secretion of insulin and glucagon by the pancreatic islet cells in response to blood glucose concentration is the primary mechanism of glucose homeostasis.[8] Impairment of the proper function of the insulin and glucagon hormonal systems, especially the former, are the underlying cause of several metabolic diseases, most notably diabetes mellitus (DM), the most common of the endocrine disorders.[9] Patients with diabetes develop hyperglycemia due to impaired insulin action and/or its unavailability. DM is classified into two categories: type 1 and type 2. Type 1 Diabetes Mellitus (T1DM) is characterized by absolute insulin deficiency, which is mainly associated with pancreatic β-cell inactivity,[10] while Type 2 Diabetes Mellitus (T2DM) is mainly due to insulin resistance and deficiency in insulin secretion.[11]

Insulin is a 51-amino acid polypeptide hormone that regulates sugar homeostasis by binding to insulin receptors (see Figure 14.1c, d).[12][13] The receptor-insulin complex activates a series of intracellular signaling events that lead to the absorption of glucose from the blood into cells, where it is utilized to provide energy and/or storage.[12][14] Glucagon is also a peptide hormone, produced by the α-cells of the pancreas, and has the opposite effect of insulin.[8] Mechanistically, glucagon binds to the glucagon receptor, a G protein–coupled receptor (see Figure 14.1e), resulting in the elevation of the concentration of glucose and fatty acids in the bloodstream.[12][15]

Current diabetes therapies include insulin and various antidiabetic agents, such as sulfonylureas and biguanides. Plant-based or natural products with known or suggested hypoglycemic properties are also used by many patients for treatment. These natural products usually possess few side effects and are relatively low cost.[16] Over 400 plant species and their various bioactive or active phytochemical components responsible for their hypoglycemic activity have been documented in the literature.[17][18] Polyphenols, glycosides, peptidoglycans, amino acids, carbohydrates, alkaloids, terpenoids, and flavonoids constitute the major classes of the phytochemicals.[19][20][21][22][23] For exhaustive lists of plants and phytochemicals and their utilization in diabetes therapy, the reader is referred to this recent review article and references therein.[23]

Plant-based extracts and specific phytochemicals are proposed to be involved in a myriad of antihyperglycemic activities that include but are not limited to the ability to protect and restore the function of pancreatic tissues, increase the secretion of insulin, inhibit intestinal glucose absorption, recover impaired peripheral nerves, eliminate free radicals, suppress key gluconeogenic enzymes, and enhance glucose disposal.[24][25] Many of these products have been studied or tested in vitro and in vivo, including clinical trials. Later we discuss the therapeutic actions of *Momordica charantia* Linnaeus (karela or cucurbitaceae), *Plantago ovata* (psyllium), *Zingiber officinale* Roscoe (ginger), *Allium sativum* L (garlic), *Cinnamomum cassia* (cinnamon), *Gymnema sylvestric* (gurmar), and *Cyamopsis tetragonolobus* (guar gum).

Momordica Charantia Linnaeus

Momordica charantia Linnaeus (karela or cucurbitaceae), also known as bitter gourd or bitter melon (see Figure 14.2a), is widely found in the tropics and subtropics, especially in Asia, Africa, and South America.[26] The bitterness is due to the saponin constituents, Momordicosides K and L (see Figure 14.2b). The fruit is green but turns orange when ripe and is used for food.[26] *M. charantia* is one of the most studied plants for its hypoglycemic effects in both animals and in the clinic.[27] Hundreds of plant species with hypoglycemic properties have been classified according to their biochemical names, country of origin, parts used, and nature of the bioactive agent(s).[28][29] Several phytochemicals have been proposed to be involved in *M. charantia* antihyperglycemic activity. Examples are saponins, glycosides, alkaloids, amino acids, and fatty acids.[29][30][31][32][33][34][35]

Scores of studies have investigated the antihyperglycemic effects of different extracts and isolated phytochemicals of *M. charantia*.[29][30][31] The results show the plant's ability to protect pancreatic β cells through down-regulation of MAPKs and NF-κB in MIN6N8 cells;[32][36] improved serum glucose levels by modulating peroxisome proliferator-activated receptor (PPAR-γ and PPAR-α) gene expression (which has been implicated in lipid and glucose homeostasis and insulin resistance);[37][38][39] lowered secretion of insulin from pancreatic β cells;[40] and decreased hepatic gluconeogenesis.[41][42] The saponins are the phytochemicals most well studied for their hypoglycemic properties.[43] For example, several analogs of momordicosides, for example Momordicoside G, K, and L (see Figure 14.2b), have been suggested to improve glucose tolerance in mice fed a high fat diet during a glucose tolerance test, prevent diabetes-associated cardiac fibrosis, and treat diabetes-induced cardiac fibrosis.[34][44][45] Other studies with saponins Mormodicine I and Momordicine II (see Figure 14.2b), using MIN6 β-cells, report significant insulin-releasing activity.[46]

Vicine (see Figure 14.2b), a glycol alkaloid, is another active phytochemical of *M. charantia* that has been reported to exhibit hypoglycemic effects in nondiabetic fasting rats.[35] A potential toxic side-effect of vicine is favism, a hemolytic anemia that occurs in individuals with

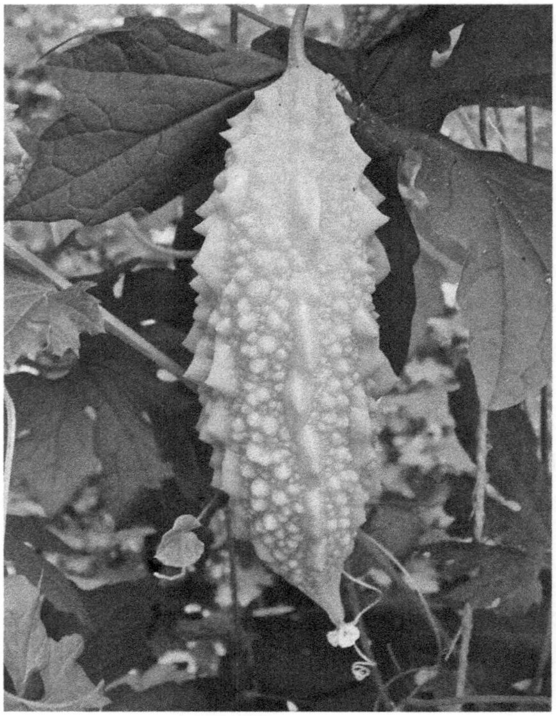

FIGURE 14.2a Bitter melon plant and fruit.

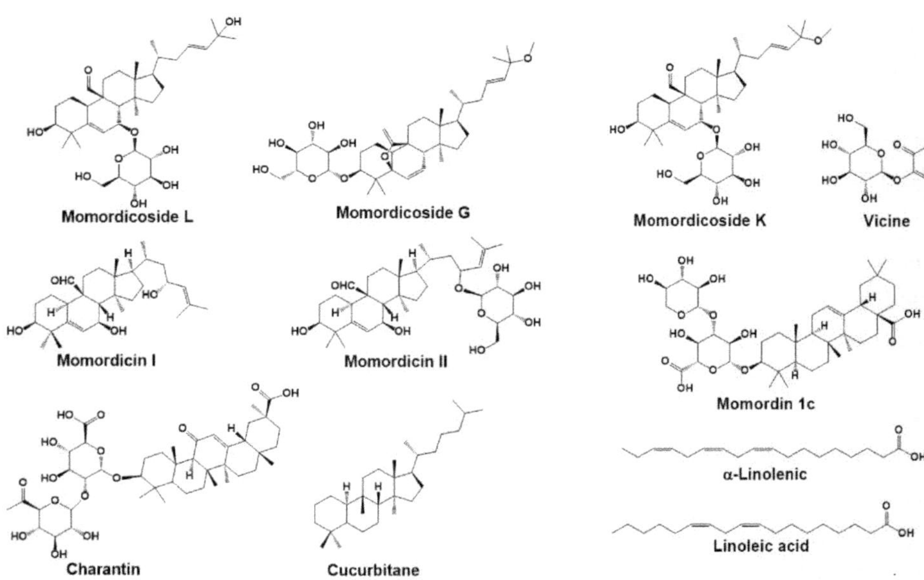

FIGURE 14.2b Chemical structures of phytochemicals.

a hereditary loss of the enzyme glucose-6-phosphate dehydrogenase.[47] Although there is no report of favism with eating bitter melon, people with this condition are advised to avoid the plant.[47]

A study by Belury et al. reported a correlation between diets high in the polyunsaturated fatty acids (see Figure 14.2b), linoleic acid (ω-6 fatty acid), and α-linolenic acid (ω-3 fatty acid) and lower risk for T2DM.[48] Consistently, the omega fatty acids isolated from *M. charantia* have been reported to show hypoglycemic activities with diverse modes of action.[48][49][50][51]

Polypeptide-P, a 166 amino-acid protein isolated from *M. charantia*, exerts potent hypoglycemic activity with significant decrease in blood sugar levels when injected subcutaneously in animals and humans by mimicking the action of human insulin.[33][52][53][54][55] Polypeptide-P is proposed as a potential plant-based insulin replacement in patients with T1DM.[56] The gene has been cloned, and the expressed recombinant polypeptide showed hypoglycemic effect in alloxan-induced diabetic mice.[57]

Several clinical studies have been conducted with *M. charantia* extract or its bioactive components, with mixed results.[51][58] For example, a 2007 double-blind randomized controlled clinical study (n = 40) to determine whether *M. charantia* capsules can decrease glycosylated hemoglobin (hemoglobin A1c or HbA1c) levels in diabetic patients did not result in a definite conclusion about its effectiveness.[59] Another controlled trial study with *M. charantia* in T2DM patients (n = 15) showed the extract to act synergistically with oral hypoglycemics, potentiating their effects in non-insulin-dependent diabetes mellitus.[60] A recent meta-analysis of clinical trials for the efficacy of *M. charantia* preparations in lowering elevated plasma glucose levels in prediabetic and T2DM patients (n = 1045) also suggested improved glycemic control.[58] However, the authors cautioned that general findings were based on low- to very low-quality evidence for the primary outcomes and sparse data for several safety outcomes.

Other human studies have been conducted to evaluate polyunsaturated fatty acid dietary enrichment on glycemic parameters.[61] A randomized controlled study by Elena Jovanovski did not observe any improvement in HbA1c, fasting blood glucose, or fasting blood insulin in people on α-linolenic acid–enriched diets.[62] Nonetheless, a recent pooled analysis of several reported studies revealed that linoleic acid is associated with dose-dependent decreases in the incidence of T2DM.[48][49] Despite the potential pharmacological benefit of *M. charantia*, there are also reports of adverse effects that limit its wider application.[26][63] For example, *M. charantia* has been suggested to induce hypoglycemic coma in children, abortion, and in some instances, death in laboratory animals.[26] It is therefore important that diabetic patients being treated with medications containing hypoglycemic drugs should use caution when taking *M. charantia* and, importantly, should be under the close supervision of a physician, as the dosage of hypoglycemic drug will need to be modified in accordance with bitter gourd juice consumption.

Cyamopsis Tetragonolobus (Guar Gum)

Cyamopsis tetragonolobus, a source of guar gum (see Figure 14.3a), is found mostly in India, Pakistan, the United States, and Africa.[64] The gum is a yellowish-white flour (see Figure 14.3b) and a good source of fiber. Its ability to hydrogen-bond with water makes it a useful thickening agent (about eight times the water-thickening potency of cornstarch) and stabilizer or additive in foods, pharmaceuticals, paper, textiles, explosives, and cosmetics.[64] Pharmacologically, *C. tetragonolobus* has been shown to be beneficial in the control of many health problems, including diabetes.[64][65] The main active ingredient associated with the hypoglycemic activity of *C. tetragonolobus* is galactomannan, a hetero-polysaccharide composed of a mannanose core and lactofuransyl side-chain (see Figure 14.3c).[64][66][67] Galactomannan has been shown to reduce postprandial blood glucose levels by delaying the intestinal absorption of carbohydrates and slowing gastric emptying.[64] Other phytochemicals, including flavonoids (e.g., quercetin, kaempferol), tannins (gallic), and coumarins (see Figure 14.3c), have also been suggested as contributing to the hypoglycemic property of the plant.[64][66] Subacute treatment with the aqueous extract of *Cyamopsis tetragonoloba* on alloxan-induced hyperglycemic rats produced a consistent reduction in blood glucose levels, which the authors attributed to the presence of flavonoids.[66]

In a clinical study involving T2DM patients, the addition of partially hydrolyzed guar gum (PHGG) to the diet was reported to improve cardiovascular and metabolic profiles by reducing HbA1c, urinary albumin excretion and serum trans-fatty acids.[68] Additionally, two recent clinical studies showed that guar gum, when used in conjunction with whey protein, reduced postprandial glycemia and HbA1c levels in T2DM patients; the results were associated with stimulation of glucagon-like peptide-1 (GLP-1) and/or slowing of gastric emptying.[69] In another reported randomized study (n = 60), galactomannan (BTI320) administration resulted in the reduction of postprandial rise in blood glucose.[70]

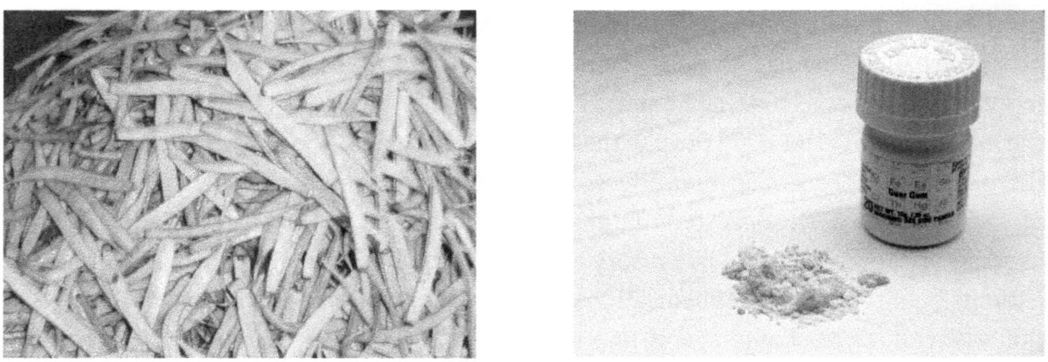

(a) **(b)**

FIGURES 14.3a and 14.3b Guar gum fruit and guar gum powder.

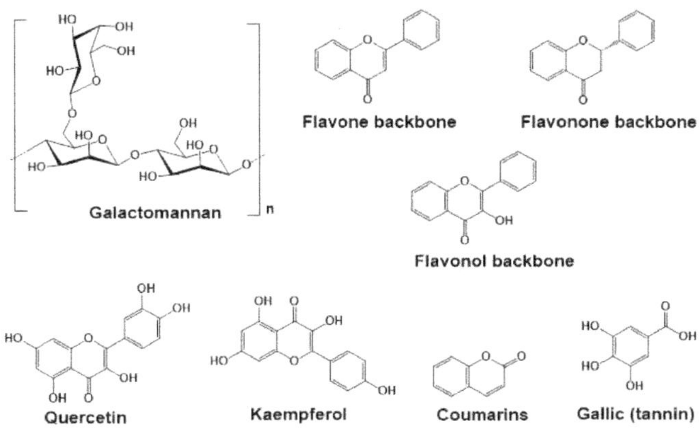

FIGURE 14.3c Chemical structures of phytochemicals.

Gymnema Sylvestric (Gurmar)

Gymnema sylvestre is a perennial woody vine that grows in tropical areas of India and Africa, China, Malaysia, and Sri Lanka (see Figure 14.4a).[71] *G. sylvestre* is used in traditional systems of medicine for diabetes, stomach ailments, liver diseases, and cardiac disorders. Several phytochemicals extracted from the plant and claimed to have antidiabetic activities have been reported. Examples are the saponins, ziziphin, and gymnemic acids (Gymnemic acids I–VII, Gymnemosides A–F) (see Figure 14.4b),[72][73][74][75] as well as a 35 amino acid peptide, gurmarin (see Figure 14.4c).[76][77] In addition to their antidiabetic activities, gymnemic acids and gurmarin have also been associated with sugar suppression activity by interacting with taste receptors on the tongue, which temporarily suppresses the taste of varicus sweets.[74][78]

Sugihara et al. reported that Gymnemic acid IV (see Figure 14.4b) increases plasma insulin levels in STZ-diabetic mice and decreases blood glucose levels by as much as 60 percent within six hours of administration compared to glibenclamide.[75] Al-Romaiyan et al. reported a high molecular weight fraction isolated from a *G. sylvestre* leaf extract (termed OSA®) to be effective in alleviating the abnormal glucose tolerance in an animal model of obesity and insulin-resistant diabetes.[79] The authors attributed the pharmacological effect of OSA® to a direct stimulatory effect on islet β-cells to promote the release of insulin, as well as the ability of OSA® to maintain insulin stores by promoting insulin biosynthesis through the elevation of prepro-insulin (PPI) mRNA. Other studies also suggest that *G. sylvestre* delays glucose absorption in the blood and prevents the absorption of sugar molecules by the intestine, which leads to reductions in blood sugar levels.[74] In a recent study, saponin extract of *G. sylvestre* (EEGS) was reported to show protection against H2O2-induced ROS generation and to increase glucose-stimulated insulin secretion in a dose-dependent manner relative to the standard antidiabetic drug glibenclamide.[80]

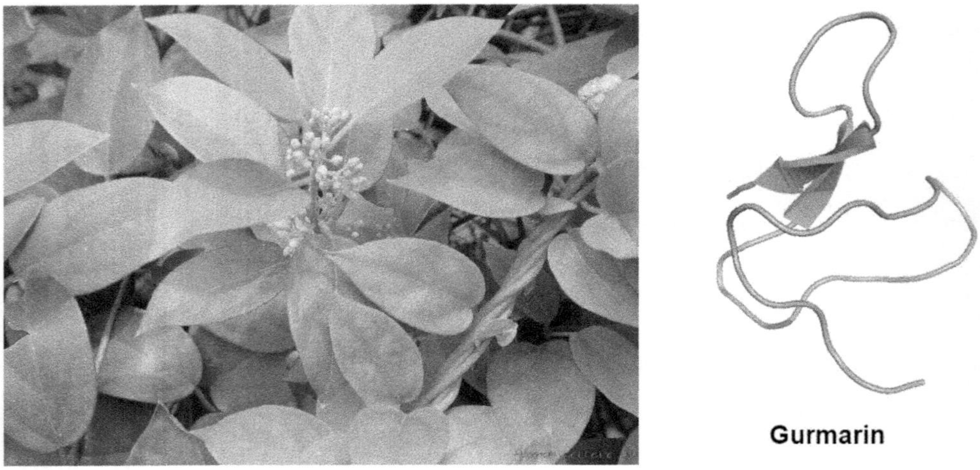

(a) (c)

FIGURES 14.4a and 14.4c Guarma plant and Gurmarin (plant insulin).

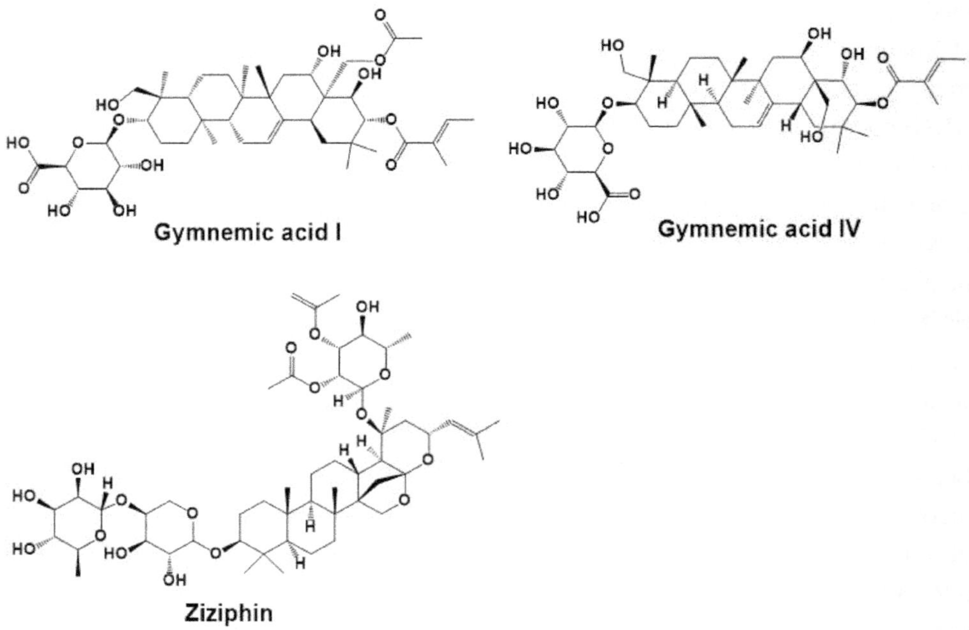

FIGURE 14.4b Chemical structures of phytochemicals.

Cinnamomum Cassia (Cinnamon)

Cinnamomum cassia (cinnamon) is a genus of the Lauraceae family (see Figures 14.5a & 14.5b). Several species are notable for their spice products. Most of the world supply of cinnamon comes from China and Indonesia. Several preclinical and clinical studies have investigated cinnamon extracts for their antidiabetic activities, and a number of cinnamon phytochemicals (see Figure 14.5c), including cinnamic acid, cinnamaldehyde, hydrocinnamic acids, and flavonoids (e.g., proanthocyanidins, rutin, catechin, quercetin, and kaempferol), have been shown to demonstrate this pharmacological effect.[81][82][83][84][85][86]

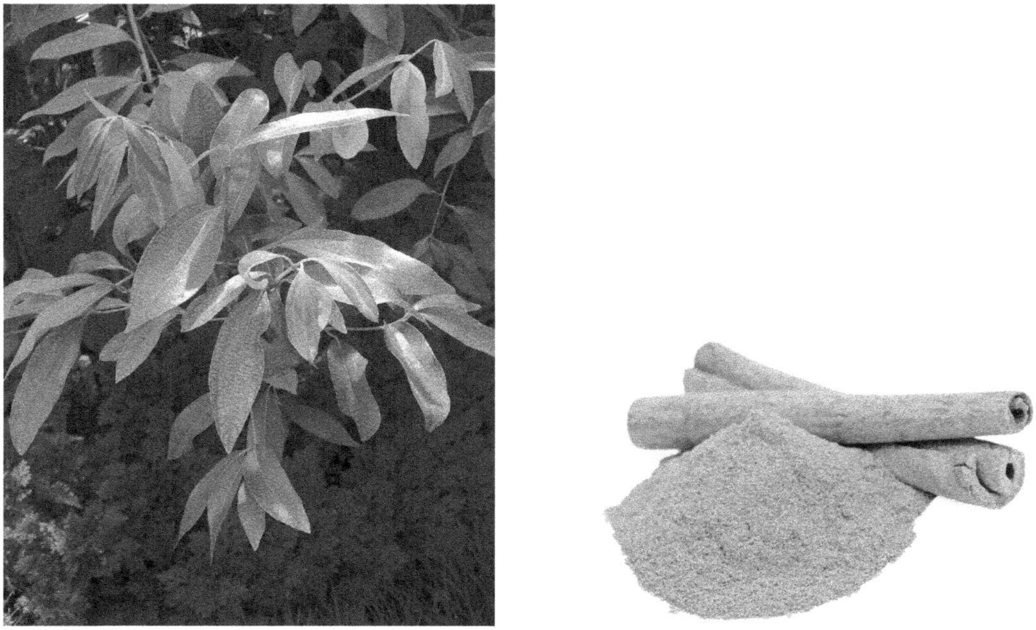

(a) (b)

FIGURES 14.5a and 14.5b Cinnamon plant and Cinnamon powder.

Cinnamaldehdye has been associated with modulating the activities of several enzymes (e.g., pyruvate kinase, phosphoenolpyruvate carboxykinase, glucose 6-phosphatase) that are involved in gluconeogenesis,[86][87] as well as enhancement of insulin release from pancreatic islets and glucose uptake in skeletal muscle tissues.[86][87] A recent study with a rat model also associated the antidiabetic properties of cinnamaldehyde with increased insulin secretion and sensitivity through activation of the antioxidant defense system, suppressing pro-inflammatory cytokine production and upregulating PPARγ gene expression.[88] Cinnamic acid was reported to contribute to hypoglycemic effects by stimulating glucose uptake and

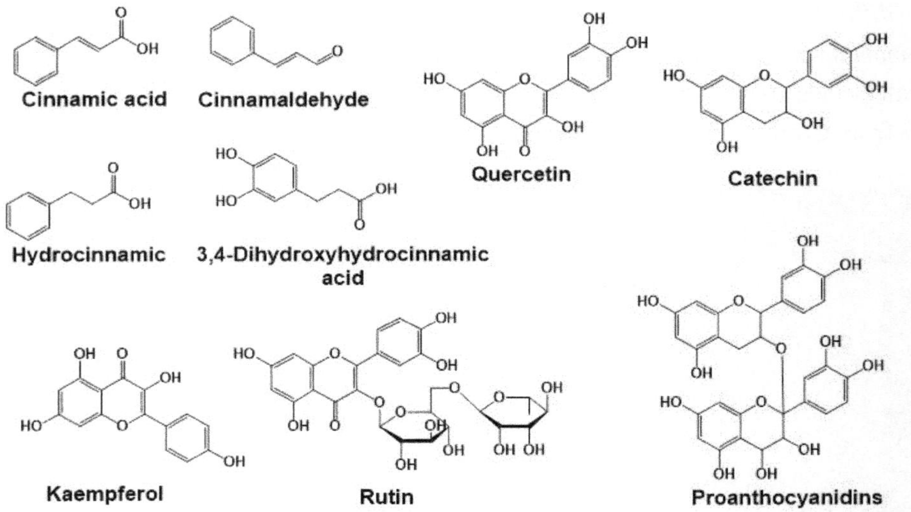

FIGURE 14.5c Chemical structures of phytochemicals.

alleviating insulin resistance through the promotion of insulin receptor tyrosyl phosphorylation and up-regulation of insulin signal–associated protein expression.[89] Hydrocinnamic acid has been reported to increase glucose disposal by enhancing translocation of glucose transporter 4.[90] Several derivatives of hydrocinnamic acid have been reported, with one of the compounds, 3,4-dihydroxyhydrocinnamic acid (see Figure 14.5c), showing significant hypoglycemic effects.[89]

Analysis of a randomized, placebo-controlled clinical trial with cinnamon extracts showed significant effects on lowering fasting plasma glucose.[91] However, an earlier study conducted on diabetic postmenopausal women receiving cinnamon supplements showed poor glycemic control.[92] A recent study suggests a combination of cinnamon with black cumin (*Nigella stavia*) acts as an adjunct therapy for diabetes mellitus, as it showed a significant reduction in blood glycemic levels in diabetic animals compared to a control group.[93]

Allium Sativum L. (Garlic)

Allium sativum L. (garlic) is a perennial plant of the Amaryllidaceae family (see Figure 14.6a).[94] It is native to central Asia and widely used as food, as well as a medicine to treat diabetes.[95] The antidiabetic potential of garlic has been associated with several mechanisms of action, including hyperinsulinemia, hypoglycemia, hypotriglyceridemia, antiglycation and antilipid-peroxidation effects.[96] The active phytochemicals attributed to *A. sativum* hypoglycemic activity are alliin, allicin, diallyl disulfide, diallyl trisulfide, diallyl sulfide, *S*-allyl cysteine, ajoene, and allyl mercaptan (see Figure 14.6b).[97][98]

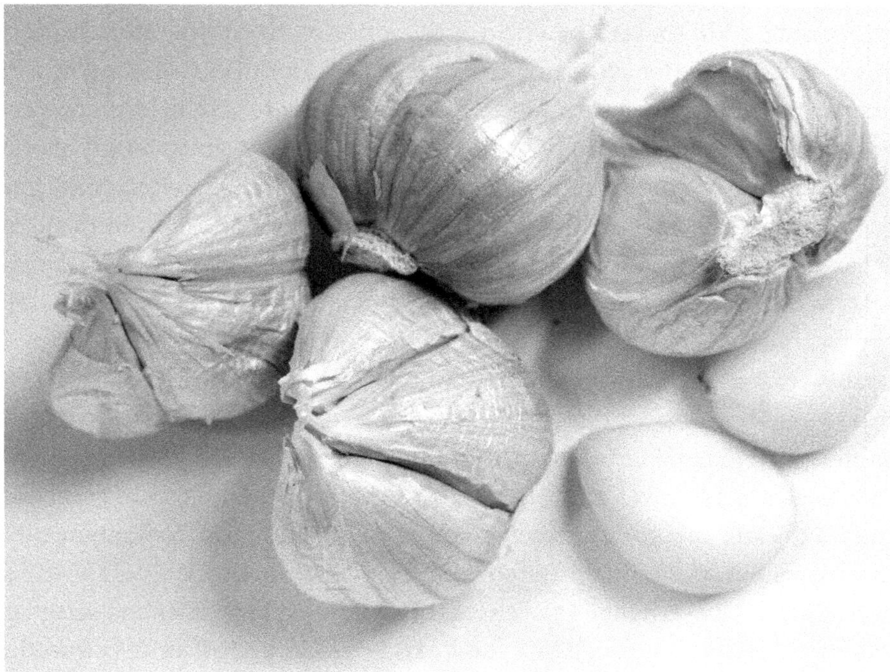

FIGURE 14.6a Garlic bulb.

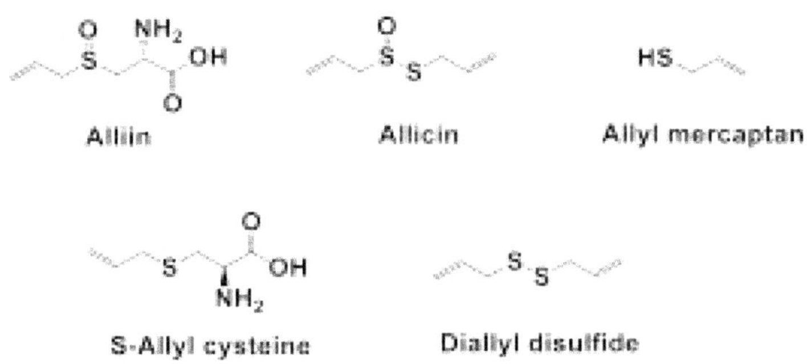

FIGURE 14.6b Chemical structures of phytochemicals.

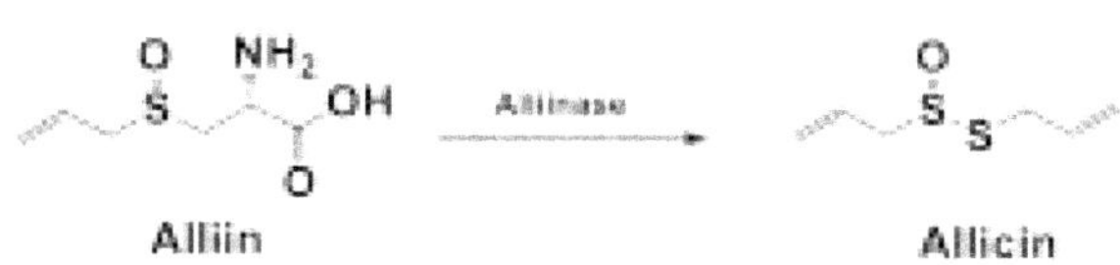

FIGURE 14.6c Enzymatic conversion of alliin to allicin.

During processing, alliin converts to allicin by the action of the enzyme allinase (see Figure 14.6c), which is responsible for garlic aroma.[99] Supplementation of alliin in the diet of diabetic rats was reported to decrease fasting glucose level and increase insulin level comparable to treatment with glibenclamide, gliclazide, or insulin.[100] A recent similar study also showed that supplementation with alliin in the diet of induced obese mice for eight weeks improved glucose homeostasis, insulin sensitivity, and improved lipid profiles.[101] Alliin's mechanism of action has been attributed to changes in intestinal bacterial composition and the ability to digest polysaccharides.[101] The antioxidant activities of these phytochemicals have also been associated with garlic's antidiabetic activities,[102][103] as oxidative stress is known to induce inflammatory responses that play an important role in the pathogenesis of T2DM.[104][105]

Clinical studies have shown that T2DM patients receiving garlic supplementation have lower fasting blood glucose levels and HbA1c compared to patients receiving placebo.[106] A meta-analysis of randomized clinical trials for the efficacy and safety of garlic in T2DM management indicated that garlic extract increased insulin secretion from pancreatic β-cells and decreased insulin resistance.[99] Moreover, meta-analysis of articles (published between 1988 and 2016) reporting studies of the effects of garlic on lipid profiles and serum glucose in patients with diabetes concluded that garlic extract is safe and effective in lowering lipid profiles and glucose in patients who are intolerant to conventional medications.[107]

Zingiber Officinale Roscoe (Ginger)

Zingiber officinale Roscoe (ginger) is a perennial plant widely used as a cooking spice for its fragrance and flavor (see Figure 14.7a).[108] Among the numerous suggested pharmacological uses of ginger[109][110] is its ability to improve the glycemic index in people with T2DM.[111]

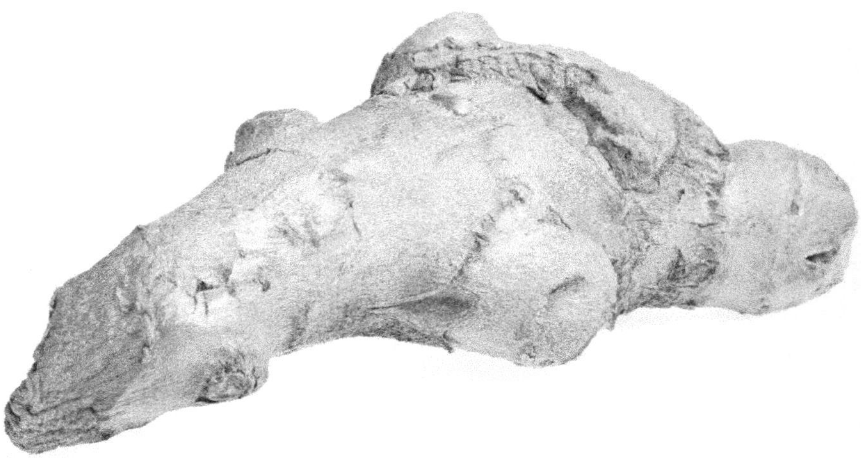

FIGURE 14.7a Ginger root.

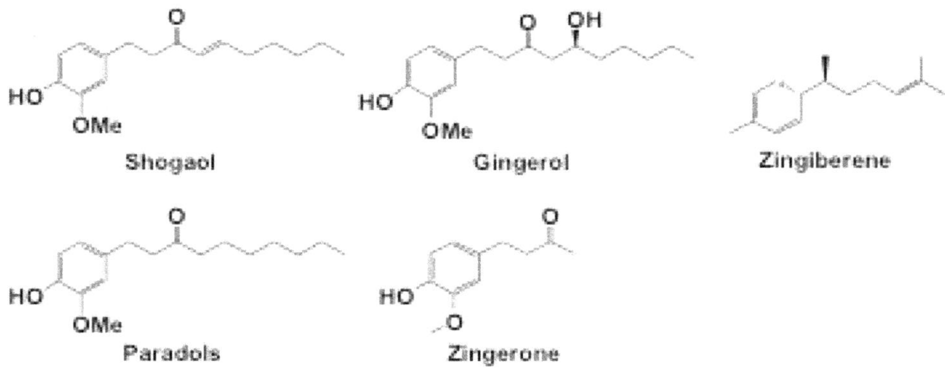

FIGURE 14.7b Chemical structures of phytochemicals.

Ginger's components, gingerols, shogaols, zingerone, and paradols, have been associated with its hypoglycemic activity (see Figure 14.7b).[112] Gingerol and shogaols are suggested to inhibit α-glucosidase and α-amylase enzymes, both of which are involved in carbohydrate digestion.[113] Gingerols, shogaols, paradols, and zingiberene are also known to exhibit anti-oxidative effects and anti-inflammatory effects; the former is suggested to be mediated by inhibition of the activity of cyclooxygenase, inducible NO synthase, and interference in cytokine signaling.[114][115]

Studies with diabetic rats have shown that ginger extract significantly increases insulin levels and decreases fasting glucose levels.[116] Clinical studies have also demonstrated that ginger significantly improved insulin sensitivity and reduced blood glucose levels in patients with T2DM versus placebo groups.[114][117] Moreover, recent meta-analysis of randomized controlled trials have shown that ginger positively affects glucose control and insulin sensitivity.[118][119]

Plantago Ovata (Psyllium)

Plantago ovata (psyllium) belongs to the Plantaginaceae family. It is a water-soluble fiber derived from psyllium husk (see Figure 14.8a) and is sometimes sold under the trademark Metamucil. *P. ovata* is used as a dietary fiber and sometimes as a food thickener. Among its many known pharmacological uses, *P. ovata* also reduces blood sugar levels.[120] *P. ovata* is a mixture of polysaccharides, and these are believed to be responsible for its hypoglycemic activity.[121] The most abundant of the polysaccharides is heteroxylans (see Figure 14.8b).[122] *P. ovata* glucose-lowering mechanisms have been associated with reduction in the intestinal absorption of glucose, delayed gastric emptying, and effects on carbohydrate digestion and absorption.[23][123][124]

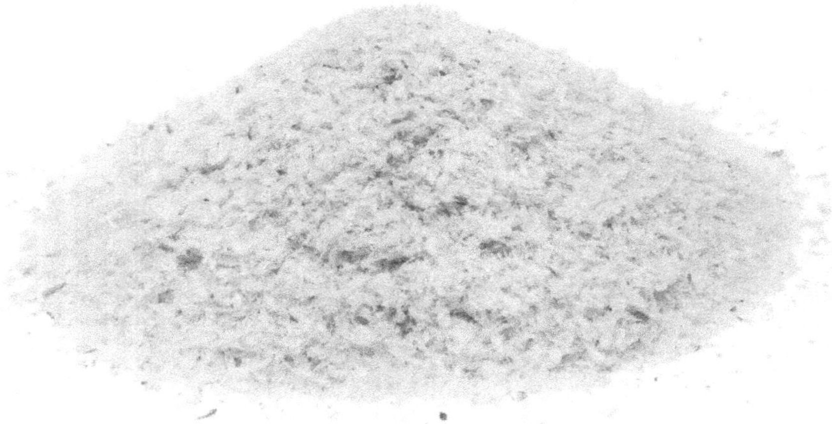

FIGURE 14.8a Psyllium husk powder.

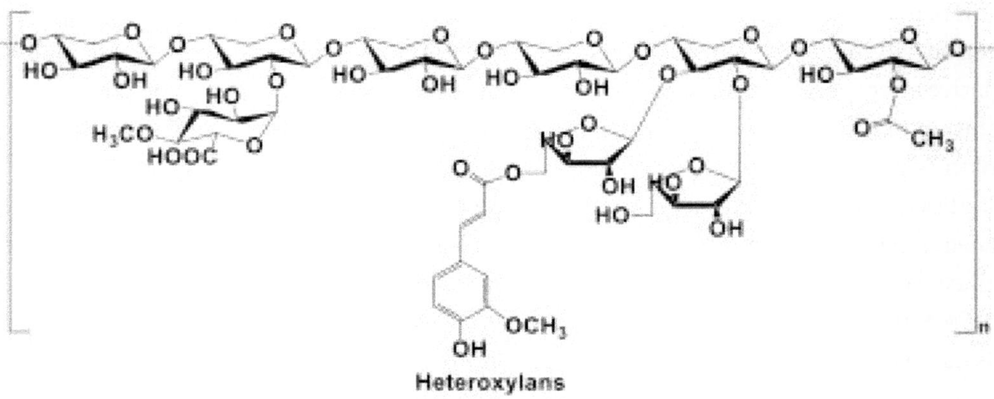

FIGURE 14.8b Chemical structure of heteroxylans.

A clinical trial with 40 T2DM patients indicated that after eight weeks of intervention, *P. ovata* supplementation provided significant improvement in fasting blood sugar and body mass index.[125] Meta-analysis of 35 randomized controlled clinical studies conducted by Procter & Gamble and Duke University reported that psyllium supplementation is associated with lowering elevated fasting blood glucose levels and HbA1c.[126] Another meta-analysis to assess the effectiveness of dietary *P. ovata* on T2DM showed that daily psyllium supplementation leads to a decrease in the incidence of developing T2DM, small reduction in fasting blood glucose levels, and reduction in HbA1c.[127]

Hormone Imbalance Disorders and Medicinal Plants

Hormones are crucial to overall health status, as they control vital biological functions, including cardiovascular, neuroendocrine, vascular, skeletal, respiratory, digestive, reproductive, cerebral, and immune system health.[128][129] Expectedly, hormonal imbalance can lead to several health issues, such as infertility, obesity, osteoporosis, endometriosis, a variety of cancers, cardiovascular diseases, and autoimmune disease.[129][130]

In women, the onset of menopause is associated with changes in hormonal balance that involve a decrease in both estrogen and progesterone levels.[131] Estrogen is responsible for secondary sex characteristics and cell growth by binding to and modulating the activities of estrogen receptor alpha (ERα) and estrogen receptor beta (ERβ).[132] Progesterone balances estrogen's proliferative effect by binding to and modulating the activity of androgen receptor.

Hot flashes and night sweats are the most commonly experienced menopausal symptoms resulting from hormonal imbalance in women.[133] Naturally occurring steroidal estrogens (see Figure 14.9a), for example, β-estradiol, equilin, equilenin, and other synthetic selective estrogen receptor modulators (SERMs), either alone or in combination with a progestin, are the most commonly used hormone replacement therapies.[134] Due to the potential side effects of these traditional medications (e.g., increased risk of breast cancer, coronary heart disease, stroke, and pulmonary embolism), women are increasingly turning to phytoestrogens and/or phytoprogesterones in medicinal plants. These are classes of plant-derived compounds that are structural mimics of estrogen and progesterone.[130][135][136][137] Phytoestrogens

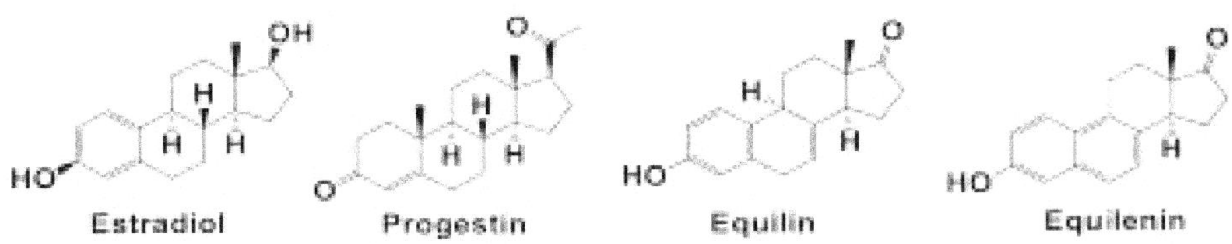

FIGURE 14.9a Naturally occurring steroidal estrogens.

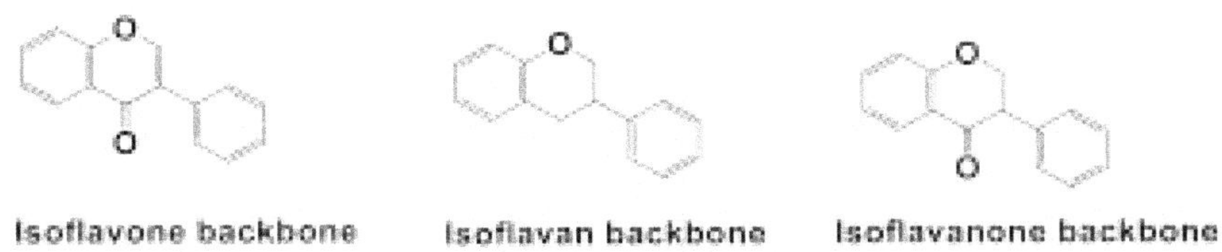

FIGURE 14.9b Hormone balancing isoflavonoids.

are suggested to be weak agonists of estrogen receptors but are capable of providing stronger estrogenic effects when the level of estrogen in the body is low.[138] Some herbal extracts are also suggested to improve sleep and memory symptoms in menopausal women by activating specific neurotransmitters.[139][140]

Several plants have been identified for their estrogenic activities,[129][140] but later we will focus on botanicals from *Cimicifuga racemose*, *Glycine max*, *Vitex agnus-castus*, and *Trifolium pretense*, respectively. Isoflavonoids (e.g., isoflavones, isoflavan; see Figure 14.9b), a class of flavonoid phenolic compounds with biological effects on estrogen receptors, are the most extensively studied phytoestrogens in these plant extracts.[141]

Cimicifuga Racemose (Black Cohosh)

Cimicifuga racemose (black cohosh) is an indigenous North American perennial herb from the buttercup family (see Figure 14.10a). It is one of the most popular botanicals for menopausal symptom relief and is commonly used to treat perimenopausal and menopausal symptoms, such as hot flashes, moodiness, vaginal dryness, and excessive sweating.[130][142] Triterpene glycosides, such as actein, 23-epi-26-deoxyactein, and cimicifugoside, are some of the active compounds found in black cohosh roots, which account for its activity (see Figure 14.10b).[143] These phytochemicals have been suggested to have selective estrogen receptor modulator properties.[144] The mechanism of action includes binding to estrogen receptors and suppressing the secretion of luteinizing hormone (LH). High levels of LH and low levels of estrogen in postmenopausal women have been implicated in higher body core temperature and the characteristic hot flashes.[145]

The black cohosh product Remifemin has been studied in at least four randomized trials, with reported efficacy in alleviating menopausal symptoms.[146][147] A meta-analysis in 2010 showed that menopausal women taking black cohosh experienced a 26 percent reduction in symptoms such as hot flashes and night sweating.[148] Other studies have shown that black cohosh may alleviate hot flashes after endocrine therapy or chemotherapy for breast and prostate cancer.[149][150]

Some studies have suggested that black cohosh is not estrogenic and may in fact have anti-estrogenic properties in breast tissue.[151][152][153] Einbond exposed a number of human breast cancer cell lines to black cohosh extracts and showed inhibition of growth.[151] A clinical trial reported that women taking black cohosh had no change in mammographic density or endometrial thickness over six months of admnistration,[153] consistent with a lack of estrogenic effect on breast and uterine tissue. Obi et al. also reported that the use of black cohosh to manage menopausal symptoms was associated with a decreased risk of breast cancer.[152]

Of note, concerns have been raised about occasional reports of hepatotoxicity associated with black cohosh usage. However, Teschke has reviewed the cases and cast doubt on this association.[154]

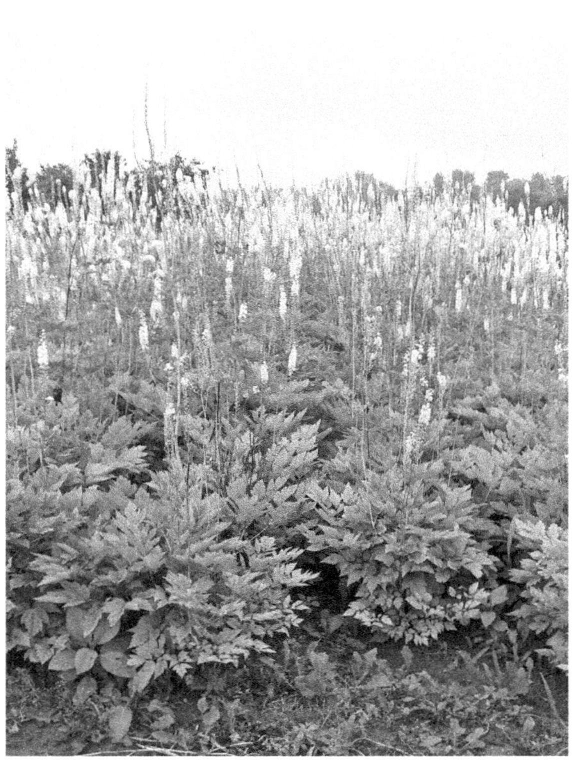

FIGURE 14.10a Black cohosh plant.

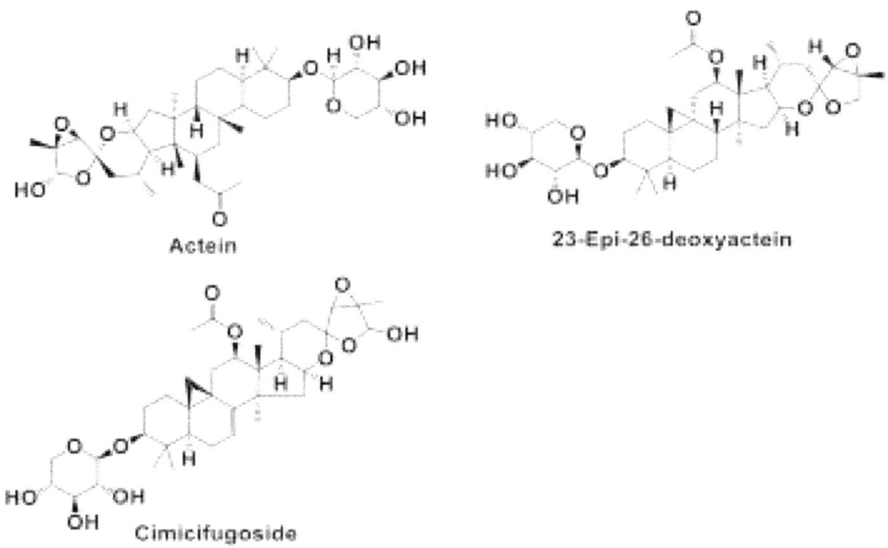

FIGURE 14.10b Chemical structures of phytochemicals.

Glycine Max (Soy)

Soybean is the protein-rich seed of *Glycine max* (see Figures 14.11a & 14.11b). Soy has been known for its health benefits in chronic diseases, such as cardiovascular, T2DM, certain types of cancer and immune and metabolic disorders.[155][158] Due to its hormone balancing effect, soy has been suggested to improve bone mass in peri- and postmenopausal women[159] and alleviate hot flashes and night sweating.[155]

Glycine max contains high concentrations of isoflavonoids such as genistein, daidzin, and coumestans, all of which are reported to exhibit estrogenic effects (see Figure 14.11c).[160][161] Another class of phytoestrogens are sterols (e.g., β-sitosterol and stigmasterol) (see Figure 14.11c). These compounds are structurally similar to β-estradiol and mimic the hormone's action.[161][162] Other phytochemicals that are known to exhibit estrogenic activity are the fatty acids α-Linolenic acid and linoleic acid (see Figure 14.11c).[161][162] A study feeding ovariectomized mice with soy reported that almost all metabolic parameters were normalized by restoring estrogen receptor alpha (ERα) deficiency.[163]

In a three-year randomized controlled clinical trial, Hodis et al. reported that soy protein supplementation reduced the progression of subclinical atherosclerosis in women.[164] Meta-analysis of 19 trials concluded that six weeks to 12 months of supplementation with soy isoflavones resulted in a 20 to 26 percent reduction of severity of hot flashes compared

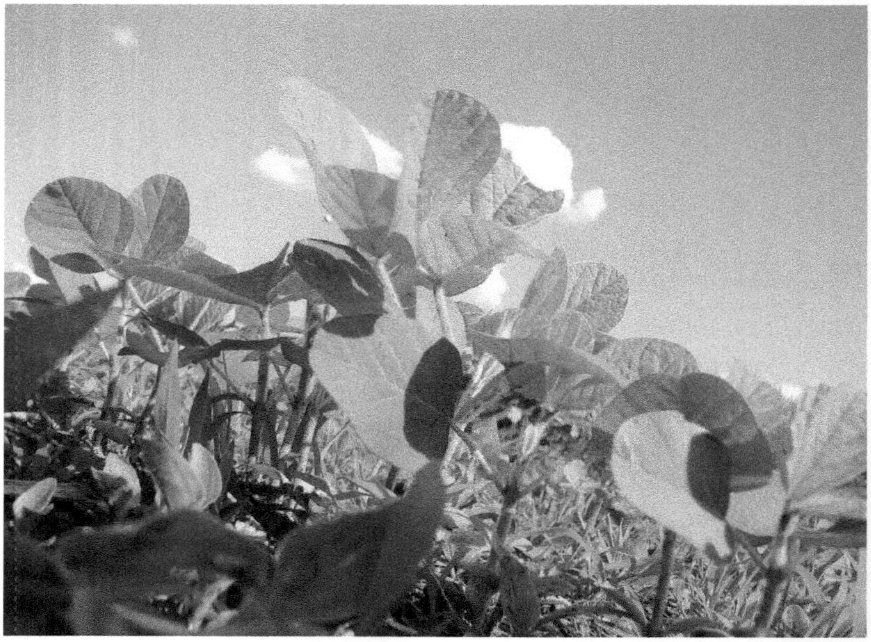

FIGURE 14.11a Soy plant.

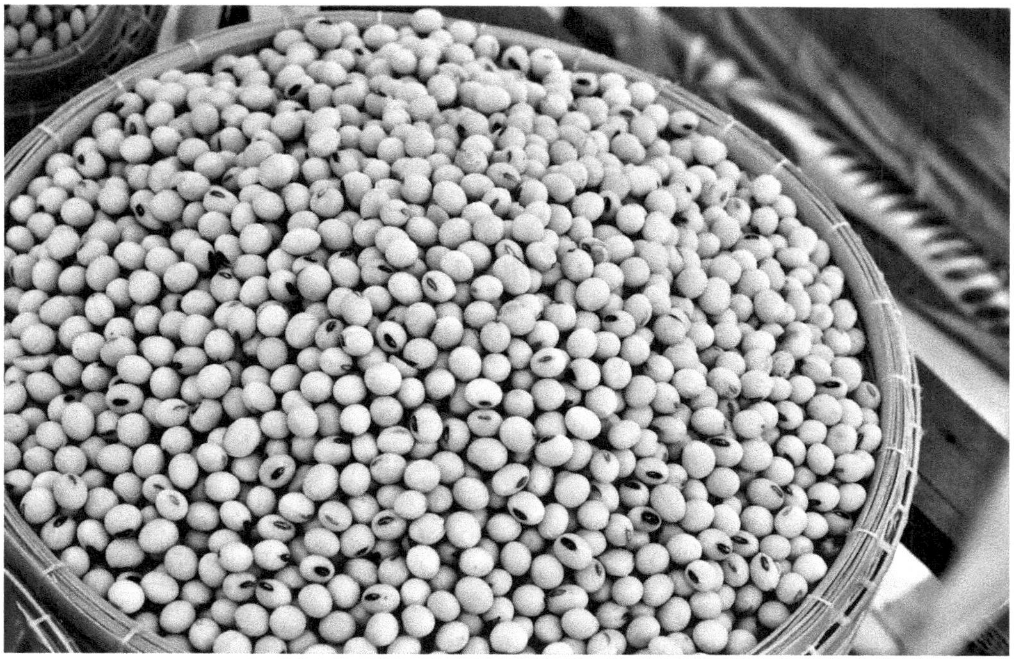

FIGURE 14.11b Soy seeds.

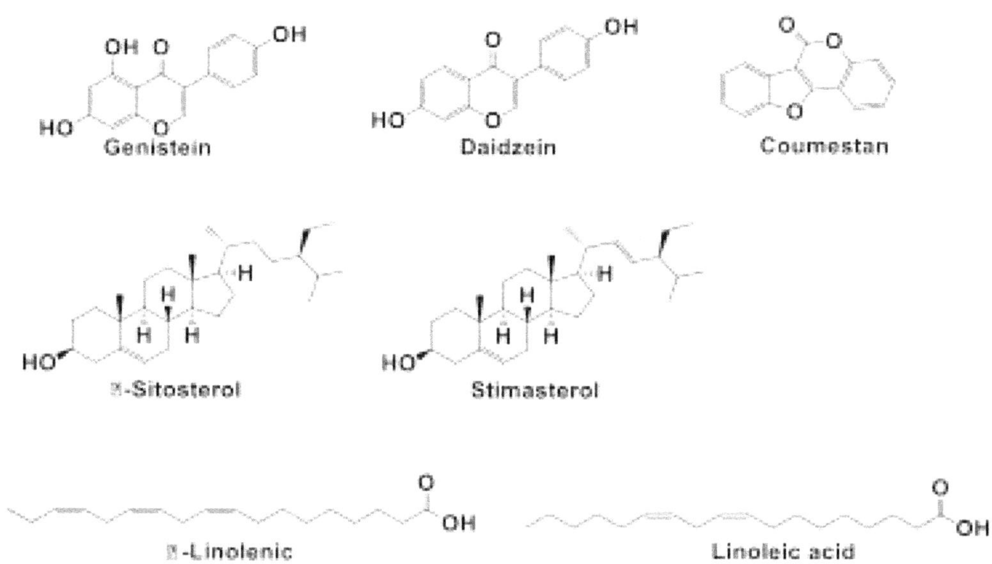

FIGURE 14.11c Chemical structures of phytochemicals.

with placebo.[165] A recent meta-analysis combining direct and indirect estimates demonstrated that soy isoflavone vaginal gel was effective in treating atrophic vaginitis (vaginal dryness).[166] However, another recent systematic review and meta-analysis cast doubt on its effectiveness on dyspareunia (painful sexual intercourse) and other sexual disorders.[167]

There are concerns that soy may be harmful to breast cancer patients based on a rodent research.[168] However, subsequent analysis of 9,514 breast cancer survivors who were followed for over seven years found no such correlation, and that higher post-diagnosis soy intake even led to a significant 25 percent reduction in tumor recurrence.[168]

Trifolium Pretense (Red clover)

Trifolium pretense (red clover) is a perennial flowering plant in the Fabaceae family (see Figure 14.12a). It is native to Europe, west Asia, and northwest Africa. *T. pretense* has been used in traditional medicine for skin diseases, cancer prevention, and cough. The identification of isoflavones and other phytoestrogens in red clover extract have made this plant useful as an alternative therapy for estrogen replacement to treat menopausal symptoms.[169] The most common phytoestrogens are genistein, daidzein, glycitein, formononetin, biochanin, coumestrol, and apigenin (see Figure 14.12b).

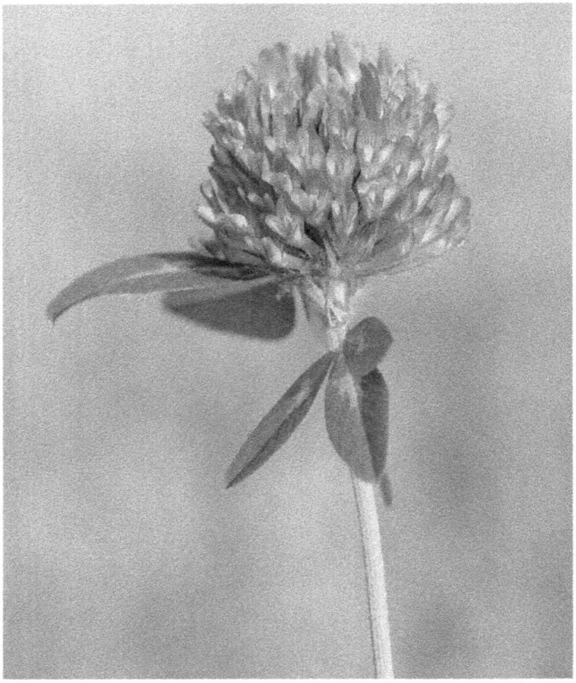

FIGURE 14.12a Red clover plant.

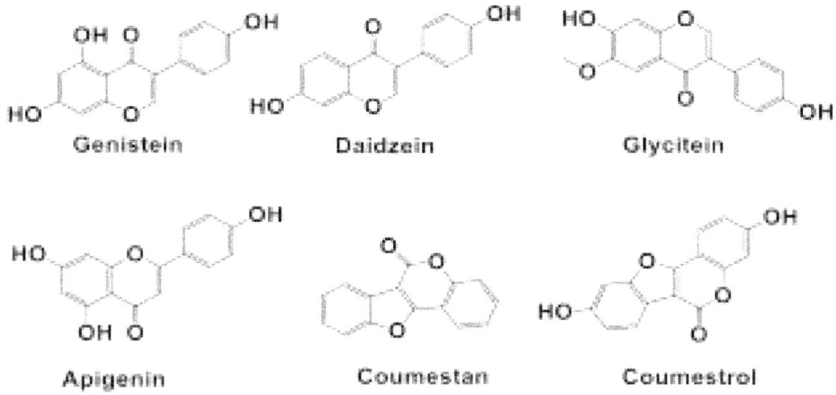

FIGURE 14.12b Chemical structures of phytochemicals.

A 12-week study in 2005 that investigated the effectiveness and safety of red clover isoflavone dietary supplementation on the frequency of hot flashes in menopausal women reported that consumption of the botanical is safe and resulted in a significant reduction of the complication in the treated group.[170] A 2015 meta-analysis also concluded that red clover had a positive effect on alleviating hot flashes in menopausal women by a slight change in follicle-stimulating hormone (FSH), LH, testosterone, and sex hormone binding globulin (SHBG) and significant effect on estrogen concentration.[171] Other studies, however, found the effects of red clover isoflavone to be similar to placebo. For example, a randomized, triple-blind, placebo-controlled clinical trial with 72 menopausal women taking 45 mg of red clover isoflavones or placebo for eight weeks resulted in no significant outcome differences, although both the red clover supplementation and the placebo resulted in a desirable effect on menopausal women's quality of life.[172]

Vitex Agnus- Castus (Chasteberry)

Vitex Agnus- Castus (chasteberry), also known as monk's pepper, is the fruit of the chaste tree (see Figure 14.13a), which is native to central Asia, eastern Europe, and the Mediterranean region. It belongs to the *Vitex* genus in the Verbenaceae plant family.[173] *V. agnus* is reported to have positive effects on female's reproductive system conditions, such as premenstrual syndrome, menstrual and menopausal symptoms, and infertility.[174] *V. agnus* exerts a hormone-balancing effect through stimulating the pituitary gland release of LH, which helps to normalize the ratio of progesterone-to-estrogen levels in the body.[174]

V. agnus contains glycosides, flavonoids, terpenes, and alkaloids, with agnuside as the main active ingredient (see Figure 14.13b).[174] One study reported that the daily intake of

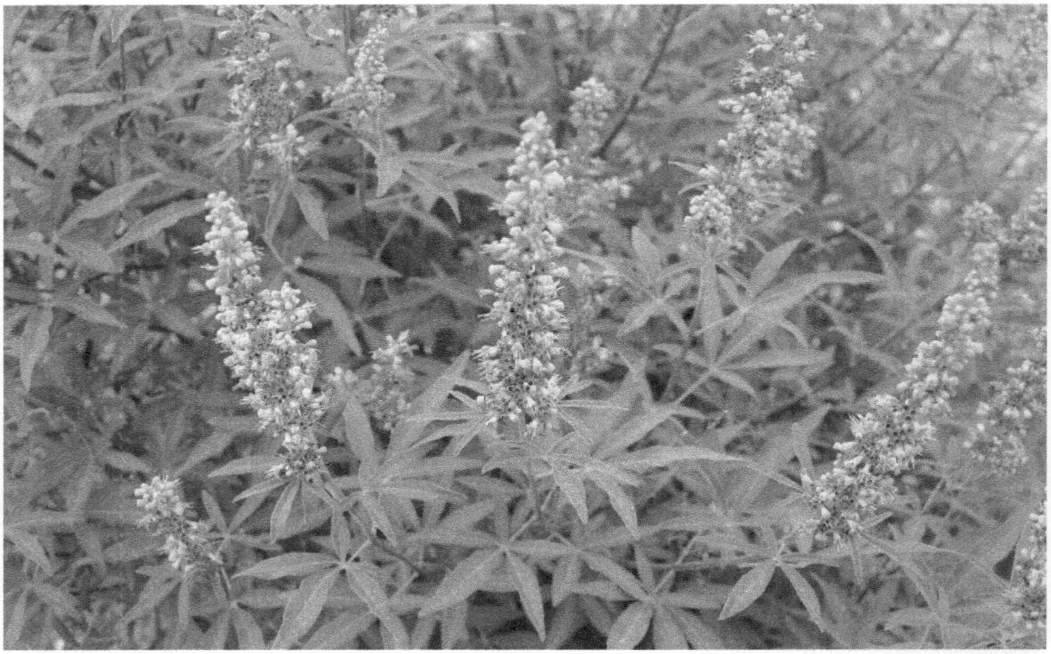

FIGURE 14.13a Chasteberry plant.

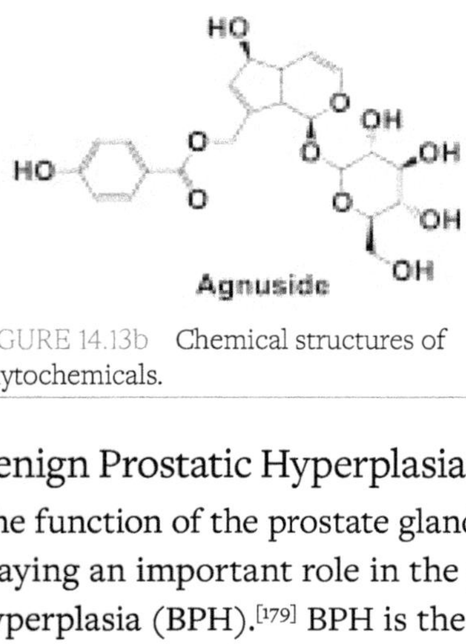

FIGURE 14.13b Chemical structures of phytochemicals.

V. agnus for three menstrual cycles led to reduction in the intensity of premenstrual symptoms, such as bloating, irritability, headache, and skin problems.[175] Meta-analysis of four randomized clinical trials concluded that *V. agnus* reduced premenstrual symptoms compared to placebo.[176] Other studies also suggest that *V. agnus* may improve menopausal symptoms.[177]

Benign Prostatic Hyperplasia and Medicinal Plants

The function of the prostate gland is androgen dependent,[178] with levels of testosterone playing an important role in the pathogenesis of prostate cancer and benign prostatic hyperplasia (BPH).[179] BPH is the most common genital problem in males and becomes prevalent with aging.[180] Estrogen is suggested to act in synergy with testosterone in the development of BPH.[181] Elevated levels of dihydrotestosterone (DHT), which is converted from testosterone by the enzyme 5-α-reductase type 2, is associated with an increased risk of developing BPH with lower urinary symptoms (LUTS).[182][183] Medical treatment for

LUTS/BPH involves the use of α-blockers (e.g., tamsulosin) and 5-α-reductase inhibitors (e.g., finasteride and dutasteride) to manage the condition in the long term, with surgery recommended for patients with moderate-to-severe LUTS/BPH or those with BPH-related complications.[184] Phytochemicals are increasingly becoming popular in the treatment of BPH and associated LUTS and have been used as first-line treatment for mild to moderate symptoms of these conditions.[185][186]

On the basis of preclinical studies, several mechanisms of action have been postulated for these phytochemicals, including α-reductase inhibition, α-adrenergic antagonism, and dihydrotestosterone and estrogen receptor inhibition.[187] The therapeutic properties of the most widely used plants, *Serenoa repens* and *Urtica dioica*, in improving uncontrolled growth of the prostate gland and/or urinary tract symptoms associated with BPH will be discussed.[188]

Serenoa Repensis (Saw Palmetto)

Serenoa repens (saw palmetto) is a small palm tree (see Figure 14.14a) native to the eastern region of North America.[189] The ripe berries of the plant have been the most popular source of phytochemicals used in the treatment of BPH/LUTS.[181] A report in 2011 suggested that

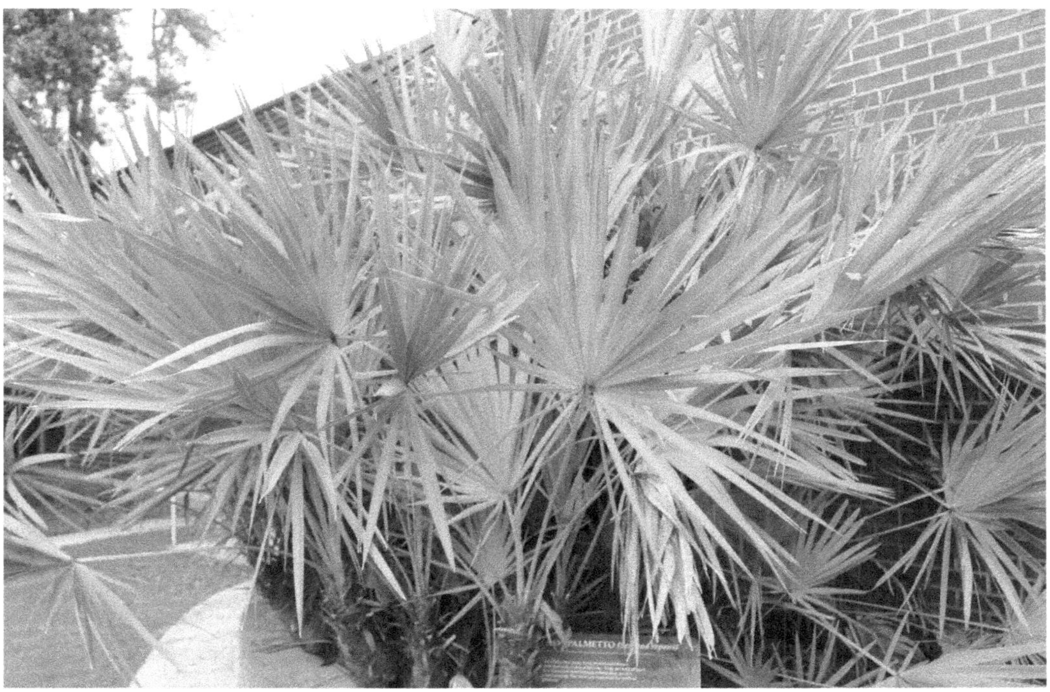

FIGURE 14.14a Saw palmetto plant.

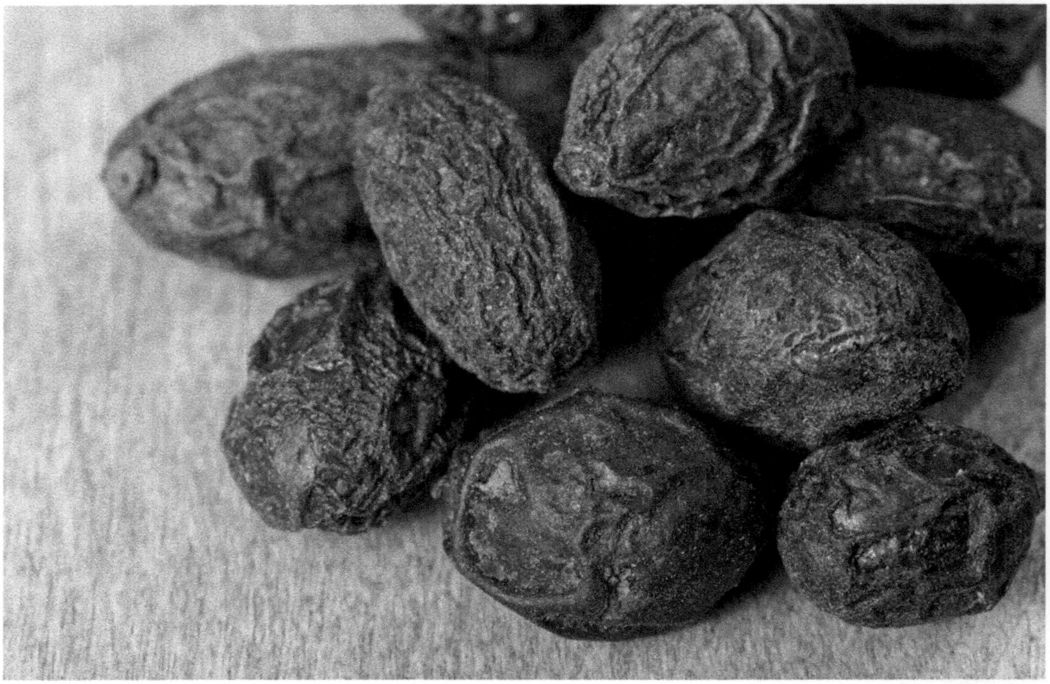

FIGURE 14.14b Saw palmetto dried seed.

more than 100 products containing *Serenoa repens* extracts were available on the market worldwide, some registered as drugs and others as food supplements.[190]

The pharmacological properties of *S. repens* extract include antiandrogenic, anti-inflammatory, and antiproliferative effects that inhibit the development and progression of LUTS/BPH.[189][191] Extracts of *S. repens* have been shown to inhibit 5α-reductase activity, the enzyme that converts testosterone to dihydrotestosterone (see Figure 14.14c),[192] in coculture epithelial and fibroblast cell models for BPH.[193] The free fatty acids (lauric acid, oleic acid, myristic acid, palmitic acid, and linoleic acid) (see Figure 14.14d) have been proposed as responsible for the inhibition of 5α-reductase. Phytosterols (e.g., β-sitosterol, campesterol, and stigmasterol) (see Figure 14.14d) have also been proposed to exhibit antiandrogenic activity.[189]

In a mouse model of BPH, Bernichtein et al. demonstrated that *S. repens* extract downregulated the prostate proinflammatory cytokine profile and significantly reduced CCR7, CXCL6, IL-6, and IL-17 expression.[194] *S. repens* extract has also been shown to be more effective than tamsulosin in the reduction of inflammation biomarkers in LUTS/BPH.[195]

A 1998 study by Wilt et al. involving 2,939 patients administered different extracts of *S. repens* reported improved urologic symptoms, similar to finasteride but with fewer side effects.[196] A meta-analysis of 14 randomized placebo control trials and three open-label

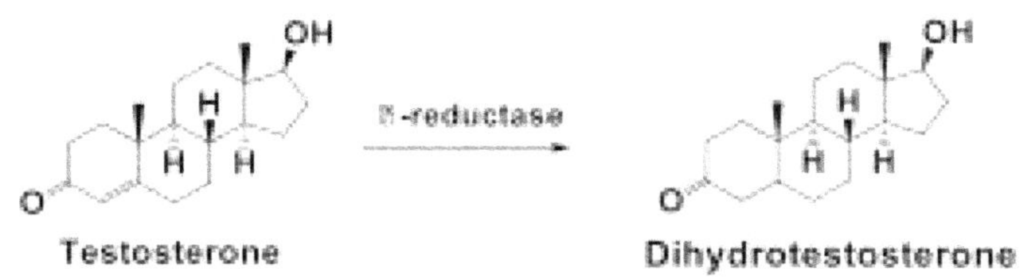

FIGURE 14.14c Biosynthesis of dihydrotestosterone from testosterone by 5-α-reductase.

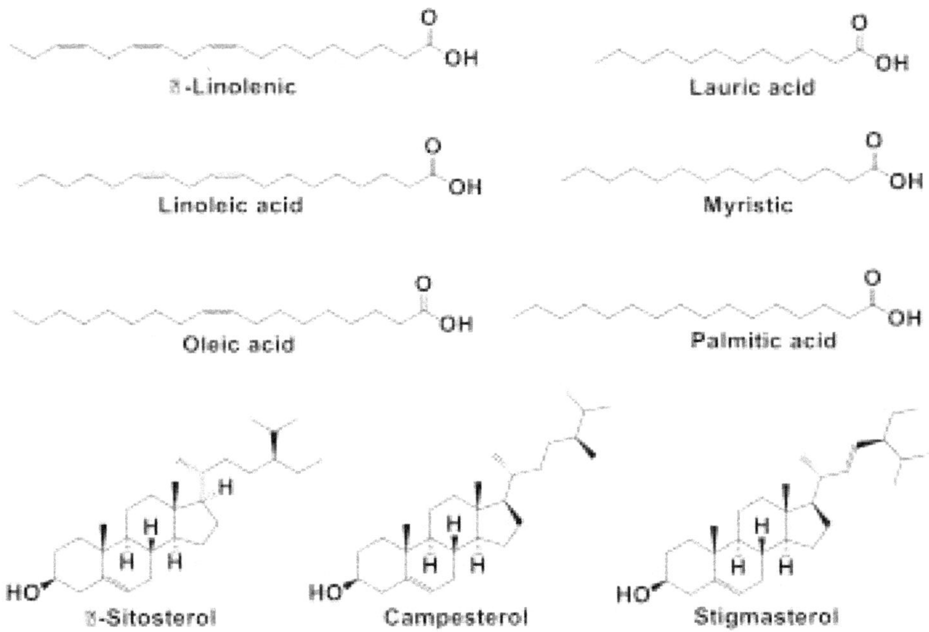

FIGURE 14.14d Chemical structures of phytochemicals.

trials with 4,280 patients also suggested that *S. repens* significantly improved several symptoms of BPH.[197] However, a more recent randomized, double-blind study that assessed the effects of *S. repens* extract in men with BPH over one year found no improvement in the symptoms of enlarged prostate.[198] Also, a 2012 report, published in the Cochrane database, of the systematic review of 32 randomized control trials involving 5,666 men found *S. repens* to be ineffective in treating LUTS in BPH.[199] A more recent review article by Ooi & Pak on the efficacy of *S. repens* on LUTS/BPH as a monotherapy, as well as in combination therapies, indicated mixed results.[191]

Several clinical trials with *S. repens* as a combination therapy have also been reported. Russo et al. showed that a combination of *S. repens* with Selenium and lycopene (SeR-Se-Ly) has greater efficacy than *S. repens* alone in the management of LUTS.[200] Ryu et al. showed that *S. repens*, when given with tamsulosin for one year, was more effective than tamsulosin monotherapy in reducing symptoms in BPH patients.[201] However, a previous but similar study showed that the combined therapy did not provide extra benefits when compared to corresponding monotherapies.[202] A study by Suardi et al., using a combination of *S. repens*, quercetin, and β-sitosterol versus control treatment for three months also showed no statistically significant improvement.[203] The extracts of *S. repens* and *Urtica dioica* (nettle root) (PRO 160/120) have also been studied in a randomized, multicenter, double-blind clinical trial involving 543 patients with the early stages of BPH.[204] The study showed that the efficacy of both PRO 160/120 and finasteride was equivalent and unrelated to prostate volume; however, PRO 160/120 had better tolerability than finasteride.

Urtica Dioica (Nettle)

Urtica dioica, commonly referred to as nettle or stinging nettle, is a plant belonging to the Urticaceae family (see Figure 14.15a). It is widely distributed across the globe in regions where the climate is humid and temperate.[205] *U. dioica* is used as a preservative and consumed by both humans and animals,[205] but the most recognized health benefits of nettles are treatment of BPH and urinary tract infections.[206]

Several diverse mechanisms of action through which *U. dioica* interferes with BPH pathogenesis have been proposed. The root extract of *U. dioica* and steroidal components stigmast-4-en-3-one, stigmasterol, and campesterol (see Figure 14.15b) have been reported to inhibit membrane Na(+)/K(+)-ATPase activity of the prostate that is expected to suppress prostate cell metabolism and growth.[207] The phytochemicals scopoletin and β-sitosterol (see Figure 14.15b) have also been proposed to inhibit 5-α-reductase activity; this is the enzyme responsible for the conversion of testosterone to dihydrotestosterone (see Figure 14.14c).[187][208] Lignans, also a component of *U. dioica* root extract, have been proposed to inhibit the binding of androgens to sex hormone–binding globulin that is involved in the pathogenesis of BPH.[209] Extract of *U. dioica* has also been reported to inhibit aromatase, a key enzyme in the biosynthesis of testosterone into estrogen in prostate tissue (see Figure 14.15c), which is also associated with prostate disease.[210][211] In BPH therapy, *U. dioica* is usually used in combination with saw palmetto (*S. repens*).[204][212]

In a randomized, controlled, double-blind study, Safarinejad reported that *U. dioica* root aqueous extract (120 mg three times/day) resulted in significant improvement in LUTS, prostate symptom score, and maximal urinary flow rate, and in moderate reduction of the

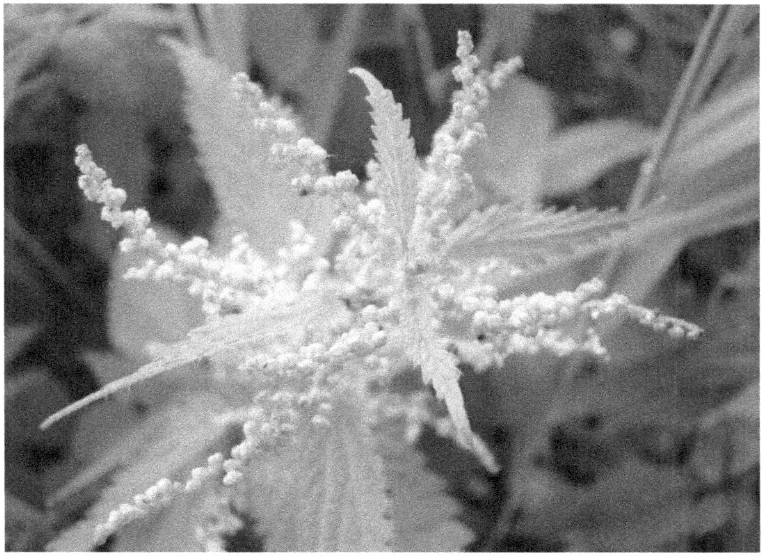

FIGURE 14.15a Nettle plant.

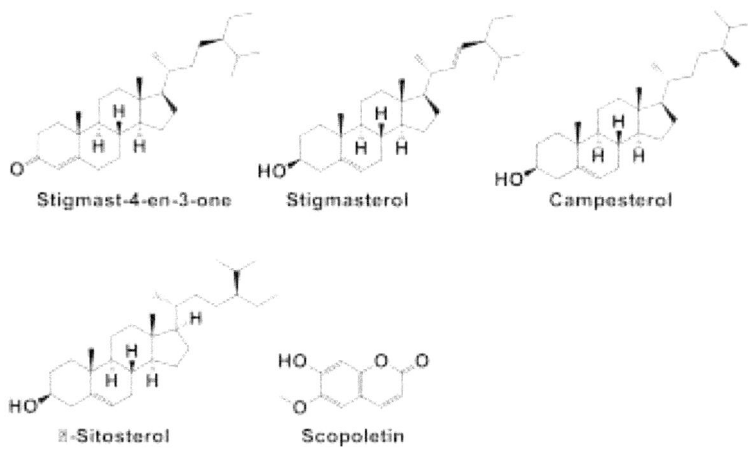

FIGURE 14.15b Chemical structures of phytochemicals.

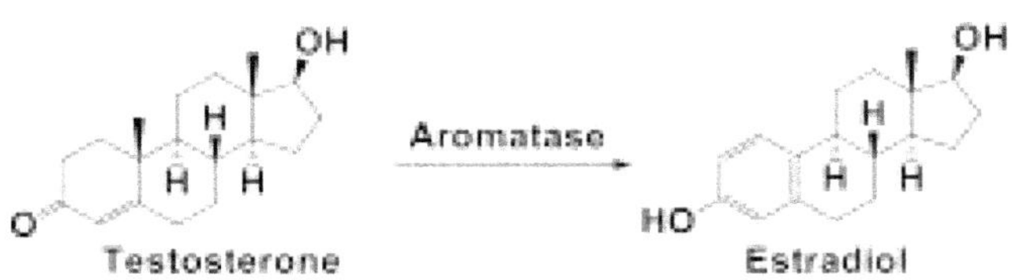

FIGURE 14.15c Biosynthesis of estrogen from testosterone by aromatase.

prostate size after six months of treatment.[213] Another study carried out by Schneider and Rübben with a higher dose of *U. dioica* (459 mg) did not confirm the previous finding.[214]

U. dioica extract is reported to be generally well tolerated[213] but is known to cause occasional diarrhea and respiratory system diseases of moderate intensity, but the effects do not differ significantly from those observed in placebo control groups.[215]

Conclusion

It is clear that plant extracts and phytochemicals can impact the regulation of several endocrine-related diseases. Indeed, there is a significant body of data in the literature covering both preclinical and clinical studies that have evaluated the efficacies of plant extracts and phytochemicals in treating various endocrine disorders. Nonetheless, the results are mixed and sometimes controversial. The mechanisms of action of some of the phytochemicals are yet to be established, and there are questions about those that have even been reported. Uncertain study outcomes or mixed results with medicinal plants can be attributed to several factors:

1. Oftentimes the outcomes from these botanicals are not different from placebo, although patients report positive effects.[216] Patients' expectations can potentially exert a greater impact on the clinical outcomes than a drug's pharmacologic activity. This "placebo effect" has even been suggested to explain the increased use of botanical dietary supplements.[216]
2. Flawed clinical findings, as they involve only short-term follow up, small sample size, absence of a placebo arm, technical or methodological problems, or poorly controlled study designs.
3. Variability in extraction procedures and/or herbal formulation, as well as natural variability in plants with significant impact on the phytochemical profile of the plant material. The quality of the botanical dietary supplements also sometimes complicate current efforts to study the clinical efficacies of botanical supplements.[217][218]
4. Incorrect authentication or misidentifications of plant source or plant material.[219][220]
5. False-positive results by some phytochemicals because of nonspecific enzyme or protein interactions, formation of aggregates that may bind to protein targets, membrane disruption, cytotoxicity in cell-based assays, precipitation of an analyte, and interference with detection methods.[221][222]
6. Active compounds are not clearly identified. Often, a single compound is not solely responsible for the activity of the extract, but rather, several phytochemicals lead to the observed overall activity through interactive processes, for example, having additive, synergistic, or antagonistic effects.[223]

7. Numerous mechanisms of action have been proposed for the plant extract and phytochemicals; however, the in vitro studies to determine the mechanisms of action of these agents often use mega physiologic doses, questioning the significance of the results.[186][224]

Clearly, more studies, including both in vitro and in vivo, are warranted to validate the phytochemicals' mechanism of action, efficacy, and safety, and large, well-designed, randomized, double-blind, placebo-controlled clinical studies also need to be carried out before their use can be recommended for treatment and/or prevention of diseases.

References

1. Carolyn C. Johnstone et al., "Endocrine System: Part 1," *Nursing Standard*, 28, no. 38 (2014): 42–49.
2. Charles Hendry et al., "Endocrine System: Part 2," *Nursing Standard*, 28, no. 39 (2014): 43–48.
3. J. G. Betts et al., "Hormones," in *Anatomy and Physiology* (Houston: Openstax, 2013).
4. Rosa Lauretta et al., "Endocrine Disrupting Chemicals: Effects on Endocrine Glands," *Frontiers in Endocrinology* (*Lausanne*) 10 (2019): 178.
5. Ana Paula Santos-Silva et al., "Frontiers in Endocrine Disruption: Impacts of Organotin on the Hypothalamus-Pituitary-Thyroid Axis," *Molecular and Cellular Endocrinology* 460 (2018): 246–57.
6. Lindsay Brown, "Editorial [Hot Topic: Targets of Research in the Metabolic Syndrome (Guest Editor: Lindsay Brown)]," *Endocrine, Metabolic and Immune Disorders—Drug Targets* 11, no. 3 (2011): 181.
7. Tânia R. Dias et al., "Emerging Potential of Natural Products as an Alternative Strategy to Pharmacological Agents Used Against Metabolic Disorders," *Current Drug Metabolism* 17, no. 6 (2016): 582–97.
8. Johan H. Koeslag et al., "A Reappraisal of the Blood Glucose Homeostat Which Comprehensively Explains the Type 2 Diabetes Mellitus-Syndrome X Complex," *The Journal of Physiology* 549, Pt. 2 (2003): 333–46.
9. Disease Control Center, *National Diabetes Statistics Report, 2017 Estimates of Diabetes and Its Burden in the United States Background* (Washington, DC: CDC, 2017).
10. Juan J. Chillarón et al., "Type 1 Diabetes, Metabolic Syndrome and Cardiovascular Risk," *Metabolism* 63, no. 2 (2014): 181–87.
11. Ralph A. DeFronzo, "Pathogenesis of Type 2 Diabetes Mellitus," *Medical Clinics of North America* 88, no. 4 (2004): 787–835.

12. Vladimir Igoravich Timofeev et al., "X-Ray Investigation of Gene-Engineered Human Insulin Crystallized from a Solution Containing Polysialic Acid," *Acta Crystallographica Section F Structural Biology and Crystallization Communications* 66, Pt. 3 (2010): 259–63.
13. John G. Menting et al., "Protective Hinge in Insulin Opens to Enable Its Receptor Engagement," *Proceedings of the National Academy of Sciences* 111, no. 33 (2014): E3395–404.
14. Pia V. Röder et al., "Pancreatic Regulation of Glucose Homeostasis," *Experimental and Molecular Medicine* 48, no. 3 (2016): e219.
15. Haonan Zhang et al., "Structure of the Glucagon Receptor in Complex with a Glucagon Analogue," *Nature* 553, no. 7686 (2018): 106–10.
16. Abha Saxena and Naval Vikram, "Role of Selected Indian Plants in Management of Type 2 Diabetes: A Review," *The Journal of Alternative and Complementary Medicine* 10, no. 2 (2004): 369–78.
17. D. K. Patel et al., "An Overview on Antidiabetic Medicinal Plants Having Insulin Mimetic Property," *Asian Pacific Journal of Tropical Biomedicine* 2, no. 4 (2012): 320–30.
18. Sudanshu Kumar Bharti et al., "Antidiabetic Phytoconstituents and Their Mode of Action on Metabolic Pathways," *Therapeutic Advances in Endocrinology and Metabolism* 9, no. 3 (2018): 81–100.
19. Neelesh Malviya et al., "Antidiabetic Potential of Medicinal Plants," *Acta Poloniae Pharmaceutica* 67, no. 2 (2010): 113–18.
20. Shanti Bhushran Mishra et al., "An Analytical Review of Plants For Anti Diabetic Activity With Their Phytoconstituent and Mechanism of Action," *International Journal of Pharmaceutical Sciences and Research* 1, no. 1 (2017): 29–46.
21. Mohamed Bnouham et al., "Medicinal Plants with Potential Antidiabetic Activity-A Review of Ten Years of Herbal Medicine Research (1990–2000)," *International Journal of Diabetes and Metabolism* 14, no. 1 (200): 1–25.
22. Jie-Qing Liu et al., "New Cucurbitane Triterpenoids and Steroidal Glycoside from Momordica Charantia," *Molecules* 14, no. 12 (2009): 4804–13.
23. Ajda Ota and Nataša P. Ulrih, "An Overview of Herbal Products and Secondary Metabolites Used for Management of Type Two Diabetes," *Frontiers in Pharmacology* 8 (2017): 436.
24. Dallas L. Clouatre, Sadanand N. Rao, and Harry G. Preuss, "Bitter Melon Extracts in Diabetic and Normal Rats Favorably Influence Blood Glucose and Blood Pressure Regulation," *Journal of Medicinal Food* 14, no. 12 (2011): 1496–504.
25. Ajay Kumar Shetty, Suresh Kumar Gurusiddaiah, and Veeresh Salimath, "Bitter Gourd (Momordica Charantia) Modulates Activities of Intestinal and Renal Disaccharidases in Streptozotocin-Induced Diabetic Rats," *Molecular Nutrition and Food Research* 49, no. 8 (2005): 791–96.
26. J. K. Grover, Satyapal Singh Yadav, "Pharmacological Actions and Potential Uses of Momordica Charantia: A Review," *Journal of Ethnopharmacology* 93, no. 1 (2004): 123–32.

27. R. V. Yin et al., "The Effect of Bitter Melon (Mormordica Charantia) in Patients with Diabetes Mellitus: A Systematic Review and Meta-Analysis," *Nutrition and Diabetes* 4, no. 12 (2014): e145.
28. Hasan, I.; Khatoon, S. "Effect of Momordica Charantia (Bitter Gourd) Tablets in Diabetes Mellitus: Type 1 and Type 2," *Prime Research on Medicine* 2, no. 2 (2012): 72–74.
29. Leslie Taylor, "Bitter Melon (Momordica Charantia)," in *Herbal Secrets of the Rainforest: Over 50 Powerful Herbs and Their Medicinal Uses* (Austin, TX: Sage Press, 2002).
30. F. E. Wehash, I. I. Abpo-Ghanema, and Rasha M. Saleh, "Some Physiological Effects of Momordica Charantia and Trigonella Foenum-Graecum Extracts in Diabetic Rats as Compared with Cidophage®," *World Academy of Science, Engineering, and Technology International Journal of Animal and Veterinary Sciences* 64, no. 1 (2012): 1206–14.
31. Anjana Fuangchan et al., "Hypoglycemic Effect of Bitter Melon Compared with Metformin in Newly Diagnosed Type 2 Diabetes Patients," *Journal of Ethnopharmacology* 134, no. 2 (2011): 422–28.
32. Naseh Pahlavani et al., "Possible Molecular Mechanisms of Glucose-lowering Activities of *Momordica Charantia* (Karela) in Diabetes," *Journal of Cellular Biochemistry* 120, no. 7 (2019): 10921–29.
33. Miao Tian et al., "Molecular Diversity and Hypoglycemic Polypeptide-P Content of *Momordica Charantia* in Different Accessions and Different Seasons," *Journal of the Science of Food and Agriculture* 95, no. 6 (2015): 1328–35.
34. Min-Jia Tan et al., "Antidiabetic Activities of Triterpenoids Isolated from Bitter Melon Associated with Activation of the AMPK Pathway," *Cell Chemical Biology* 15, no. 3 (2008): 263–73.
35. Haixia Zhang et al., "Analysis of Vicine in Bitter Melon with High Performance Liquid Chromatography," *Analytical Letters* 36, no. 8 (2003): 1597–605.
36. Kyong Kim and Hye Young Kim, "Bitter Melon (Momordica Charantia) Extract Suppresses Cytokineinduced Activation of MAPK and NF-κB in Pancreatic β-Cells," *Food Science and Biotechnology* 20, no. 2 (2011): 531–35.
37. Vidya Gadang et al., "Dietary Bitter Melon Seed Increases Peroxisome Proliferator-Activated Receptor-γ Gene Expression in Adipose Tissue, Down-Regulates the Nuclear Factor-KB Expression, and Alleviates the Symptoms Associated with Metabolic Syndrome," *Journal of Medicinal Food* 14, no. 1–2, (2011): 86–93.
38. Hui-Ling Huang et al., "Bitter Melon (*Momordica Charantia L.*) Inhibits Adipocyte Hypertrophy and down Regulates Lipogenic Gene Expression in Adipose Tissue of Diet-Induced Obese Rats," *British Journal of Nutrition* 99, no. 2 (2008): 230–39.
39. Chun-Ching Shih, Cheng-Hsiu Lin, and Wei-Li Lin, "Effects of Momordica Charantia on Insulin Resistance and Visceral Obesity in Mice on High-Fat Diet," *Diabetes Research and Clinical Practice* 81, no. 2 (2008): 134–43.
40. J. Jeong et al., "Effect of Bitter Melon (Momordica Charantia) on Anti-Diabetic Activity in C57BLI/6J Db/Db Mice," *Korean Journal of Veterinary Research* 48, no. 3 (2008): 327–36.

41. B. A. Shibib, L. A. Khan, R. Rahman, "Hypoglycaemic Activity of *Coccinia Indica* and *Momordica Charantia* in Diabetic Rats: Depression of the Hepatic Gluconeogenic Enzymes Glucose-6-Phosphatase and Fructose-1,6-Bisphosphatase and Elevation of Both Liver and Red-Cell Shunt Enzyme Glucose-6-Phosphate Dehydrogenase," *Biochemical Journal* 292, no. 1 (1993): 267–70.
42. Chung-Huang Tsai et al., "Wild Bitter Gourd Improves Metabolic Syndrome: A Preliminary Dietary Supplementation Trial," *Nutrition Journal* 11, no. 1 (2012): 4.
43. Sutthaya Poolperm and Wannee Jiraungkoorskul, "An Update Review on the Anthelmintic Activity of Bitter Gourd, Momordica Charantia," *Pharmacognosy Reviews* 11, no. 21 (2017): 31–34.
44. Po-Yuan Chen et al., "Inhibitory Effects of Momordicine I on High-Glucose-Induced Cell Proliferation and Collagen Synthesis in Rat Cardiac Fibroblasts," *Oxidative Medicine and Cellular Longevity* 2018 (2018): 1–11.
45. Liva Harinantenaina et al., "Momordica Charantia Constituents and Antidiabetic Screening of the Isolated Major Compounds," *Chemical and Pharmaceutical Bulletin (Tokyo)* 54, no. 7 (2006): 1017–21.
46. Amy C. Keller et al., "Saponins from the Traditional Medicinal Plant Momordica Charantia Stimulate Insulin Secretion in Vitro," *Phytomedicine: International Journal of Phytotherapy and Phytopharmacology* 19, no. 1 (2011): 32–37.
47. Ethan Basch, Steven Gabardi, and Catherine Ulbricht, "Bitter Melon (Momordica Charantia): A Review of Efficacy and Safety," *American Journal of Health-System Pharmacy* 60, no. 4 (2003): 356–59.
48. Martha A. Belury et al., "Linoleic Acid, Glycemic Control and Type 2 Diabetes," *Prostaglandins, Leukotrienes, and Essential Fatty Acids* 132 (2018): 30–33.
49. Jason H. Y. Wu et al., "Omega-6 Fatty Acid Biomarkers and Incident Type 2 Diabetes: Pooled Analysis of Individual-Level Data for 39 740 Adults from 20 Prospective Cohort Studies," *The Lancet Diabetes and Endocrinoogy* 5, no. 12 (2017): 965–74.
50. Ulf Risérus, Walter C. Willett, and Frank B. Hu, "Dietary Fats and Prevention of Type 2 Diabetes," *Progress in Lipid Research* 48, no. 1 (2009): 44–51.
51. Emanuel L. Peter et al., "Safety and Efficacy of Momordica Charantia Linnaeus in Pre-Diabetes and Type 2 Diabetes Mellitus Patients: A Systematic Review and Meta-Analysis Protocol," *Systematic Reviews* 7, no. 1 (2018): 192.
52. Baby Joseph and D. Jini, "Antidiabetic Effects of Momordica Charantia (Bitter Melon) and Its Medicinal Potency," *Asian Pacific Journal of Tropical Disease* 3, no. 2 (2013): 93–102.
53. Jaipaul Singh et al., "Medicinal Chemistry of the Anti-Diabetic Effects of Momordica Charantia: Active Constituents and Modes of Actions," *The Open Medicinal Chemistry Journal* 5, no. S2 (2011): 70–77.
54. Pushpa Khanna et al., "Hypoglycemic Activity of Polypeptide-p From a Plant Source," *Journal of Natural Products* 44, no. 6 (1981): 648–55.

55. V. S. Baldwa et al., "Clinical Trial in Patients with Diabetes Mellitus of an Insulin-like Compound Obtained from Plant Source," *Upsala Journal of Medical Sciences* 82, no. 1 (1977): 39–41.
56. Ananya Paul and Sen Sarmistha Raychaudhuri, "Medicinal Uses and Molecular Identification of Two Momordica Charantia Varieties-a Review," *Electronic Journal of Biology* 6, no. 2 (2010): 43–51.
57. Bi-lian Wang et al., "Gene Cloning and Expression of a Novel Hypoglycaemic Peptide from Momordica Charantia," *Journal of the Science of Food and Agriculture* 91, no. 13 (2011): 2443–48.
58. Emanuel L. Peter et al., "Momordica charantia L. Lowers Elevated Glycaemia in Type 2 Diabetes Mellitus Patients: Systematic Review and Meta-Analysis," *Journal of Ethnopharmacology* 231 (2019): 311–24.
59. Antonio M. L. Dans et al., "The Effect of Momordica Charantia Capsule Preparation on Glycemic Control in Type 2 Diabetes Mellitus Needs Further Studies," *Journal of Clinical Epidemiology* 60, no. 6 (2007): 554–59.
60. Abishek Tongia, Sudhir Kumar Tongia, and Mangala Dave, "Phytochemical Determination and Extraction of Momordica Charantia Fruit and Its Hypoglycemic Potentiation of Oral Hypoglycemic Drugs in Diabetes Mellitus (NIDDM)," *Indian Journal of Physiology and Pharmacology* 48, no. 2 (2004): 241–44.
61. Akintunde O. Akinkuolie et al., "Omega-3 Polyunsaturated Fatty Acid and Insulin Sensitivity: A Meta-Analysis of Randomized Controlled Trials," *Clinical Nutrition* 30, no. 6 (2011): 702–07.
62. Elena Jovanovski et al., "The Effect of Alpha-Linolenic Acid on Glycemic Control in Individuals with Type 2 Diabetes," *Medicine (Baltimore)* 96, no. 21 (2017): e6531.
63. Shuo Jia et al., "Recent Advances in Momordica Charantia: Functional Components and Biological Activities," *International Journal of Molecular Sciences* 18, no. 12 (2017): 2555.
64. Deepak Mudgil, Shewata Barak, and Bhupendar Khatkar, "Guar Gum: Processing, Properties and Food Applications-A Review," *Journal of Food Science and Technology* 51, no. 3 (2014): 409–18.
65. José-Luis Ríos et al., "Modulation of Diabetes by Natural Products and Medicinal Plants via Incretins," *Planta Medica* 85, no. 11–12 (2019): 825–39.
66. Hayat M. Mukhtar et al., "Effect of Aqueous Extract of Cyamopsis Tetragonoloba Linn. Beans on Blood Glucose Level in Normal and Alloxan-Induced Diabetic Rats," *Indian Journal of Experimental Biology* 42, no. 12 (2004): 1212–15.
67. Saeed Samarghandian et al., "Antihyperglycemic and Antihyperlipidemic Effects of Guar Gum on Streptozotocin-Induced Diabetes in Male Rats," *Pharmacognosy Magazine* 8, no. 29 (2012): 65.
68. Valesca Dall'Alba et al., "Improvement of the Metabolic Syndrome Profile by Soluble Fibre—Guar Gum—in Patients with Type 2 Diabetes: A Randomised Clinical Trial," *The British Journal of Nutrition* 110, no. 9 (2013): 1601–10.

69. Linda E. Watson et al., "A Whey/Guar 'Preload' Improves Postprandial Glycaemia and Glycated Haemoglobin Levels in Type 2 Diabetes: A 12-Week, Single-Blind, Randomized, Placebo-Controlled Trial," *Diabetes, Obesity and Metabolism* 21, no. 4 (2019): 930–38.
70. Andrea O. Y. Luk et al., "A Proof-of-Concept Study to Evaluate the Efficacy and Safety of BTI320 on Post-Prandial Hyperglycaemia in Chinese Subjects with Pre-Diabetes," *BMC Endocrine Disorders* 18, no. 1 (2018): 59.
71. Vinay Kumar Singh et al., "*Gymnema sylvestre* for Diabetics," *Journal of Herbs, Spices and Medicinal Plants* 14, no. 1–2 n(2008): 88–106.
72. Matthew J. Leach, "*Gymnema sylvestre* for Diabetes Mellitus: A Systematic Review," *Journal of Alternative and Complementary Medicine* 13, no. 9 (2007): 977–83.
73. V. A. Khramov, A. A. Spasov, and M. P. "Samokhina, Chemical Composition of Dry Extracts of Gymnema Sylvestre Leaves," *Pharmaceutical Chemistry Journal* 42, no. 1 (2008): 29–31.
74. Pragya Tiwari, B. N. Mishra, and Neelam S. Sangwan, "Phytochemical and Pharmacological Properties of Gymnema Sylvestre: An Important Medicinal Plant," *Biomed Research International* 2014, no. 1 (2014): 830285.
75. Yoshitaka Sugihara et al., "Antihyperglycemic Effects of Gymnemic Acid IV, a Compound Derived from *Gymnema Sylvestre* Leaves in Streptozotocin-Diabetic Mice," *Journal of Asian Natural Products Research* 2, no. 4 (2000): 321–27.
76. Ashutosh Kumar Verma et al., "Genetic and Chemical Profiling of Gymnema Sylvestre Accessions from Central India: Its Implication for Quality Control and Therapeutic Potential of Plant," *Pharmacognosy Magazine* 12, no. S4 (2016): 407–13.
77. Toshiaki Imoto et al., "A Novel Peptide Isolated from the Leaves of Gymnema Sylvestre—I. Characterization and Its Suppressive Effect on the Neural Responses to Sweet Taste Stimuli in the Rat," *Comparative Biochemistry and Physiology Part A: Physiology* 100, no. 2 (1991): 309–14.
78. Keisuke Sanematsu et al., "Molecular Mechanisms for Sweet-Suppressing Effect of Gymnemic Acids," *Journal of Biological Chemistry* 289, no. 37 (2014): 25711–20.
79. A. Al-Romaiyan et al., "A Novel Extract of *Gymnema Sylvestre* Improves Glucose Tolerance *In Vivo* and Stimulates Insulin Secretion and Synthesis *In Vitro*," *Phytotherapy Research* 27, no. 7 (2013): 1006–11.
80. Rashmi S. Shenoy, Harish Prashanth, and H. K. Manonmani, "*In Vitro* Antidiabetic Effects of Isolated Triterpene Glycoside Fraction from *Gymnema sylvestre*," *Evidence-Based Complementary and Alternative Medicine* 2018, no. 7 (2018): 1–12.
81. Rajadurai Akilen et al., "Cinnamon in Glycaemic Control: Systematic Review and Meta Analysis," *Clinical Nutrition* 31, no. 5 (2012): 609–15.
82. Bolin Qin, Kiran S. Panickar, and Richard A. Anderson, "Cinnamon: Potential Role in the Prevention of Insulin Resistance, Metabolic Syndrome, and Type 2 Diabetes," *Journal of Diabetes Science and Technology* 4, no. 3 (2010): 685–93.

83. Hua-Bin Li et al., "Antioxidant Properties in Vitro and Total Phenolic Contents in Methanol Extracts from Medicinal Plants," *LWT—Food Science and Technology* 41, no. 3 (2008): 385–90.
84. Zhoalian Lu et al., "Hypoglycemic Activities of A- and B-Type Procyanidin Oligomer-Rich Extracts from Different Cinnamon Barks," *Phytomedicine* 18, no. 4 (2011): 298–302.
85. Liang Chen et al., "Diverse Mechanisms of Antidiabetic Effects of the Different Procyanidin Oligomer Types of Two Different Cinnamon Species on *Db/Db* Mice," *Journal of Agricultural and Food Chemistry* 60, no. 36 (2012): 9144–50.
86. Diana M.Cheng et al., "In Vivo and in Vitro Antidiabetic Effects of Aqueous Cinnamon Extract and Cinnamon Polyphenol-Enhanced Food Matrix," *Food Chemistry* 135, no. 4 (2012): 2994–3002.
87. Prachi Anand et al., "Insulinotropic Effect of Cinnamaldehyde on Transcriptional Regulation of Pyruvate Kinase, Phosphoenolpyruvate Carboxykinase, and GLUT4 Translocation in Experimental Diabetic Rats," *Chemico-Biological Interactions* 186, no. 1 (2010): 72–81.
88. Ahmed A. Hosni et al., "Cinnamaldehyde Potentially Attenuates Gestational Hyperglycemia in Rats through Modulation of PPARγ, Proinflammatory Cytokines and Oxidative Stress," *Biomedicine and Pharmacotherapy* 88 (2017): 52–60.
89. Da-WeiHuang, Szu-Chuan Shen, and James Swi-Bea Wu, "Effects of Caffeic Acid and Cinnamic Acid on Glucose Uptake in Insulin-Resistant Mouse Hepatocytes," *Journal of Agricultural and Food Chemistry* 57, no. 17 (2009): 7687–92.
90. Wi Kim et al., "Naphthalenemethyl Ester Derivative of Dihydroxyhydrocinnamic Acid, a Component of Cinnamon, Increases Glucose Disposal by Enhancing Translocation of Glucose Transporter 4," *Diabetologia* 49, no. 10 (2006): 2437–48.
91. Paul A. Davis and Wallace Yokoyama, "Cinnamon Intake Lowers Fasting Blood Glucose: Meta-Analysis," *Journal of Medicinal Food* 14, no. 9 (2011): 884–89.
92. Kristof Vanschoonbeeket al., "Cinnamon Supplementation Does Not Improve Glycemic Control in Postmenopausal Type 2 Diabetes Patients," *Journal of Nutrition* 136, no. 4 (2006): 977–80.
93. Ginpreet Kaur et al., "A Nutraceutical Combination of Cinnamomum Cassia & Nigella Sativa for Type 1 Diabetes Mellitus," *Journal of Ayurveda and Integrative Medicine* 9, no. 1 (2018): 27–37.
94. Malgorzata Iciek, Inga Kwiecień, and Lidia Włodek, "Biological Properties of Garlic and Garlic-Derived Organosulfur Compounds," *Environmental and Molecular Mutagenesis* 50, no. 3 (2009): 247–65.
95. Hafiz Ansar Suleria et al., "Garlic (Allium Sativum): Diet Based Therapy of 21st Century–A Review," *Asian Pacific Journal of Tropical Disease* 5, no. 4 (2015): 271–78.
96. Martha Thomson et al., "Anti-Diabetic and Anti-Oxidant Potential of Aged Garlic Extract (AGE) in Streptozotocin-Induced Diabetic Rats," *BMC Complementary and Alternative Medicine* 16, no. 1 (2015): 17.
97. Layla Bayan, Peir Hossain Koulivand, and Ali Gorji, "Garlic: A Review of Potential Therapeutic Effects," *Avicenna Journal of Phytomedicine* 4, no. 1 (2014): 1–14.

98. Raju Padiya and Sanjay K. Banerjee, "Garlic as an Anti-Diabetic Agent: Recent Progress and Patent Reviews," *Recent Patents on Food, Nutrition and Agriculture* 5, no. 2 (2013): 105–27.
99. Juan Wang et al., "Effect of Garlic Supplement in the Management of Type 2 Diabetes Mellitus (T2DM): A Meta-Analysis of Randomized Controlled Trials," *Food and Nutrition Research* 61, no. 1 (2017): 1377571.
100. Ganapathy Saravanan et al., "Antidiabetic Properties of S-Allyl Cysteine, a Garlic Component on Streptozotocin-Induced Diabetes in Rats," *Journal of Applied Biomedicine* 7, no. 3 (2009): 151–59.
101. Baiqiang Zhai, et al., "Hypoglycemic and Hypolipidemic Effect of S-Allyl-Cysteine Sulfoxide (Alliin) in DIO Mice," *Scientific Reports* 8, no. 1 (2018): 3527.
102. Hana Drobiova et al., "Garlic Increases Antioxidant Levels in Diabetic and Hypertensive Rats Determined by a Modified Peroxidase Method," *Evidence-Based Complementary and Alternative Medicine* 2011 (2011): 703049.
103. Nasrin Ziamajidi et al., "Ameliorative Effects of Allium Sativum Extract on INOS Gene Expression and NO Production in Liver of Streptozotocin + Nicotinamide-Induced Diabetic Rats," *Indian Journal of Clinical Biochemistry* 33, no. 2 (2018): 147–53.
104. Marc Y. Donath and Steven E. Shoelson, "Type 2 Diabetes as an Inflammatory Disease," *Nature Reviews Immunology* 11, no. 2 (2011): 98–107.
105. Cheng Ye and John P. Driver, "Suppressors of Cytokine Signaling in Sickness and in Health of Pancreatic β-Cells," *Frontiers in Immunology* 7 (2016): 169.
106. Raju Padiya et al., "Garlic Improves Insulin Sensitivity and Associated Metabolic Syndromes in Fructose Fed Rats," *Nutrition and Metabolism* (*London*) 8, no. 1 (2011): 53.
107. Ehsan Shabani, Korosh Sayemiri, and Mohammadtaghi Mohammadpour, "The Effect of Garlic on Lipid Profile and Glucose Parameters in Diabetic Patients: A Systematic Review and Meta-Analysis," *Primary Care Diabetes* 13, no. 1 (2019): 28–42.
108. Mathew Attokaran, "Ginger," in *Natural Food Flavors and Colorants* (Chichester, UK: John Wiley & Sons, Ltd., 2017), 209–14.
109. Renhard Grzanna, Lars Lindmark, and Carmelita G. Frondoza, "Ginger—An Herbal Medicinal Product with Broad Anti-Inflammatory Actions," *Journal of Medicinal Food* 8, no. 2 (2005): 125–32.
110. Eun Jung Park and John M. Pezzuto, "Botanicals in Cancer Chemoprevention," *Cancer Metastasis Reviews* 21, no. 3–4 (2002): 231–55.
111. Jing Wang et al., "Beneficial Effects of Ginger *Zingiber Officinale Roscoe* on Obesity and Metabolic Syndrome: A Review," *Annals of the New York Academy of Sciences* 1398, no. 1 (2017): 83–98.
112. Masood Sadiq Butt, and Muhammad Tauseef Sultan, "Ginger and Its Health Claims: Molecular Aspects," *Critical Reviews in Food Science and Nutrition* 51, no. 5 (2011): 383–93.

113. Manjeet Priya Rani et al., "Inhibitory Potential of Ginger Extracts Against Enzymes Linked to Type 2 Diabetes, Inflammation and Induced Oxidative Stress," *International Journal of Food Sciences and Nutrition* 62, no. 2 (2011): 106–10.
114. Tahereh Arablou et al., "The Effect of Ginger Consumption on Glycemic Status, Lipid Profile and Some Inflammatory Markers in Patients with Type 2 Diabetes Mellitus," *International Journal of Food Sciences and Nutrition* 65, no. 4 (2014): 515–20.
115. Badreldin Ali, et al., "Some Phytochemical, Pharmacological and Toxicological Properties of Ginger (Zingiber Officinale Roscoe): A Review of Recent Research," *Food and Chemical Toxicology* 46, no. 2 (2008): 409–20.
116. Sanjay P. Akhani, Santosh Vishwakarma, and Ramesh Goyal, "Anti-Diabetic Activity of *Zingiber Officinale* in Streptozotocin-Induced Type I Diabetic Rats," *Journal of Pharmacy and Pharmacology* 56, no. 1 (2004): 101–5.
117. Sepide Mahluji et al., "Effects of Ginger (*Zingiber officinale*) on Plasma Glucose Level, HbA1c and Insulin Sensitivity in Type 2 Diabetic Patients," *International Journal of Food Sciences and Nutrition* 64, no. 6 (2013): 682–86.
118. Jie Zhu et al., "Effects of Ginger (*Zingiber officinale* Roscoe) on Type 2 Diabetes Mellitus and Components of the Metabolic Syndrome: A Systematic Review and Meta-Analysis of Randomized Controlled Trials," *Evidence-Based Complementary and Alternative Medicine* 2018, no. 1 (2018): 5692962.
119. Fang-yan Huang et al., "Dietary Ginger as a Traditional Therapy for Blood Sugar Control in Patients with Type 2 Diabetes Mellitus," *Medicine (Baltimore)* 98, no. 13 (2019): e15054.
120. Roger Gibb et al., "Psyllium Fiber Improves Glycemic Control Proportional to Loss of Glycemic Control: A Meta-Analysis of Data in Euglycemic Subjects, Patients at Risk of Type 2 Diabetes Mellitus, and Patients Being Treated for Type 2 Diabetes Mellitus," *American Journal of Clinical Nutrition* 102, no. 6 (2015): 1604–14.
121. Sandra Gonçalves and Anabela Romano, "The Medicinal Potential of Plants from the Genus Plantago (Plantaginaceae)," *Industrial Crops and Products* 83 (2016): 213–26.
122. Vijay Kumar Thakur and Manu Kumari Thakur, "Recent Trends in Hydrogels Based on Psyllium Polysaccharide: A Review," *Journal of Cleaner Production* 82 (2014): 1–15.
123. J. G. Pastors et al., "Psyllium Fiber Reduces Rise in Postprandial Glucose and Insulin Concentrations in Patients with Non-Insulin-Dependent Diabetes," *American Journal of Clinical Nutrition* 53, no. 6 (1991): 1431–35.
124. James W. Anderson et al., "Effects of Psyllium on Glucose and Serum Lipid Responses in Men with Type 2 Diabetes and Hypercholesterolemia," *American Journal of Clinical Nutrition* 70, no. 4 (1999): 466–73.

125. Ayman S. Abutair, Ihab N. Naser, and Amin T. Hamed, "Soluble Fibers from Psyllium Improve Glycemic Response and Body Weight Among Diabetes Type 2 Patients (Randomized Control Trial)," *Nutrition Journal* 15, no. 1 (2016): 86.
126. Mark N. Feinglos et al., "Psyllium Improves Glycemic Control in Patients with Type-2 Diabetes Mellitus," *Bioactive Carbohydrates and Dietary Fibre* 1, no. 2 (2013): 156–61.
127. Marc McRae, "Dietary Fiber Intake and Type 2 Diabetes Mellitus: An Umbrella Review of Meta-Analyses," *Journal of Chiropractic Medicine* 17, no. 1 (2018): 44–53.
128. Katherine A. Burns and Kenneth S. Korach, "Estrogen Receptors and Human Disease: An Update," *Archives of Toxicology* 86, no. 10 (2012), 1491–504.
129. Birgit M. Dietz et al., "Botanicals and Their Bioactive Phytochemicals for Women's Health," *Pharmacological Reviews* 68, no. 4 (2016): 1026–73.
130. Maida Taylor, "Complementary and Alternative Approaches to Menopause," *Endocrinology and Metabolism Clinics of North America* 44, no. 3 (2015): 619–48.
131. James J. Brokaw et al., "The Teaching of Complementary and Alternative Medicine in U.S. Medical Schools: A Survey of Course Directors," *Academic Medicine* 77, no. 9 (2002): 876–81.
132. Katherine J. Hamilton et al., "Estrogen Hormone Biology," in *Current Topics in Developmental Biology* 125 (2017): 109–46.
133. Heidi D. Nelson, "Menopause," *Lancet* 371, no. 9614 (2008): 760–70.
134. Bhagu R. Bhavnani and Frank Z. Stanczyk, "Pharmacology of Conjugated Equine Estrogens: Efficacy, Safety and Mechanism of Action," *Journal of Steroid Biochemestry and Molecular Biology* 142 (2014): 16–29.
135. Ivonne M. Rietjens, Jochem Louisse, and Karsten Beekmann, "The Potential Health Effects of Dietary Phytoestrogens," *British Journal of Pharmacology* 174, no. 11 (2017): 1263–80.
136. Qixing Nie et al., "Metabolism and Health Effects of Phyto-Estrogens," *Critical Reviews in Food Science and Nutrition* 57, no. 11 (2017): 2432–54.
137. Harini Anandhi Senthilkumar, Jimmy E. Fata, and Edward J. Kennelly, "Phytoestrogens: The Current State of Research Emphasizing Breast Pathophysiology," *Phytotherapy Research* 32, no. 9 (2018): 1707–19.
138. Liselotte Krenn, Iris Unterrieder, and Renate Ruprechter, "Quantification of Isoflavones in Red Clover by High-Performance Liquid Chromatography," *Journal of Chromatography B.* 777, no. 1–2 (2002): 123–28.
139. Katrien Vandecasteele et al., "Evaluation of the Efficacy and Safety of Salvia Officinalis in Controlling Hot Flashes in Prostate Cancer Patients Treated with Androgen Deprivation," *Phytotherapy Research* 26, no. 2 (2012): 208–13.
140. Rahele Kargozar, Hoda Azizi, and Roshanak Salari, "A Review of Effective Herbal Medicines in Controlling Menopausal Symptoms," *Electronic Physician* 9, no. 11 (2017): 5826–33.

141. Hye-Rim Lee et al., "Molecular Mechanism(s) of Endocrine-Disrupting Chemicals and Their Potent Oestrogenicity in Diverse Cells and Tissues That Express Oestrogen Receptors," *Journal of Cellular and Molecular Medicine* 17, no. 1 (2013): 1–11.
142. M. Taylor, "Complementary and Alternative Medicine Preparations Used to Treat Symptoms of Menopause," *Menopausal Medicine* 20 (2012): S1–S8.
143. S. O. Kruse et al., "Fukiic and Piscidic Acid Esters from the Rhizome of *Cimicifuga racemosa* and the in Vitro Estrogenic Activity of Fukinolic Acid," *Planta Medica* 65, no. 8 (1999): 763–64.
144. Carla M. Lopes, A. Dourado, and R. Oliveira, "Phytotherapy and Nutritional Supplements on Breast Cancer," *BioMed Research International* 2017, no. 12 (2017): 1–42.
145. Patricia Jane Murphy and Scott S. Campbell, "Sex Hormones, Sleep, and Core Body Temperature in Older Postmenopausal Women," *Sleep* 30, no. 12 (2007): 1788–94.
146. Rossella E. Nappi et al., "Efficacy of Cimicifuga Racemosa on Climacteric Complaints: A Randomized Study versus Low-Dose Transdermal Estradiol," *Gynecological Endocrinology* 20, no. 1 (2005): 30–35.
147. Ralf Uebelhack et al., "Black Cohosh and St. John's Wort for Climacteric Complaints," *Obstetrics and Gynecology* 107, no. 2, Part 1 (2006): 247–55.
148. Taghreed Shams et al., "Efficacy of Black Cohosh-Containing Preparations on Menopausal Symptoms: A Meta-Analysis," *Alternative Therapies in Health Medicine* 16, no. 1 (2010): 36–44.
149. Brian Hutton et al., "Comparison of Physical Interventions, Behavioral Interventions, Natural Health Products, and Pharmacologics to Manage Hot Flashes in Patients with Breast or Prostate Cancer: Protocol for a Systematic Review Incorporating Network Meta-Analyses," *Systematic Reviews* 4, no. 1 (2015): 114.
150. Shairoz Merchant and Justin Stebbing, "Black Cohosh, Hot Flushes, and Breast Cancer," *Lancet Oncology* 16, no. 2 (2015): 137–38.
151. Linda Saxe Einbond et al., "Growth Inhibitory Activity of Extracts and Compounds from Cimicifuga Species on Human Breast Cancer Cells," *Phytomedicine* 15, no. 6–7 (2008): 504–11.
152. Nadia Obi et al., "The Use of Herbal Preparations to Alleviate Climacteric Disorders and Risk of Postmenopausal Breast Cancer in a German Case-Control Study," *Cancer Epidemiology Biomarkers and Prevention* 18, no. 8 (2009): 2207–13.
153. Angelica Lindén Hirschberg et al., "An Isopropanolic Extract of Black Cohosh Does Not Increase Mammographic Breast Density or Breast Cell Proliferation in Postmenopausal Women," *Menopause* 14, no. 1 (2007): 89–96.
154. Rolf Teschke, "Black Cohosh and Suspected Hepatotoxicity," *Menopause* 17, no. 2 (2010): 426–40.
155. Chisato Nagata et al., "Soy Product Intake and Hot Flashes in Japanese Women: Results from a Community-Based Prospective Study," *American Journal of Epidemiology* 153, no. 8 (2001): 790–93.

156. John R. Crouse et al., "A Randomized Trial Comparing the Effect of Casein with That of Soy Protein Containing Varying Amounts of Isoflavones on Plasma Concentrations of Lipids and Lipoproteins," *Archives of Internal Medicine* 159, no. 17 (1999): 2070–76.
157. Mark J. Messina et al., "Soy Intake and Cancer Risk: A Review of the in Vitro and in Vivo Data," *Nutrition and Cancer* 21, no. 2 (1994): 113–31.
158. Nathalie Dijsselbloem et al., "Soy Isoflavone Phyto-Pharmaceuticals in Interleukin-6 Affections. Multi-Purpose Nutraceuticals at the Crossroad of Hormone Replacement, Anti-Cancer and Anti-Inflammatory Therapy," *Biochemical Pharmacology* 68, no. 6 (2004): 1171–85.
159. Deborah Lee Alekel et al., "Isoflavone-Rich Soy Protein Isolate Attenuates Bone Loss in the Lumbar Spine of Perimenopausal Women," *American Journal of Clinical Nutrition* 72, no. 3 (2000): 844–52.
160. Atieh Hajirahimkhan, Birgit Dietz, and Judy L. Bolton, "Botanical Modulation of Menopausal Symptoms: Mechanisms of Action?" *Planta Medica* 79, no. 7 (2013): 538–53.
161. Silvina Levis, Marcio L. Griebeler, "The Role of Soy Foods in the Treatment of Menopausal Symptoms," *Journal of Nutrition* 140, no. 12 (2010): 2318S–21S.
162. Zhigang Wu, Ryan P. Rodgers, and Alan G. Marshall, A. G. "Characterization of Vegetable Oils: Detailed Compositional Fingerprints Derived from Electrospray Ionization Fourier Transform Ion Cyclotron Resonance Mass Spectrometry," *Journal of Agricultural and Food Chemistry* 52, no. 17 (2004): 5322–28.
163. Heba M. A. Abdelrazek et al., "Soy Isoflavones Ameliorate Metabolic and Immunological Alterations of Ovariectomy in Female Wistar Rats: Antioxidant and Estrogen Sparing Potential," *Oxidative Medicine and Cellular Longevity* 2019 (2019): 5713606.
164. Howard N. Hodis et al., "Isoflavone Soy Protein Supplementation and Atherosclerosis Progression in Healthy Postmenopausal Women," *Stroke* 42, no. 11 (2011): 3168–375.
165. Kyoko Taku et al., "Extracted or Synthesized Soybean Isoflavones Reduce Menopausal Hot Flash Frequency and Severity," *Menopause* 19, no. 7 (2012): 776–90.
166. Arum Lee et al., "Therapeutic Approaches to Atrophic Vaginitis in Postmenopausal Women: A Systematic Review with a Network Meta-Analysis of Randomized Controlled Trials," *Journal of Menopausal Medicine* 24, no. 1 (2018): 1–10.
167. M. Najaf Najafi, and M. Ghazanfarpour, "Effect of Phytoestrogens on Sexual Function in Menopausal Women: A Systematic Review and Meta-Analysis," *Climacteric* 21, no. 5 (2018): 437–45.
168. Mark Messina, "Soy and Health Update: Evaluation of the Clinical and Epidemiologic Literature," *Nutrients* 8, no. 12 (2016): 754.
169. Marijana Tucak et al., "Forage Legumes as Sources of Bioactive Phytoestrogens for Use in Pharmaceutics: A Review," *Current Pharmaceutical Biotechnology* 19, no. 7 (2018): 537–44.

170. Cathy R. Kessenich, "Review: Plant Based Oestrogens Do Not Relieve Hot Flushes or Other Menopausal Symptoms," *Evidence-Based Nursing* 8, no. 3 (2005): 83.
171. Masumeh Ghazanfarpour et al., "Effects of Red Clover on Hot Flash and Circulating Hormone Concentrations in Menopausal Women: A Systematic Review and Meta-Analysis," *Avicenna Journal of Phytomedicine* 5, no. 6 (2015): 498–511.
172. Soheila Ehsanpour et al., "The Effects of Red Clover on Quality of Life in Post-Menopausal Women," *Iranian Journal of Nursing and Midwifery Research* 17, no. 1 (2012): 34–40.
173. Angela Mari et al., "Metabolic Profiling of Vitex Agnus Castus Leaves, Fruits and Sprouts: Analysis by LC/ESI/(QqQ)MS and (HR) LC/ESI/(Orbitrap)/MSn," *Journal of Pharmaceutical and Biomedical Analysis* 102 (2015): 215–21.
174. Diana van Die et al., "Vitex Agnus-Castus Extracts for Female Reproductive Disorders: A Systematic Review of Clinical Trials," *Planta Medica* 79, no. 7 (2013): 562–75.
175. Mikio Momoeda et al., "Efficacy and Safety of Vitex Agnus-Castus Extract for Treatment of Premenstrual Syndrome in Japanese Patients: A Prospective, Open-Label Study," *Advances in Therapy* 31, no. 3 (2014): 362–73.
176. Giulia Dante and Fabio Facchinetti, "Herbal Treatments for Alleviating Premenstrual Symptoms: A Systematic Review," *Journal of Psychosoatic Obstetrics and Gynecology* 32, no. 1 (2011): 42–51.
177. Diana van Die et al., "*Vitex Agnus-Castus* (Chaste-Tree/Berry) in the Treatment of Menopause-Related Complaints," *Journal of Alternative and Complementary Medicine* 15, no. 8 (2009): 853–62.
178. Gerald R. Cunha et al., "The Endocrinology and Developmental Biology of the Prostate," *Endocrine Reviews* 8, no. 3 (1987): 338–62.
179. Natasha Kyprianou, Huacheng Tu, and Stephen C. Jacobs, "Apoptotic versus Proliferative Activities in Human Benign Prostatic Hyperplasia," *Human Pathology* 27, no. 7 (1996): 668–75.
180. Mark Emberton, M et al., "Benign Prostatic Hyperplasia: A Progressive Disease of Aging Men," *Urology* 61, no. 2 (2003): 267–73.
181. Mar Royuela et al., "Estrogen Receptors Alpha and Beta in the Normal, Hyperplastic and Carcinomatous Human Prostate," *Journal of Endocrinology* 168, no. 3 (2001): 447–54.
182. Herbert Lepor, "Pathophysiology, Epidemiology, and Natural History of Benign Prostatic Hyperplasia," *Reviews in Urology* 6, no. 9 (2004): S3–S10.
183. J. Kellogg Parsons et al., "Prospective Study of Serum Dihydrotestosterone and Subsequent Risk of Benign Prostatic Hyperplasia in Community Dwelling Men: The Rancho Bernardo Study," *Journal of Urology* 184, no. 3 (2010): 1040–44.
184. Ryan Pearson and Pamela Williams, "Common Questions About the Diagnosis and Management of Benign Prostatic Hyperplasia," *American Family Physician* 90, no. 11 (2014): 769–74.
185. F. Di Silverio et al., "Plant Extracts in BPH," *Minerva Urologica e Nefrologica* 45, no. 4 (1993): 143–49.

186. A. C. Buck, "Phytotherapy for the Prostate," *British Journal of Urology* 78, no. 3 (1996): 325–36.
187. Olta Allkanjari and Annabella Vitalone, "What Do We Know about Phytotherapy of Benign Prostatic Hyperplasia?" *Life Sciences* 126 (2015): 42–56.
188. B. Veeresha et al., "Lauric Acid and Myristic Acid Prevent Testosterone Induced Prostatic Hyperplasia in Rats," *European Journal of Pharmacology* 626, no. 2–3 (2010): 262–65.
189. Mayumi Suzuki et al., "Pharmacological Effects of Saw Palmetto Extract in the Lower Urinary Tract," *Acta Pharmacologica Sinica* 30, no. 3 (2009): 271–81.
190. Petrisor Geavlete, Rasvan Multescu, and Bogdan Geavlete, "Serenoa Repens Extract in the Treatment of Benign Prostatic Hyperplasia," *Therapeutic Advances in Urology* 3, no. 4 (2011): 193–98.
191. Soo Liang Ooi and Sok Cheon Pak, "*Serenoa repens* for Lower Urinary Tract Symptoms/Benign Prostatic Hyperplasia: Current Evidence and Its Clinical Implications in Naturopathic Medicine," *Journal of Alternative and Complementary Medicine* 23, no. 8 (2017): 599–606.
192. Kavitha Penugonda and Brian L. Lindshield, "Fatty Acid and Phytosterol Content of Commercial Saw Palmetto Supplements," *Nutrients* 5, no. 9 (2013): 3617–33.
193. Daniela Buonocore et al., "*Serenoa repens* Extracts: In Vitro Study of the 5α-Reductase Activity in a Co-Culture Model for Benign Prostatic Hyperplasia," *Archivio Italiano di Urologia e Andrologia* 90, no. 3 (2018): 199.
194. Sophie Bernichtein et al., "Anti-Inflammatory Properties of Lipidosterolic Extract of Serenoa Repens (Permixon®) in a Mouse Model of Prostate Hyperplasia," *Prostate* 75, no. 7 (2015): 706–22.
195. Alain Latil et al., "Effects of Hexanic Extract of Serenoa Repens (Permixon® 160 Mg) on Inflammation Biomarkers in the Treatment of Lower Urinary Tract Symptoms Related to Benign Prostatic Hyperplasia," *Prostate* 75, no. 16 (2015): 1857–67.
196. Timothy J. Wilt et al., "Saw Palmetto Extracts for Treatment of Benign Prostatic Hyperplasia: A Systematic Review," *JAMA* 280, no. 18 (1998): 1604–9.
197. P. Boyle et al., "Updated Meta-Analysis of Clinical Trials of Serenoa Repens Extract in the Treatment of Symptomatic Benign Prostatic Hyperplasia," *BJU International* 93, no. 6 (2004): 751–56.
198. Michael J. Barry et al., "Effect of Increasing Doses of Saw Palmetto Extract on Lower Urinary Tract Symptoms: A Randomized Trial," *JAMA* 306, no. 12 (2011): 1344–51.
199. James Tacklind et al., "*Serenoa repens* for Benign Prostatic Hyperplasia," *Cochrane Database of Systematic Reviews* 12, no. 12 (2012): CD001423.
200. Andrea Russo et al., "*Serenoa repens*, Selenium and Lycopene to Manage Lower Urinary Tract Symptoms Suggestive for Benign Prostatic Hyperplasia," *Expert Opinion on Drug Safety* 15, no. 12 (2016): 1661–70.

201. Young Woo Ryu et al., "Comparison of Tamsulosin plus Serenoa Repens with Tamsulosin in the Treatment of Benign Prostatic Hyperplasia in Korean Men: 1-Year Randomized Open Label Study," *Urologia Internationalis* 94, no. 2 (2015): 187–93.
202. Fatih Hizli and M. Cemil Uygur, "A Prospective Study of the Efficacy of Serenoa Repens, Tamsulosin, and Serenoa Repens plus Tamsulosin Treatment for Patients with Benign Prostate Hyperplasia," *International Urology and Nephrology* 39, no. 3 (2007): 879–86.
203. Nazareno Suardi et al., "Effects of Difaprost® on Voiding Dysfunction, Histology and Inflammation Markers in Patients with Benign Prostatic Hyperplasia Who Are Candidates for Surgical Treatment," *Minerva Urologica e Nefrologica* 66, no. 2 (2014): 119–25.
204. J. Sökeland, "Combined Sabal and Urtica Extract Compared with Finasteride in Men with Benign Prostatic Hyperplasia: Analysis of Prostate Volume and Therapeutic Outcome," *BJU International* 86, no. 4 (2000): 439–42.
205. Dorota Kregiel, Ewelina Pawlikowska, and Hubert Antolak, H. "*Urtica* Spp.: Ordinary Plants with Extraordinary Properties," *Molecules* 23, no. 7 (2018): 1664.
206. Johannes J. Lichius, and C. Muth, "The Inhibition Effects of *Urtica Dioica* Root Extracts on Experimentally Induced Prostatic Hyperplasia in the Mouse," *Planta Medica* 63, no. 4 (1997): 307–10.
207. T. Hirano, M. Homma, and K. Oka, "Effects of Stinging Nettle Root Extracts and Their Steroidal Components on the Na^+, K^+-ATPase of the Benign Prostatic Hyperplasia," *Planta Medica* 60, no. 1 (1994): 30–33.
208. M. Sajfrtová et al., "Near-Critical Extraction of β-Sitosterol and Scopoletin from Stinging Nettle Roots," *Journal of Supercritical Fluids* 35, no. 2 (2005): 111–18.
209. Matthias Schöttner, Dietmar Ganßer, and Gerhard Spiteller, "Lignans from the Roots of *Urtica Dioica* and Their Metabolites Bind to Human Sex Hormone Binding Globulin (SHBG)," *Planta Medica* 63, no. 6 (1997): 529–32.
210. Julia E. Chrubasik et al., "Comprehensive Review on the Stinging Nettle Effect and Efficacy Profiles. Part II: Urticae Radix," *Phytomedicine* 14, no. 7–8 (2007): 568–79.
211. Rupert Kraus, Gerhard Spiteller, and Wilfried Bartsch, "(10E,12Z)-9-Hydroxy-10,12-octadecadienoic Acid, an Aromatase Inhibitor from Roots of Urtica Dioica," *European Journal of Organic Chemistry* 1991, no. 4 (1991): 335–39.
212. Egon Koch, "Extracts from Fruits of Saw Palmetto (Sabal Serrulata) and Roots of Stinging Nettle (Urtica Dioica): Viable Alternatives in the Medical Treatment of Benign Prostatic Hyperplasia and Associated Lower Urinary Tracts Symptoms," *Planta Medica* 67, no. 6 (2001): 489–500.
213. Mohammed Reza Safarinejad, "Urtica Dioica for Treatment of Benign Prostatic Hyperplasia: A Prospective, Randomized, Double-Blind, Placebo-Controlled, Crossover Study," *Journal of Herbal Pharmacotherapy* 5, no. 4 (2005): 1–11.

214. T. Schneider and H. Rübben, "[Stinging Nettle Root Extract (Bazoton-Uno) in Long Term Treatment of Benign Prostatic Syndrome (BPS). Results of a Randomized, Double-Blind, Placebo Controlled Multicenter Study after 12 Months]," *Urologe A.* 43, no. 3 (2004): 302–6.
215. Nicolai Lopatkin et al., "Efficacy and Safety of a Combination of Sabal and Urtica Extract in Lower Urinary Tract Symptoms—Long-Term Follow-up of a Placebo-Controlled, Double-Blind, Multicenter Trial," *International Urology and Nephrology* 39, no. 4 (2007): 1137–46.
216. Veronica Chi Ken Wong et al., "Current Alternative and Complementary Therapies Used in Menopause," *Gynecological Endocrinology* 25, no. 3 (2009): 166–74.
217. Elliot Fagelman and Franklin C. Lowe, "Herbal Medications in the Treatment of Benign Prostatic Hyperplasia (BPH)," *Urologic Clinics of North America* 29, no. 1 (2002): 23–29.
218. Eva-Maria Pferschy-Wenzig and Rudolf Bauer, "The Relevance of Pharmacognosy in Pharmacological Research on Herbal Medicinal Products," *Epilepsy and Behavior* 52, no. B (2015): 344–62.
219. Birgit Dietz and Judy L. Bolton, "Botanical Dietary Supplements Gone Bad," *Chemical Research in Toxicology* 20, no. 4 (2007): 586–90.
220. Charlotte Simmler et al., "Metabolite Profiling and Classification of DNA-Authenticated Licorice Botanicals," *Journal of Natural Products* 78, no. 8 (2015): 2007–22.
221. C. E. Piersen et al., "Chemical and Biological Characterization and Clinical Evaluation of Botanical Dietary Supplements: A Phase I Red Clover Extract as a Model," *Current Medicinal Chemistry* 11, no. 11 (2004): 1361–74.
222. Jonathan Bisson et al., "Can Invalid Bioactives Undermine Natural Product-Based Drug Discovery?" *Journal of Medicinal Chemistry* 59, no. 5 (2016): 1671–90.
223. Jürg Gertsch, "Botanical Drugs, Synergy, and Network Pharmacology: Forth and Back to Intelligent Mixtures," *Planta Medica* 77, no. 11 (2011): 1086–98.
224. F. C. Lowe and E. Fagelman, "Phytotherapy in the Treatment of Benign Prostatic Hyperplasia: An Update," *Urology* 53, no. 4 (1999): 671–78.

Credits

Fig 14.2a: Copyright © 2009 by H. Zell, (CC BY-SA 3.0) at https://commons.wikimedia.org/wiki/File:Momordica_charantia_003.JPG.

Fig 14.3a: Source: https://commons.wikimedia.org/wiki/File:Cluster_bean-guar-Cyamopsis_psoralioides-Cyamopsis_tetragonolobus-TAMIL_NADU74.jpg.

Fig 14.3b: Copyright © 2007 by Quintinz, (CC BY 3.0) at https://commons.wikimedia.org/wiki/File:Guargum.jpg.

Fig 14.4a: Copyright © 2010 by Lalithamba, (CC BY 2.0) at https://commons.wikimedia.org/wiki/File:Gymnema_sylvestre_R.Br_-_Flickr_-_lalithamba.jpg.

Fig 14.5a: Copyright © 2009 by H. Zell, (CC BY-SA 2.0) at https://commons.wikimedia.org/wiki/File:Cinnamomum_verum_002.JPG#mw-jump-to-license.
Fig 14.5b: Copyright © 2018 Depositphotos/deeaf.
Fig 14.6a: Copyright © 2018 Depositphotos/Handini.
Fig 14.7a: Copyright © 2015 Depositphotos/domnitsky.yar.
Fig 14.8a: Copyright © 2013 Depositphotos/Ispace.
Fig 14.10a: Copyright © 2009 by H. Zell, (CC BY-SA 3.0) at https://commons.wikimedia.org/wiki/File:Actaea_racemosa_005.JPG.
Fig 14.11a: Copyright © 2014 by Voggacom. Reprinted with permission.
Fig 14.11b: Copyright © 2018 by Tris T7, (CC BY 3.0) at https://commons.wikimedia.org/wiki/File:Soy_Beans_Photographed_by_Trisorn_Triboon_02.jpg.
Fig 14.12a: Copyright © 2016 by Ivar Leidus, (CC BY-SA 4.0) at https://commons.wikimedia.org/wiki/File:Trifolium_pratense_-_Keila2.jpg.
Fig 14.13a: Copyright © 2006 by Sten Porse, (CC BY-SA 3.0) at https://commons.wikimedia.org/wiki/File:Vitex-agnus-castus-foliage.JPG.
Fig 14.14a: Copyright © 2016 by Michael Rivera, (CC BY-SA 4.0) at https://commons.wikimedia.org/wiki/File:Saw_Palmetto,_Florida_Museum_of_Natural_History.jpg.
Fig 14.14b: Copyright © 2012 Depositphotos/Quasarphoto.
Fig 14.15a: Copyright © 2008 by Adampauli, (CC BY-SA 3.0 DE) at https://commons.wikimedia.org/wiki/File:Urtica_dioica_flowers.jpg.

Chapter 15

Natural Products Used for the Treatment of Cancers

Keith C. Ellis, John M. Saathoff, and Jacqueline L. West

Since the beginning of recorded history, societies and cultures have used preparations from natural sources to treat the spectrum of ailments that affect the human body. Using a process of trial and error, natural remedies to directly treat ailments such as infections, inflammation, respiratory conditions, or skin irritations could be discovered and then consistently applied to therapy. Cancer, however, is a disease that only came to prevalence in the 20th century, as a leading cause of death for modern populations in which other diseases, such as infectious diseases (influenza, tuberculosis, bacterial infections, etc.) and cardiac diseases, had been addressed with reliable therapy. As a result, the investigation of natural products for use in the treatment of cancers was carried out in the modern scientific environment of the 20th century, resulting in numerous natural products (or semisynthetic derivatives) being FDA approved for use in the human population. While this collection of FDA-approved natural products for the treatment of cancer represents only a small fraction of the number of natural products investigated, they are a disproportionately large fraction of the total number of FDA-approved oncology agents. Overall, investigations of natural products are in some way responsible for the discovery of three out of every four FDA-approved oncology drugs.

Historic Importance of Natural Products for Oncology Drug Discovery and as Oncology Drugs

Investigators David J. Newman and Gordon M. Cragg of the National Cancer Institute have published multiple literature studies on the impact of natural products as a source of new drugs, both overall and specifically in oncology.[1][2][3][4] In the period from the 1940s through the end of 2014, 207 small-molecule drugs have been FDA approved as oncology therapeutics.[4] Of these,

92 drugs (44%) are either natural products used as isolated directly from nature or are semi-synthetic derivatives of isolated natural products. For an additional 68 drugs (33%), natural products played a key role in the drug being developed by discovery of the molecular target, discovery of the pharmacophore, or the drug being a mimetic of a natural product. Taken together, 160 (77%) of the oncology drugs approved from the 1940s to 2014 in some way involved the use of a natural product, demonstrating the impact of these molecules in this therapeutic area.[4]

Scope of This Work

In the literature, there are hundreds of reports each year of various natural products being used as potential oncology agents. A significant number of natural products have also entered clinical trials for use as oncology agents but failed to enter the clinic. Due to the sheer volume of literature that reports the anticancer activity of natural products, this chapter will be limited in scope to only those natural products or their derivatives that are approved by the FDA for use in human patients.

FDA-Approved Natural Products and Natural Product Derivatives for the Treatment of Cancer

Natural products were an area of intense focus for oncology drug discovery in the 20th century, with all but three of the FDA-approved natural products (NPs) and NP derivatives being approved prior to the year 2000. Aligning with oncology drug discovery trends in the 20th century, the majority of these natural products and/or NP-derivative oncology agents act as cytotoxic kinetic poisons using one of two mechanisms of action: modulation of microtubule function or inhibition of DNA synthesis and function. Not to be left out of 21st-century approaches to oncology therapy, natural products have also crossed over into the targeted therapeutics realm with the inhibitors of mTORC kinase function.

Natural Products and Drugs Targeting Microtubule Function

Microtubules are hollow, cylindrical structural filaments in cells that play an important role in many processes, including intracellular transport. Microtubules are formed by the polymerization of two protein subunits, α-tubulin and β-tubulin, which form a heterodimer subunit. Most importantly for natural products and NP-derivative oncology agents, microtubules form the mitotic spindle, which separates the two pairs of daughter chromosomes produced during replication and allows for cell division to occur. Blocking the formation or depolymerization of the mitotic spindle can arrest cell division at the metaphase stage of the cell cycle and induce cell death.[5][6]

The natural products and NP-derivative oncology agents in this section all either inhibit microtubule formation, thus preventing separation of the daughter chromosomes, or stabilize the microtubules forming the mitotic spindle, thus preventing budding of the dividing cell into two separate daughter cells. As this molecular target (microtubules) and the mechanisms of action for these drugs can occur in both tumor and healthy cells, all of the natural products and NP-derivative oncology agents in this section are cytotoxic and act as kinetic poisons, killing tumor cells at a faster rate than normal cells. Off-target toxicity in rapidly dividing normal tissues, such as hair and the lining of the GI tract, lead to the side effects of hair loss and nausea commonly experienced by patients.[7]

Inhibitors of Microtubule Formation

Vinca Alkaloids. The vinca alkaloid natural products are components of the extracts of the Madagascar periwinkle plant *Catharanthus roseus* (also known as *Vinca rosea*). This periwinkle plant, originally native to Madagascar but now found growing in most countries, has long been used by multiple societies as a traditional medicinal remedy.[8] In Europe and Jamaica, the extracts have been used as a treatment for diabetes, while Chinese culture has used these extracts as diuretics and a cough remedy.[9] The vinca alkaloids transitioned from traditional folk remedy to oncology agent when *C. roseus* extracts were screened by the pharmaceutical company Eli Lilly, where they were discovered to inhibit growth in cancer cell lines. Following bioassay-guided isolation, structural elucidation, and advanced testing of the natural products, vincristine and vinblastine, Eli Lilly took both drugs to market as oncology drugs.[10]

Structurally, the vinca alkaloids are highly complex dimeric alkaloids that contain two polycyclic subunits known as catharanthine and vindoline (see Figure 15.1), both of which are required for high-affinity binding to microtubules.[11] The two vinca alkaloid natural products that are FDA-approved drugs, vincristine and vinblastine, differ solely by the substituent on the N1 vindoline indole nitrogen (CHO in vincristine vs. Me in vinblastine). In addition to these two natural products, two semisynthetic derivatives of the vinca alkaloids, vindesine and vinorelbine, have been developed and introduced into the clinic. Relative to vincristine, vindesine has been modified to remove the C4 acetate (leaving the C4 hydroxyl) and transform the C3 methyl ester into the amide. Again relative to vincristine, vinorelbine has been modified to truncate the C6' to C9' ethylene bridge to a methylene and dehydrated the C4' hydroxyl to form the C3'–C4' olefin. While all the structural changes between these four compounds are small and subtle, these modifications lead to significant differences in potency, toxicity, and clinical utility.[12]

At the molecular level, the vinca alkaloids bind with high affinity to β-tubulin at a site near the guanosine triphosphate (GTP) binding site. This vinca alkaloid binding site is at

TABLE 15.1 Natural Products and Drugs Targeting Microtubule Function

Mechanism of Action	Drug Class	Source	Species	Natural Product or Generic Name	Brand Name	Molecule Type	FDA Approval Year
Inhibition of Microtubule Formation	Vinca Alkaloids	Plant	*Catharanthus roseus*	Vincristine	Oncovin	Natural Product	1963
				Vinblastine	Velbe	Natural Product	1965
				Vindesine	Eldisine	Semisynthetic NP Derivative	N/A[a]
				Vinorelbine	Navelbine	Semisynthetic NP Derivative	1994
Microtubule Stabilizer	Taxanes	Plant	*Taxus brevafolia* or *Taxus baccata*	Paclitaxel	Taxol	Natural Product	1992
				Docetaxel	Taxotere	Semisynthetic NP Derivative	1996
				10-Deacetyl Baccatin III	N/A	Natural Product	N/A
	Epothilones	Bacteria	*Sorangium cellulosum*	Epothilone B	N/A	Natural Product	N/A
				Ixabepilone	Ixempra	Semisynthetic NP Derivative	2007

a. Not approved for clinical use in the United States.

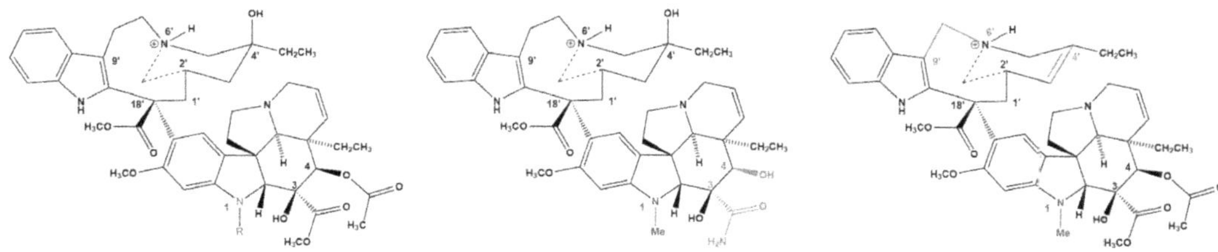

FIGURE 15.1 Structures and analysis of the vinca alkaloid oncology drugs vincristine, vinblastine, vindesine, and vinorelbine.

the interface of two α-β tubulin heterodimers, and drug binding leads to decreased binding of GTP as well as changes in microtubule conformation that leads to inhibition of microtubule polymerization. As a result of the lost ability to polymerize microtubules, the mitotic spindle is unable to separate daughter chromosome sets during replication, ultimately leading to clumping of chromosomes into unnatural shapes (balls and stars) and cell death.[13][14]

Microtubule Stabilizers

Taxanes. The development of the taxane class of oncology drugs is regarded as one of the greatest success stories of the development of natural products into clinically useful drugs. The development of the taxane drugs began in the 1960s with the isolation of the natural product taxol from the Pacific Yew tree (*Taxus brevafolia*) and discovery that this natural product has cytotoxicity not only against a commonly used mouse model of leukemia but also against solid tumors and a melanoma cell line. While this highly sought biological activity was known immediately for this natural product, several things delayed its development into a clinical drug. First, due to the extremely complicated structure of taxol and the limited analytical tools available at the time, elucidation of the structure of taxol required many years. Second, the supply of taxol was very limited due to the small amounts that could be isolated—isolation of 0.5 g of taxol required starting the extraction procedure with 12 kg of Pacific Yew tree bark. Taken together, these factors led to a cooling of interest in taxol as an oncology agent, despite its interesting and highly desirable biological activity.[15][16]

Over time, two new discoveries were made that overcame the supply limitation and rejuvenated interest in taxol as a potential oncology drug. The compound supply issue was addressed when it was discovered that a natural precursor in the biosynthesis of taxol, 10-deacetylbaccatin III, could be isolated from the needles of the English Yew tree (*Taxus baccata*), as opposed to the bark of the Pacific Yew tree (*Taxus brevafolia*). 10-Deacetylbaccatin III could then be isolated from this new, renewable natural source and could be converted semisynthetically to taxol. This discovery opened the door not only to the synthesis of adequate amounts of taxol for preclinical and clinical studies but also for the preparation and biological evaluation of additional taxol analogues.[17]

The second discovery that led to renewed interest in taxol was the determination that taxol had a unique mechanism of action compared to other microtubule inhibitors such as vincristine and colchichine. While taxol does inhibit mitosis, it acts by stabilizing the already-formed microtubules and inhibiting their depolymerization to soluble tubulin. The vinca alkaloids, on the other hand, bind to soluble tubulin and inhibit its polymerization into microtubules.[18][19]

The parent natural product taxol was taken to market by Bristol-Meyers Squibb as Paclitaxel (Taxol®) and approved by the FDA in 1993.[15] Structurally, paclitaxel is a highly functionalized and complex diterpenoid with a 15-membered tricyclic rings system, 11 stereocenters, and functional groups ranging from esters and hydroxyls to an amide and an epoxide.[20] The overall rigidity of the tricyclic ring system and fixed stereochemistry of the 11 stereocenters create a precise and specific three-dimensional conformation that is essential for binding to microtubules. The β-phenylisoserine ester side chain at C13 is also critical for taxol's antitumor effect.[21] Cleavage of this side chain results in the inactive compound 10-acetylbaccatin III. As can be seen from comparing the structures, 10-deacetylbaccatin III can be converted biosynthetically or semisynthetically to paclitaxel by acylation of the C10 hydroxyl and installation of the C13 β-phenylisoserine ester side chain. Following the identification of 10-deacetylbaccatin III and the completion of the total synthesis of taxol by several groups, extensive structure-activity relationship studies were carried out. From this extensive medicinal chemistry work, Docetaxel (Taxotere®) was the second taxane drug to enter the clinic. Docetaxel can also be made semisynthetically from 10-deacetylbaccatin III by simple installation of the C13 sidechain. Docetaxel differs from Paclitaxel in that it has the C10 hydroxyl (vs. the C10 acetate in paclitaxel), and the C13 sidechain contains a tert-butyl carbamate (vs. the phenyl amide in paclitaxel). These modifications make docetaxel slightly more water soluble than paclitaxel. However, both drugs are administered by the intravenous route.[22][23][24]

The taxanes bind in a hydrophobic binding site composed of the 31 N-terminal amino acids of β-tubulin. This binding site is unique from and does not overlap with the binding site on β-tubulin for the vinca alkaloids or GTP. Taxane binding to assembled microtubules promotes a stable conformation, which prevents depolymerization and promotes additional polymerization in excess of that required for mitosis. The inability of the mitotic spindle to disassemble interrupts the normal process of cell division and leads to cell death.[21]

Epothilones. In an effort to build on the success of the taxanes, the epothilone family of natural products has also been investigated and developed into a clinical drug. When initially investigated, the epothilones displayed high potency and a similar mechanism of

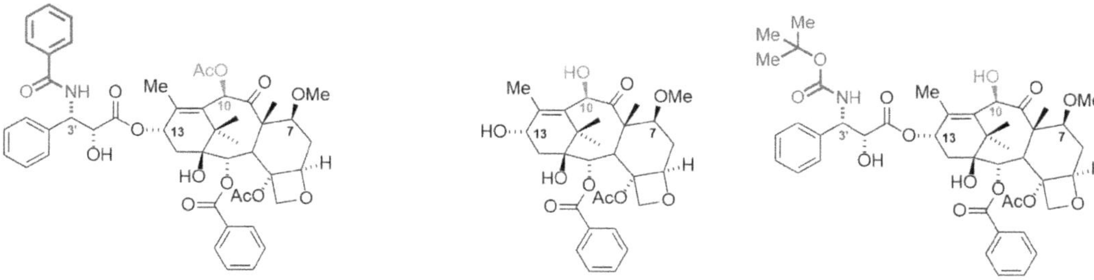

Paclitaxel (Taxol) **10-Deacetylbaccatin III** **Docetaxel (Taxotere)**

FIGURE 15.2 Taxane natural products and FDA-approved drugs. Drawings of taxol, 10-deacetylbaccatin iii, and taxotere.

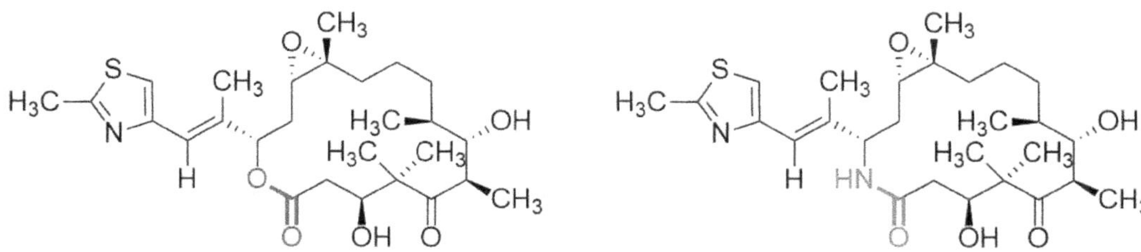

Epothilone B **Ixabepilone (Ixempra)**

FIGURE 15.3 Epothilone B and ixabepilone (Ixempra®). Drawings of epothilone B and ixabepilone.

action to the taxanes in an NIH COMPARE assay analysis.[25] Epothilone B was determined to bind with high affinity to the same hydrophobic binding site on β-tubulin. Epothilone B is produced by the mycobacteria *Sorangium cellulosum* and can be isolated in large quantities by fermentation. Importantly, epothilone B displays increased water solubility compared to the taxanes.[26]

Structurally, epothilone B is a 16-membered polyketide macrolide with a α,β-unsaturated thiazole side chain, 8 stereocenters, and functional groups including hydroxyls, a ketone, and an epoxide.[27] The ester functionality in the epothilone B macrolide makes the natural product susceptible to hydrolysis and inactivation in vivo. To develop this natural product lead into a clinical candidate, the ester of the macrolide was converted semisynthetically into amide to form the macrolactam.[28] This new molecule was taken to market by Bristol-Meyers Squibb as ixabepilone (Ixempra®), which was FDA approved in 2007.[25]

Natural Products and Drugs Targeting DNA Function

The replication of DNA is a vital process in the cell cycle and cellular division. Due to the rapidly growing nature of tumors, cancer cells are disproportionately dependent on their ability to replicate DNA. Natural products and NP-derivative oncology agents that can disrupt

TABLE 15.2 Natural Products and Drugs Targeting DNA Function

Mechanism of Action	Drug Class	Source	Species	Natural Product or Generic Name	Brand Name	Molecule Type	FDA Approval Year
TopoII Inhibition	Anthracyclines	Bacteria	*Streptomyces peucetius*	Doxorubicin	Adriamycin	Natural Product	1985
				Daunorubicin	Cerubidine	Natural Product	1979
				Idarubicin	Idamycin	Semisynthetic NP Derivative	1990
				Epirubicin	Ellence	Semisynthetic NP Derivative	1999
				Valrubicin	Valstar	Semisynthetic NP Derivative	1998
	Epipodo-phyllotoxins	Plant	*Podophyllum peltarum*	Podophyllotoxin	Podofilox	Natural Product	N/A[a]
				Etoposide	VePesid	Semisynthetic NP Derivative	1983
				Etoposide Phosphate	Etopophos	Semisynthetic NP Derivative	1983
				Teniposide	Vumon	Semisynthetic NP Derivative	1992
TopoI Inhibition	Camptothecins	Plant	*Camptotheca acuminata*	Camptothecin	N/A	Natural Product	N/A
				SN-38	N/A	Active Metabolite	N/A
				Irinotecan	Camptosar	Semisynthetic NP Derivative	1996
				Topotecan	Hycamtin	Semisynthetic NP Derivative	1996
DNA Alkyla-tion	Mitomycins	Bacteria	*Streptomyces caespitosus*	Mitomycin C	Mutamycin	Natural Product	1988
DNA Inter-calation	Bleomycins	Bacteria	*Streptomyces verticillus*	Bleomycin	Blenoxane	Natural Product	1973
	Actinomycin D	Bacteria	*Streptomyces parvullus*	Dactinomycin	Cosmegen	Natural Product	1964

a. Not FDA approved for use in oncology; approved FDA indication is for topical treatment of warts.

DNA replication are therefore highly effective antitumor agents. These agents kill tumor cells preferentially over normal, healthy cells due to the fact that the tumor cells grow and divide more rapidly, thereby offering selective cytotoxicity based on kinetic effects, hence why these compounds are often referred to as kinetic poisons.

The natural products and NP-derivative oncology agents in this section act either directly or indirectly on DNA and result in breaks in DNA, DNA damage by alkylation or free radicals, or DNA intercalation. Following treatment with these agents, cell death usually results from cellular responses to DNA damage caused by the drug, which induces apoptosis. Similar to the drugs targeting microtubule formation, the natural products and NP-derivative oncology agents targeting DNA replication are kinetic poisons and have off-target toxicity in rapidly dividing normal tissues, leading to the side effects of hair loss and nausea.

Topoisomerase II Inhibitors

DNA replication is a dynamic process where DNA is uncoiled from its stored form and ultimately straightened into linear stretches of nucleotides that are then separated to form the replication fork with DNA polymerase. In this process of unpacking DNA from a highly compacted and coiled form to the linear regions needed for the replication fork, additional coiling, twists, bends, kinks, and tangles can form, much like what happens when unraveling a rope or garden hose. The topoisomerase family of enzymes assists in the process of DNA replication by helping to untangle these twists, bends, and tangles. This family of enzymes accomplishes this task by making controlled cuts in DNA that can allow the DNA to uncoil or untangle.[29]

Specifically, the Topoisomease II enzyme (TopoII) cuts both strands of dsDNA and then allows other portions of the DNA strand to pass through the cut, followed by religation and closing of the cut. In this way, tangles or loops of DNA that are locked together can be freed from each other, thereby allowing DNA replication to continue and proceed more efficiently. When TopoII cuts DNA, one side of the cut DNA backbone forms a covalent bond with the enzyme while the other is held electrostatically to the surface of the enzyme by positively charged His and Arg residues. The intermediate that is formed between the enzyme and the covalently bound DNA is commonly referred to as the cleavage complex, as cleaved DNA is bound to the enzyme at this stage of the catalytic cycle.[29]

There are two classes of natural products and NP-derivative oncology agents that target TopoII, the anthracyclines and the epipodophyllotoxins.

Anthracyclines. The anthracyclines are a class of polyketide antitumor antibiotics that were first isolated from the bacteria *Streptomyces peucetius* in the 1960s. Bacteria have long been rich sources of biologically active natural products, as these organisms often synthesize complex molecules as defenses against other species of bacteria. For much of the 20th century, bacterial natural product extracts were screened for both antibacterial activity and anticancer activity. The anthracyclines possess both these biological activities, but the potent cytotoxic effects render them too toxic to be used as antibiotics, thereby relegating them to oncology treatment. The first anthracycline to be isolated and tested, daunorubicin, was found to be active against leukemia, while its companion natural product, doxorubicin, was found to have a broader spectrum of oncology activity and is active against both solid tumors and hematological cancers.[30] Similar to the vinca alkaloids vincristine and vinblastine, both doxorubicin and daunorubicin were taken directly to market as oncology drugs.

Structurally, the anthracyclines possess a tetracyclic linear ring system similar to anthracene (hence the name anthracyclines) with an appended ketone functional group and an attached L-daunosamine aminosugar. Doxorubicin and daunorubicin vary by a single functional group, located in the ketone of the anthracycline aglycone—in doxorubicin, the ketone is a simple methyl ketone, while in daunorubicin it is an α-hydroxymethyl ketone.[31] Several semisynthetic derivatives of doxorubicin and daunorubicin have also been developed. Idarubicin is a daunorubicin analogue where the 4-methoxy group has been removed from the anthracycline aglycone.[32] Epirubicin is a doxorubicin analogue where the stereochemistry of the 4'-hydroxyl of the daunosamine aminosugar has been inverted into an unnatural β-configuration.[31] Finally, Valrubicin is a doxorubicin analogue where the C14 α-hydroxymethyl ketone has been substituted as the valerate ester and the 3'-amine of the L-daunosamine aminosugar has been substituted as the trifluoromethyl amide.[33] These modifications make valrubicin more hydrophobic than its doxorubicin parent, which promotes more rapid and extensive penetration in tumor cells.[33]

At the molecular level, the anthracyclines exert their antitumor effect by binding to the covalent TopoII-DNA cleavage complex and preventing the religation of the cut in DNA.[34] Both the aglycone and amino sugar portions of the natural products or NP-derivative oncology agents are critical for binding to the cleavage complex. The aromatic B, C, and D rings of the aglycone intercalate between the DNA bases and form π-stacking interactions.[34] The oxygen hetero atoms in the aglycone form hydrogen bonding interactions with various amino acids in the TopoII enzyme.[34] The L-daunosamine aminosugar binds in the minor groove of the DNA at the TopoII-DNA interface and causes hyperstabilization of the ternary drug-TopoII-DNA complex, preventing religation of DNA. Over time, cellular DNA repair machinery detects the cut to DNA and, when the cell is unable to repair it, enters apoptosis.

While the anthracycline natural products and NP-derivative oncology agents are effective antitumor agents, they suffer from off-target cardiotoxicity, which is dose- and use-limiting. In vivo, the hydroquinone moiety of the anthracycline aglycone can be reduced to the hydroxyquinone, with the concomitant generation of cytotoxic free radicals. While these effects can contribute to and enhance the cytotoxicity of the compounds in tumor cells

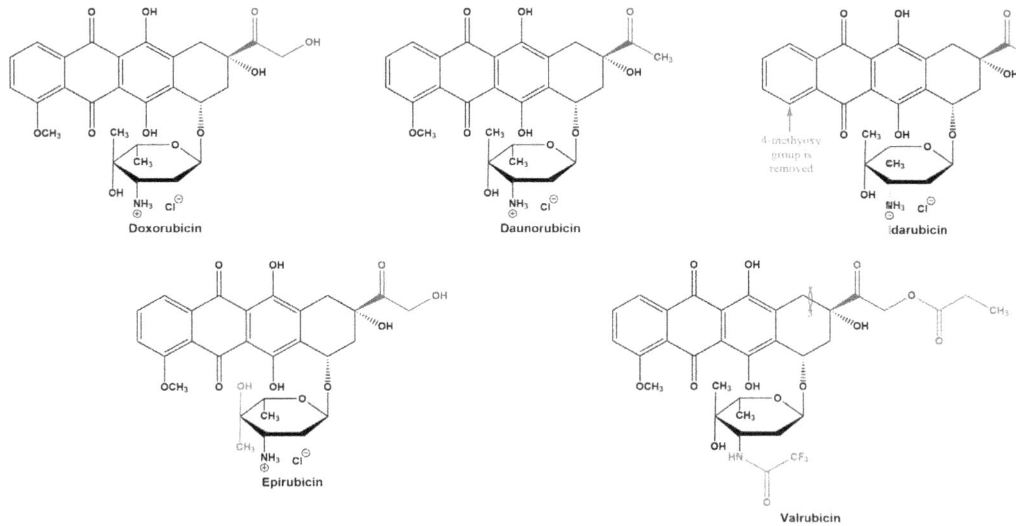

FIGURE 15.4 Anthracycline antitumor antibiotic natural products and FDA-approved drugs. Drawings of doxorubicin, daunorubicin, idarubicin, epirubicin, and valrubicin.

and increase their efficacy, when this process occurs in cardiac tissues, it can lead to both reversible short-term and irreversible chronic cardiotoxicity.[35] This use-limit side effect can be overcome with the coadministration of dexrazoxane or by use of the new liposomal formulations of doxorubicin (Doxil) and daunorubicin (DaunoXome).[35]

Epipodophyllotoxins. The epipodophyllotoxic class of oncology agents are derivatives of the natural product podophyllotoxin, which is isolated from the rhizomes of the American mandrake or mayapple (*Podophyllum peltatum*). The natural product itself has long been used by Native American tribes as a laxative, to combat intestinal worms, and to treat warts and other skin growths. The podophyllotoxin natural product itself is too toxic to be used internally but is FDA approved as a topical treatment for warts. Based on the use of podophyllotoxin extracts in traditional medicine and its activity as a tubulin-binding antimitotic agent, chemists at Sandoz Pharmaceutical company launched a program to screen extracts and make semisynthetic derivatives of these natural products. Their efforts ultimately led to the discovery of etoposide. Interestingly, etoposide and the follow-up drugs etoposide phosphate and teniposide exert their antitumor effect by inhibiting TopoII, not by binding to tubulin.[36]

Structurally, podophyllotoxin contains a mostly saturated tetracyclic linear ring system that includes a catechol and lactone, a trimethoxyphenyl substituent, and a C1 hydroxyl. Etoposide differs from the parent podophyllotoxin by containing the 4'-hydroxyl (vs. the 4'-methoxy in podophyllotoxin), the epimeric hydroxy group at the 1-position, and a methylidene glycoside substituent at the 1-position.[37] Etoposide phosphate bears a phosphate substituent on

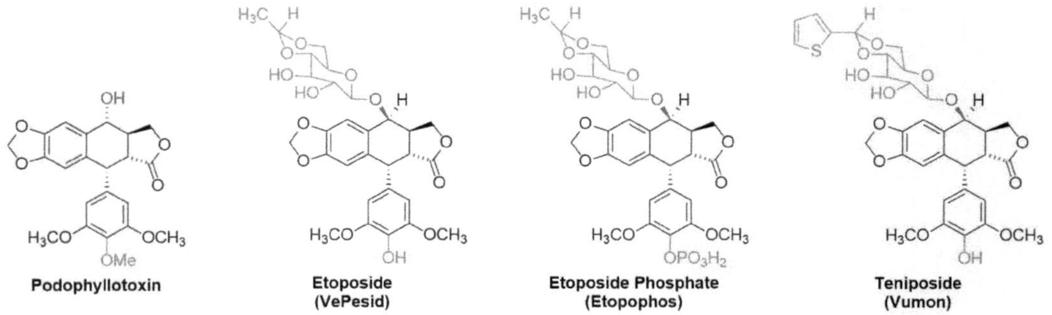

FIGURE 15.5 Epipodophyllotoxin natural products and FDA-approved drugs. Drawings of podophyllotoxin, etoposide, etoposide phosphate, and teniposide.

the 4'hydroxyl, increasing the water solubility and aiding in both formulation and administration. Teniposide is similar to etoposide except that it contains a thienylidene glycoside substituent at the 1-position (vs. the methylidene in etoposide), which results in a higher lipophilicity, cellular uptake, and potency for teniposide.[38]

Similar to the anthracyclines, the epipodophyllotoxins exert their antitumor effect by binding to the covalent TopoII-DNA cleavage complex and preventing the religation of the cut in DNA.[36] Both the aglycone and glycoside portions of the natural products and NP-derivative oncology agents are critical for binding to the cleavage complex. The aglycone portion of the drugs make contact with the TopoII enzyme and intercalate between the DNA bases while the glycone binds in the minor groove of DNA.[36]

Topoisomerase I Inhibitors

Similar to the Topoisomerase II enzyme above, the Topoisomerase I enzyme (TopoI) makes cuts in DNA to alleviate strain and tangles caused by uncoiling of DNA during replication. In the case of TopoI, this enzyme cuts only one strand of double stranded DNA (dsDNA), allowing DNA to unwind and relieve strain along the long axis of the DNA molecule. Again similar to TopoII, TopoI makes a cut in the single strand of DNA and forms an enzyme-DNA complex where one side of the DNA break is bound covalently to the enzyme while the other side of the break is free to move and alleviate supercoiling or strain. TopoI is targeted clinically by the camptothecin class of natural products and NP-derivative oncology agents.

Camptothecins. The natural product camptothecin was identified as a component of the ethanolic extracts of the Chinese *xi shu* or "happy tree" (*Camptotheca acuminata*), which displayed anticancer activity when screened against a mouse model of leukemia in the 1960s.[39] Following laborious work to identify fractions with active natural product by bioassay-directed screening and extensive work to purify the compound by liquid-liquid extraction and chromatography, the structure of camptothecin was elucidated by X-ray crystallographic analysis of a semisynthetic iodoacetate derivative.[40] Initial interest in camptothecin was high due to its activity in a mouse life-prolongation assay and against solid tumors, leading to several small clinical trials conducted in the early 1970s. While there was some response by patients taking the drugs, both poor water solubility and off-target toxicity resulted in diminished interest. Medicinal chemists, however, continued to investigate this class of natural products and determined that the 10-hydroxycamptothecin analogue was more potent than the parent natural product.[41] Interest in these natural products was reignited in 1985 when it was determined that camptothecin acts by inhibiting TopoI, offering a new molecular target and therapeutic drug class to clinical oncology treatment.[42]

Structurally, camptothecin is a conjugated pentacyclic lactone with one stereocenter. Addition of the 10-hydroxy to the scaffold affords the 10-hydroxycamptothecin analogue, which is more potent than the parent natural product.[41] In order to overcome the poor water solubility of both these natural products, basic side chains were installed in the molecules, which were developed for the clinic and FDA approved. In topotecan, the basic dimethylaminomethyl side chain was installed at C9 of 10-hydroxycamptothecin, allowing the drug to be formulated as a water-soluble HCl salt.[41] In irinotecan, a basic 4-piperdinyl-piperdine carbamate is installed on the C10-hydroxyl, resulting in a prodrug that is cleaved in the liver in vivo to afford the active metabolite SN-38.[43] Irinotecan also has an additional ethyl side chain installed at C7. The antitumor activity of all of the camptothecin natural products and NP-derived oncology drugs require the lactone ring to be in the closed, cyclized form. At physiological pH, however, this ring is in equilibrium with the ring-opened, hydroxy carboxylic acid form. The position of the equilibrium between these two forms is dictated by

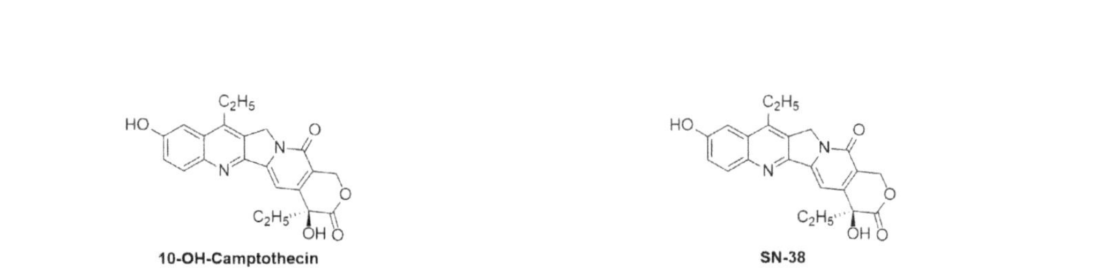

FIGURE 15.6 Camptothecin natural products and FDA-approved drugs. Drawings of camptothecin, 10-OH-camptothecin, topotecan, irinotecan, SN-38.

binding to serum albumin, with the active lactone form binding more tightly and shifting the equilibrium in favor of the active, lactone form.[44]

The camptothecins exert their antitumor effect by binding to the covalent TopoI-DNA cleavage complex and preventing the religation of the cut in DNA.[45] The flat ring system of the camptothecins intercalate the base pairs of DNA in the cut site with the enzyme. The pyridinyl nitrogen, C17 pyridine carbonyl, C20 hydroxyl, and C21 lactone carbonyl all make important contacts with residues in TopoI.[45] The bulky substituents at C7, C9, and C10 all point into the major groove of the enzyme-bound DNA.[45]

DNA Alkylating Agents

Mitomycin C. Mitomycin C is an antitumor antibiotic that was first isolated from the bacteria *Streptomyces caespitosus* in the late 1950s in Japan. Structurally, mitomycin C contains a redox reactive quinone as part of a tricyclic scaffold that also contains carbamate, methoxy, and aziridine functional groups. Mitomycin C undergoes multiple chemical transformations in vivo to become an active antitumor agent.[46] First, the quinone undergoes a two-electron bioreduction to form the hydroquinone, which then eliminates the methoxy group to form the aromatic indole ring system. The electrophilic aziridine and carbamate methylene in this active metabolite can react with amino groups on guanine and cytosine, resulting in the crosslinking of DNA and resulting in cell death.[46]

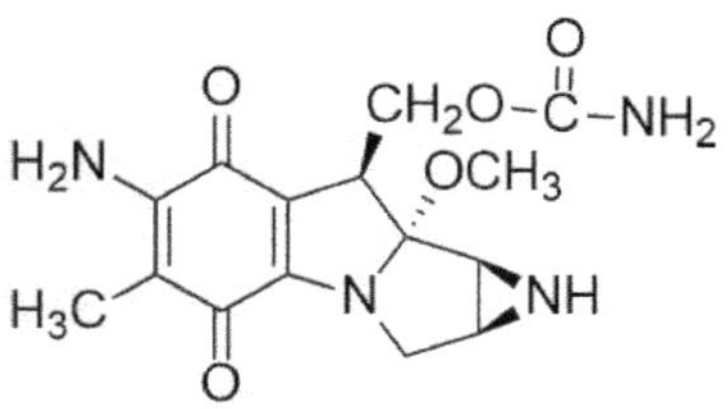

Mitomycin
(Mutamycin)

FIGURE 15.7 Mitomycin C and its in vivo activation.

DNA Intercalators

Bleomycins. The bleomycins are a family of glycopeptide antitumor antibiotics that were first isolated from the bacteria *Streptomyces verticillus* in 1962 in Japan. The clinically administered drug (Blenexane®) is a mixture of multiple bleomycin natural products, including bleomycin A2 (~60%), bleomycin B2 (~30%), and other minor components (~10%). It was first taken into clinical trials and approved in Japan in the 1960s, followed by FDA approval for use in the United States in 1973. Structurally, the bleomycins contain a peptidic core with a side chain and two sugar moieties. The bleomycin family members differ only by the functional group in the side chain, with bleomycin A2 containing a dimethylthiazonium cation and bleomycin B2 containing a methylgunanidine.[47] The antitumor effect of the bleomycins results from their first intercalating into DNA and then catalyzing iron-mediate formation of reactive oxygen radicals by a one-electron reduction mechanism, which results in single- and double-strand breaks in DNA.[47] The first step in the in vivo mechanism is

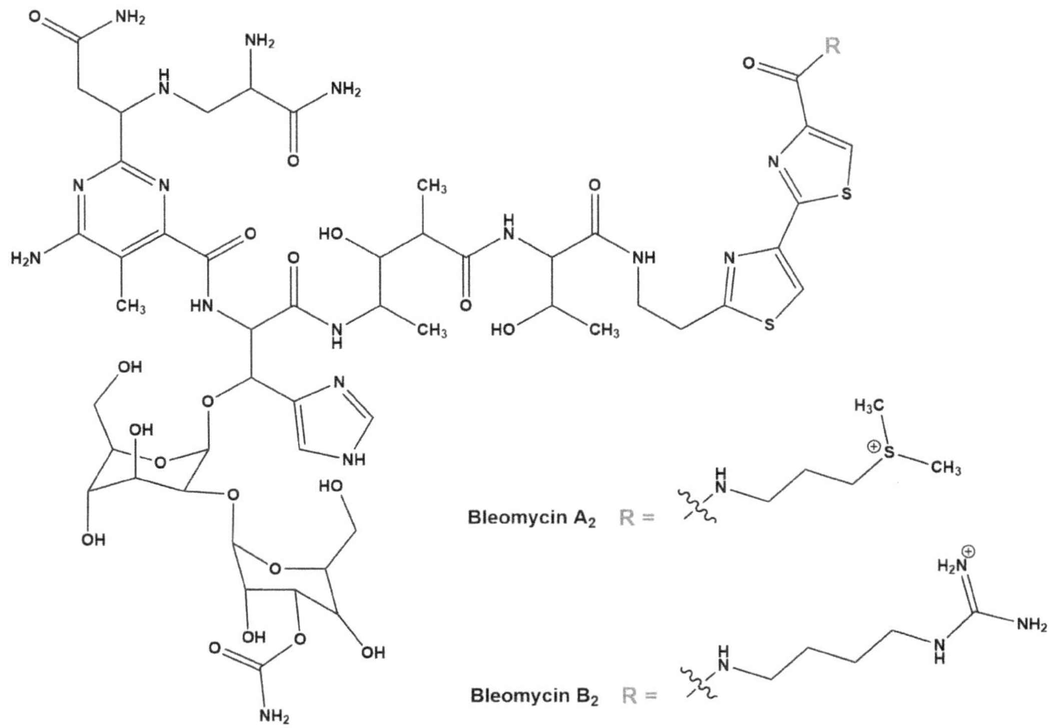

FIGURE 15.8 Bleomycin natural product oncology agents. Drawings of bleomycin scaffold with R groups for A2 and B2.

bleomycin-mediated abstraction of a hydrogen from the DNA, forming a DNA radical intermediate that then reacts through a series of steps to cleave the DNA polymer chain.[47]

Actinomycin D. Actinomycin D, which is also referred to as dactomycin, is an antitumor antibiotic first isolated in 1940 from the bacteria *Streptomyces parvullus*. Dactomycin contains an aromatic tricyclic phonoxazinone ring system that is substituted by two pentapeptide lactone rings. The aromatic tricyclic ring system intercalates with DNA, showing preference for binding between guanine and cytosine base pairs on a single DNA strand.[48] Once intercalated, dactomycin causes DNA elongation by spreading the distance between the base pairs, while the pentapeptide lactone rings bind in the minor groove of DNA, making multiple high-affinity interactions through hydrophobic interactions, hydrogen bonding, and π-stacking.[49] Binding of dactomycin to DNA is noncovalent but tight with a slow dissociation rate, leading to a pseudoirreversible effect.[49] Tight binding of dactomycin to DNA results in inhibition of transcription (and therefore translation), RNA polymerase, and the activity of topoisomerases has the cumulative effect of decreasing mRNA levels and protein synthesis, eventually leading to cell death.[48]

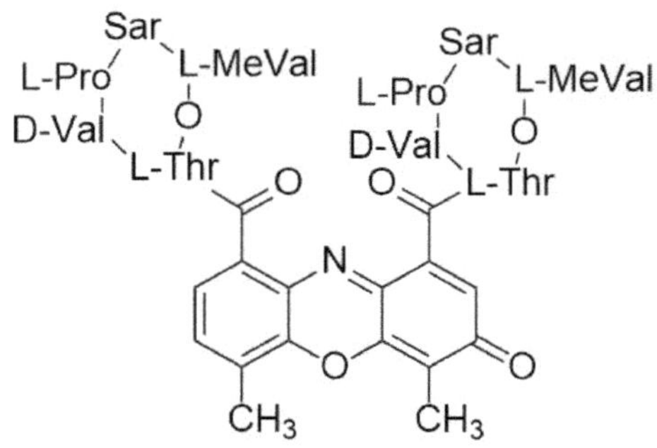

FIGURE 15.9 Dactinomycin natural product oncology agent.

Natural Products and Drugs Targeting Kinase Function

As oncology therapy has transitioned into the 21st century, development of selective and targeted therapeutics that inhibit kinases has been a major focus of research due to the importance of kinases in multiple-cell signaling pathways; their aberrant expression, activation, or mutation in various cancers; and the ability to discover inhibitors for these enzymes using high-throughput screening and rational design based on crystal structures. However, not to be left out of this new era of oncology drug development, natural products have also contributed NP-derived oncology agents to the pantheon of clinically useful kinase inhibitors.

Inhibitors of mTORC Kinase Function

Mammalian target of rapamycin (mTOR) is a serine/threonine kinase that phosphorylates and activates other kinases in cell-signaling pathways to promote de novo protein synthesis and cell growth.[50] Along with a kinase domain, mTOR possesses a macrolide binding domain containing two subunits.[50] The natural product rapamycin and the semisynthetic analogues that have been developed and introduced into the clinic bind the mTOR macrolide binding domain and inhibit the downstream phosphorylation activity of this kinase.

Rapamycin. Rapamycin is a polyketide natural product first isolated from the bacteria *Streptomyces hygroscopicus* in the 1970s. Due to its similarity to the immunosuppressant natural product FK506, rapamycin was originally developed as an immunosuppressant mTOR kinase inhibitor for use in organ transplant patients and is currently FDA approved for that activity.[51] Based on the role of mTOR in driving tumor growth and development, additional rapamycin derivatives were developed for use in oncology. Structurally, rapamycin is a 31-membered macrolide ring with 15 stereocenters, four olefins, four ketones, and pyran, piperidine, and cyclohexyl rings.[52] The two rapamycin analogues that are FDA approved

TABLE 15.3 Natural Products and Drugs Targeting Kinase Function

Mechanism of Action	Drug Class	Source	Species	Natural Product or Generic Name	Brand Name	Molecule Type	FDA Approval Year
Inhibitors of mTORC	Rapa-mycins	Bacteria	*Streptomyces hygroscopicus*	Rapamycin/ Sirolimus	Rapamune	Natural Product	N/A[a]
				Temsirolimus	Torisel	Semisynthetic NP Derivative	2007
				Everolimus	Afinitor	Semisynthetic NP Derivative	2009

a. Not FDA approved for use in oncology; approved FDA indication is for immunosuppression in transplant patients.

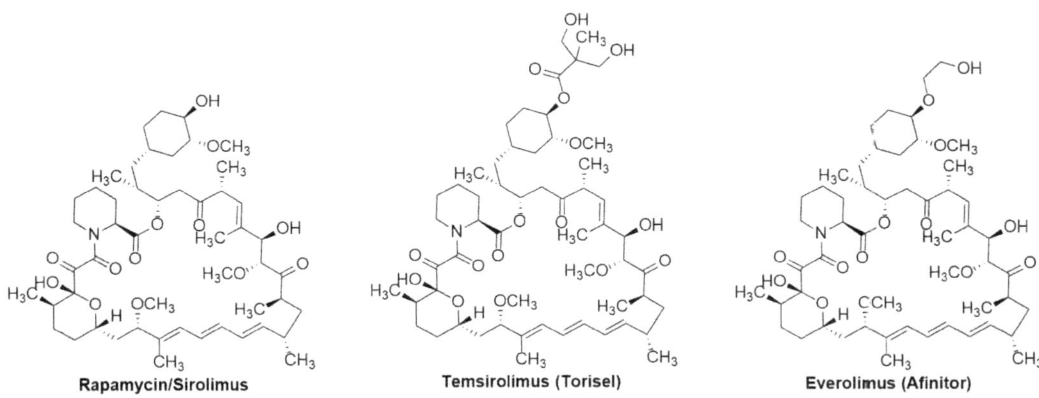

FIGURE 15.10 Rapamycin natural product and FDA-approved drugs.

for the treatment of cancer, temsirolimus,[53] and everolimus[54] differ from rapamycin only in the substitution at O13 substituent of the cyclohexyl ring. Both these NP-derived oncology agents retain their immunosuppressive activity in addition to having antitumor effect.

References

1. David J. Newman, Gordon M. Cragg, and Kenneth M. Snader, "Natural Products as Sources of New Drugs over the Period 1981–2002," *Journal of Natural Products* 66, no. 7 (2003): 1022–37.
2. David J. Newman and Gordon M. Cragg, "Natural Products as Sources of New Drugs over the Last 25 Years," *Journal of Natural Products* 70, no. 3 (2007): 461–77.

3. David J. Newman and Gordon M. Cragg, "Natural Products As Sources of New Drugs over the 30 Years from 1981 to 2010," *Journal of Natural Products* 75, no. 3 (2012): 311–35.
4. David J. Newman and Gordon M. Cragg, "Natural Products as Sources of New Drugs from 1981 to 2014," *Journal of Natural Products* 79, no. 3 (2016): 629–61.
5. Mary Ann Jordan, "Mechanism of Action of Antitumor Drugs that Interact with Microtubules and Tubulin," *Current Medicinal Chemistry: Anti-Cancer Agents* 2, no. 1 (2002): 1–17.
6. Mary Ann Jordan and Leslie Wilson, "Microtubules as a Target for Anticancer Drugs," *Nature Reviews Cancer* 4, no. 4 (2004): 253–65.
7. Federico Pellegrini and Daniel R. Budman, "Review: Tubulin Function, Action of Antitubulin Drugs, and New Drug Development," *Cancer Investigation* 23, no. 3 (2005): 264–73.
8. Leslie R. Noble, C. T. Beer, and Rosalind J. Cutts, "Role of Chance Observations in Chemotherapy: *Vinca rosea*," *Annals of the New York Academy of Sciences* 76, no. 3 (1958): 882–94.
9. Maryam Moudi et al., "Vinca Alkaloids," *International Journal of Preventive Medicine* 4, no. 11 (2013): 1231–35.
10. Homer L. Pearce and Mary Alice Miller, "The Evolution of Cancer Research and Drug Discovery at Lilly Research Laboratories," *Advances in Enzyme Regulation* 45, no. 1 (2005): 229–55.
11. Eric Rowinsky, "The Vinca Alkaloids," In *Holland-Frei Cancer Medicine*, 6th ed., edited by Robert C. Bast et al. (Hamilton, ON: BC Decker, 2003).
12. Péter Keglevich et al., "Modifications on the Basic Skeletons of Vinblastine and Vincristine," *Molecules* 17, no. 5 (2012): 5893–914.
13. Mary Ann Jordan, Douglas Thrower, and Leslie Wilson, "Mechanism of Inhibition of Cell Proliferation by Vinca Alkaloids," *Cancer Research* 51, no. 8 (1991): 2212.
14. Benoît Gigant et al., "Structural Basis for the Regulation of Tubulin by Vinblastine," *Nature* 435, no. 7041 (2005): 519–22.
15. Beth A. Weaver, "How Taxol/Paclitaxel Kills Cancer Cells," *Molecular Biology of the Cell* 25, no. 18 (2014): 2677–81.
16. Mansukhlal C. Wani et al., "Plant Antitumor Agents. VI. Isolation and Structure of Taxol, a Novel Antileukemic and Antitumor Agent from *Taxus brevifolia*," *Journal of the American Chemical Society* 93, no. 9 (1971): 2325–27.
17. Pierre Potier, "Rhône-Poulenc Lecture. Search and Discovery of New Antitumour Compounds," *Chemical Society Reviews* 21, no. 2 (1992): 113–19.
18. M. A. Jordan et al., "Mechanism of Mitotic Block and Inhibition of Cell Proliferation by Taxol at Low Concentrations," *Proceedings of the National Academy of Sciences USA* 90, no. 20 (1993): 9552.
19. Mikhail Blagosklonny, "Unwinding the Loop of Bcl-2 Phosphorylation," *Leukemia* 15, no. 6 (2001): 869–74.
20. K. C. Nicolaou et al., "Total Synthesis of Taxol," *Nature* 367, no. 6464 (1994): 630–34.

21. Srinivasa Rao et al., "Characterization of the Taxol Binding Site on the Microtubule: 2-(m-Azidobenzoyl) taxol Photolabels a Pepetide (Amino Acids 217–231) of β-Tubulin," *Journal of Biological Chemistry* 270, no. 35 (1995): 20235–38.
22. Robert A. Holton et al., "First Total Synthesis of Taxol. 1. Functionalization of the B Ring," *Journal of Am. Chemical Society* 116, no. 4 (1994): 1597–98.
23. Robert A. Holton et al., "First Total Synthesis of Taxol. 2. Completion of the C and D Rings," *Journal of the American Chemical Society* 116, no. 4 (1994): 1599–600.
24. Daniel Guenard, Francoise Gueritte-Voegelein, and Pierre Potier, "Taxol and Taxotere: Discovery, Chemistry, and Structure-Activity Relationships," *Accounts of Chemical Research* 26, no. 4 (1993): 160–67.
25. Stefano Forli, "Epothilones: From Discovery to Clinical Trials," *Current Topics in Medicinal Chemistry* 14, no. 20 (2014): 2312–21.
26. Daniel M. Bollag et al., "Epothilones, a New Class of Microtubule-stabilizing Agents with a Taxol-like Mechanism of Action," *Cancer Research* 55, no. 11 (1995): 2325.
27. Gerhard Höfle et al., "Epothilone A and B—Novel 16-Membered Macrolides with Cytotoxic Activity: Isolation, Crystal Structure, and Conformation in Solution," *Angewandte Chemie, International Edition in English* 35, no. 13–14 (1996): 1567–69.
28. K. C. Nicolaou, Frank Roschangar, and Dionisios Vourloumis, "Chemical Biology of Epothilones," *Angewandte Chemie, International Edition* 37, no. 15 (1998): 2014–45.
29. Yves Pommier et al., "DNA Topoisomerases and Their Poisoning by Anticancer and Antibacterial Drugs," *Chemistry and Biology* 17, no. 5 (2010): 421–33.
30. D. A. Gewirtz, "A Critical Evaluation of the Mechanisms of Action Proposed for the Antitumor Effects of the Anthracycline Antibiotics Adriamycin and Daunorubicin," *Biochemical Pharmacology* 57, no. 7 (1999): 727–41.
31. Alvaro Mordente et al., "New Developments in Anthracycline-Induced Cardiotoxicity," *Current Medicinal Chemistry* 16, no. 13 (2009): 1656–72.
32. Franco Zunino, Graziella Pratesi, and Paola Perego, "Role of the Sugar Moiety in the Pharmacological Activity of Anthracyclines: Development of a Novel Series of Disaccharide Analogs," *Biochemical Pharmacological* 61, no. 8 (2001): 933–38.
33. H. Barton Grossman et al., "Bacillus Calmette-Guérin Failures and Beyond: Contemporary Management of Non-Muscle-Invasive Bladder Cancer," *Reviews in Urology* 10, no. 4 (2008): 281–89.
34. Diego Dal Ben et al., "DNA Topoisomerase II Structures and Anthracycline Activity: Insights into Ternary Complex Formation," *Current Pharmaceutical Design* 13, no. 27 (2007): 2766–80.
35. Dawn Natalie Waterhouse et al., "A Comparison of Liposomal Formulations of Doxorubicin with Drug Administered in Free Form," *Drug Safety* 24, no. 12 (2001): 903–20.

36. Pradeep Kumar Naik et al., "The Binding Modes and Binding Affinities of Epipodophyllotoxin Derivatives with Human Topoisomerase IIα," *Journal of Molecular Graphics and Modelling* 29, no. 4 (2010): 546–64.
37. Ki-ho Lee et al., "Antitumor Agents, 107. New Cytotoxic 4-Alkylamino Analogues of 4'-Demethyl-Epipodophyllotoxin as Inhibitors of Human DNA Topoisomerase II," *Journal of Natural Products* 52, no. 3 (1989): 606–13.
38. Peter I. Clark and Maurice L. Slevin, "The Clinical Pharmacology of Etoposide and Teniposide," *Clinical Pharmacokinetics* 12, no. 4 (1987): 223–52.
39. Mark Kirschbaum, "Comeback for the Camptothecins?" *Leukemia and Lymphoma* 50, no. 12 (2009): 1914–15.
40. A. T. McPhail and G. A. Sim, "The Structure of Camptothecin: X-Ray Analysis of Camptothecin Iodoacetate," *Journal of the Chemical Society B* 0 (1968): 923–28.
41. William D. Kingsbury et al., "Synthesis of Water-Soluble (Aminoalkyl) Camptothecin Analogs: Inhibition of Topoisomerase I and Antitumor Activity," *Journal of Medicinal Chemistry* 34, no. 1 (1991): 98–107.
42. Bart Staker et al., "Structures of Three Classes of Anticancer Agents Bound to the Human Topoisomerase I–DNA Covalent Complex," *Journal of Medicinal Chemistry* 48, no. 7 (2005): 2336–45.
43. Y. Ando et al., "UGT1A1 Genotypes and Glucuronidation of SN-38, the Active Metabolite of Irinotecan," *Annals of Oncology* 9, no. 8 (1998): 845–47.
44. T. G. Burke and Z. Mi, "The Structural Basis of Camptothecin Interactions with Human Serum Albumin: Impact on Drug Stability," *Journal of Medicinal Chemistry* 37, no. 1 (1994): 40–46.
45. B. L. Staker, K. Hjerrild, M. D. Feese, C. A. Behnke, A. B. Burgin, and L. Stewart, "The Mechanism of Topoisomerase I Poisoning by a Camptothecin Analog," *Proceedings of the National Academy of Sciences USA* 99, no. 24 (2002): 15387.
46. Marie A. Colucci, Gavin D. Couch, and Christopher J. Moody, C. J. "Natural and Synthetic Quinones and Their Reduction by the Quinone Reductase Enzyme NQO1: From Synthetic Organic Chemistry to Compounds with Anticancer Potential," *Organic and Biomolecular Chemistry* 6, no. 4 (2008): 637–56.
47. Marina S. Chow, Lei V. Liu, and Edward I. Solomon, "Further Insights into the Mechanism of the Reaction of Activated Bleomycin with DNA," *Proceedings of the National Academy of Sciences USA* 105, no. 36 (2008): 13241.
48. Hyun-Jin Kang and Hyun-Ju Park, "Novel Molecular Mechanism for Actinomycin D Activity as an Oncogenic Promoter G-Quadruplex Binder," *Biochemistry* 48, no. 31 (2009): 7392–98.
49. Randy M. Wadkins et al., "Actinomycin D Binding to Single-stranded DNA: Sequence Specificity and Hemi-intercalation Model from Fluorescence and1H NMR Spectroscopy," *Journal of Molecular Biology* 262, no. 1 (1996): 53–68.

50. Robert A. Saxton and David M. Sabatini, "mTOR Signaling in Growth, Metabolism, and Disease," *Cell* 168, no. 6 (2017): 960–76.
51. Jing Li, Sang Gyun Kim, and John Blenis, "Rapamycin: One Drug, Many Effects," *Cell Metabolism* 19, no. 3 (2014): 373–79.
52. K. C. Nicolaou et al., "Total Synthesis of Rapamycin," *Journal of the American Chemical Society* 115, no. 10 (1993): 4419–20.
53. Brian I. Rini, "Temsirolimus, an Inhibitor of Mammalian Target of Rapamycin," *Clinical Cancer Research* 14, no. 5 (2008): 1286.
54. David Lebwohl et al., "Research and Innovation in the Development of Everolimus for Oncology," *Expert Opinion on Drug Discovery* 6, no. 3 (2011): 323–38.

Chapter 16

Natural Products Used for the Treatment of Respiratory Symptoms

Keith C. Ellis, John M. Saathoff, and Jacqueline L. West

Ailments of the respiratory tract are typically caused either by an infectious disease (bacterial or viral infection) or by an inflammatory condition such as asthma, chronic obstructive pulmonary disorder, or environmental allergies. There are also more serious respiratory conditions, such as the genetic disease cystic fibrosis, pulmonary fibrosis, and multiple forms of lung cancer. While there are no natural products or NP-derived drugs that treat the specific underlying causes of these diseases (with the exception of antibiotics, which are covered elsewhere), there are natural products and NP-derived drugs that treat the respiratory symptoms that accompany these diseases. Many of these drugs are available as over-the-counter, FDA-approved drugs, while others are typically sold as a health supplement or nutraceutical product. Natural products and NP-derived drugs are available that act as decongestants, bronchodilators, cough suppressants, and immune system stimulants to help cope with the symptoms of respiratory diseases.

Decongestants and Bronchodilators

Systemic

Ma Huang

Ma huang is an extract of the *Ephedra sinica* plant and other members of the Ephedraceae plant family that has long been used in traditional Chinese medicine as a decongestant and bronchodilator. Ma huang is the original source of ephedrine and has been traditionally been used to treat asthma and upper respiratory congestion. The major component of the natural product extract is (-)-ephedrine and also contains (+)-pseudoephedrine and other alkaloids.[1] Typically the extract is taken orally or as nasal drops, but the intact herb can also be ingested, which attenuates some of the negative side effects. Unlike pharmaceutical preparations that contain pure

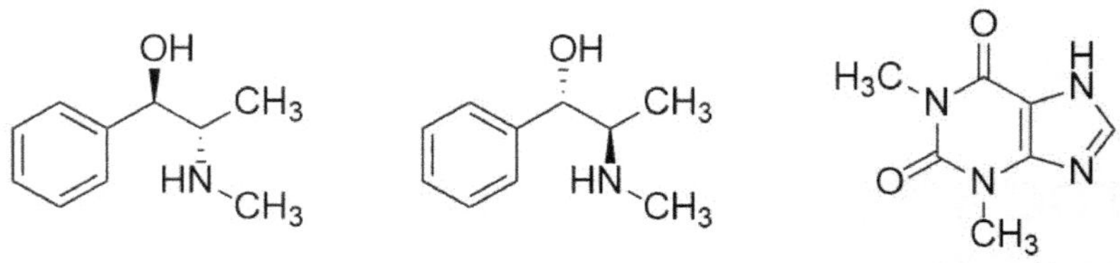

Ephedrine **Pseudoephedrine** **Theophylline**

FIGURE 16.1 Systemic decongestants and bronchodilators.

(-)-ephedrine and (+)-pseudoephedrine APIs, the concentrations of these active alkaloids can vary in the natural product extracts, leading to potentially dangerous side effects.[1] In addition to the decongestant and bronchodilation effects of ma huang, the natural product extract can cause increases in blood pressure and other adverse cardiac events, so care must be taken in patients with these diseases.

Theophylline

Theophylline is a xanthine natural product, similar to caffeine, that is isolated from cocoa, coffee, and tea plants. The natural product is typically isolated and purified from these sources and is used as a purified compound to treat asthma and other conditions with cause airway obstruction symptoms.[2] The typical dose for theophylline is 125–250 mg three times daily, but the compound has a narrow therapeutic window due to off-target toxicities, which include tachycardia, palpitations, nausea, and gastrointestinal irritation.[2]

Oils Used in Inhalants and Oral Lozenges

Eucalyptus

Eucalyptus oil is a natural liquid produced by oil glands found in the leaves of trees in the myrtle family Myrtaceae. There are several hundred species in this family, most of them native to Australia.[3] Eucalyptus oil has several traditional medicinal uses, including as a bronchodilator, expectorant, antispasmodic, and insect repellent.[3] Eucalyptus oil can be ingested in small quantities internally; in large quantities it is an irritant and causes gastrointestinal distress. Due to this, eucalyptus oil is commonly applied topically as an ointment or rub and inhaled to take advantage of the bronchodilator effects for people with colds, coughs, or bronchitis. Eucalyptus oil contains a variety of aromatic natural products, with 1,8-cineole (eucalyptol) as the major component, along with other compounds, including terpineol, α-pinene, and *p*-cymene.[3]

Camphor

Camphor is a terpenoid natural product that is isolated in pure form from the Asian camphor tree *Cinnamomum camphora*.[4] Structurally, camphor possesses a bridged cyclic ring

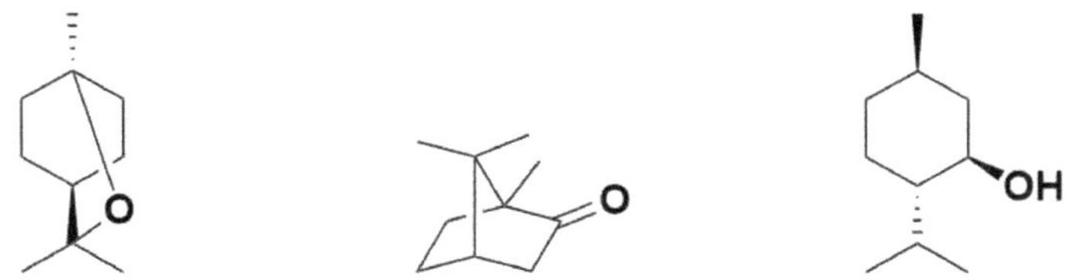

1,8-Cineole (eucalyptol) **Camphor** **(-)-Menthol**

FIGURE 16.2 Inhaled decongestants and bronchodilators.

system and has a low boiling point, contributing to its pleasant aroma and ability to be used as an inhaled therapeutic. Camphor has several medicinal uses, including as a decongestant and antiseptic.[5] While once used internally, it is now used only topically due to the fact that ingestion of high doses can cause vomiting, convulsions, and heart palpitations.[6] When used medicinally as a decongestant, camphor is typically mixed with other essential oils such as eucalyptus.

Menthol

Menthol is a monoterpene natural product that is isolated as mint oil or in pure form from multiple species of mint plants from the *Mentha* genus.[7] Whole mint oil, including peppermint oil, is often used in herbal preparations to treat respiratory infections, and pure menthol acts as a decongestant, leading to its use in many oral lozenges, nasal sprays, and inhalers.[7] Menthol can only be ingested in small quantities for therapeutic use; ingestion of pure menthol or mint oils in larger doses can cause irritation and gastrointestinal distress.[7]

Cough Suppressants

Codeine

Codeine is an opioid natural product that is found in opium and is isolated from the seeds of the poppy flower *Papaver somniferum*.[8] Structurally, codeine is an alkaloid and can be defined as the 3-methyl analogue of morphine. Codeine is found at concentrations of 1–3 percent in opium isolated from the poppy flower, but modern medicinal preparations use pure codeine that has been chemically synthesized.[8] Codeine has multiple medicinal uses, including as a cough suppressant and for pain treatment. The codeine dosage for cough suppression is typically 5–10 mg every four hours,

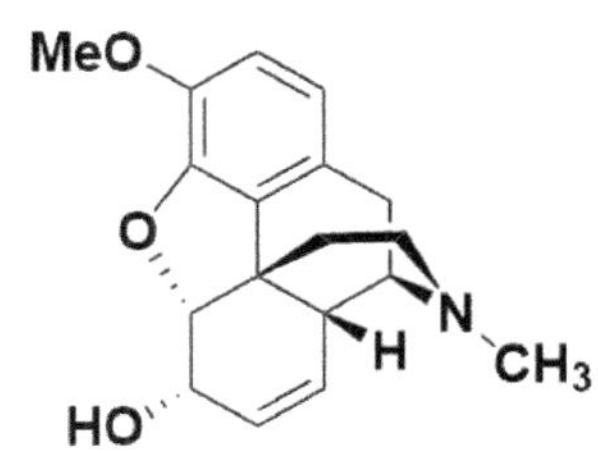

Codeine

FIGURE 16.3 The cough suppressant codeine.

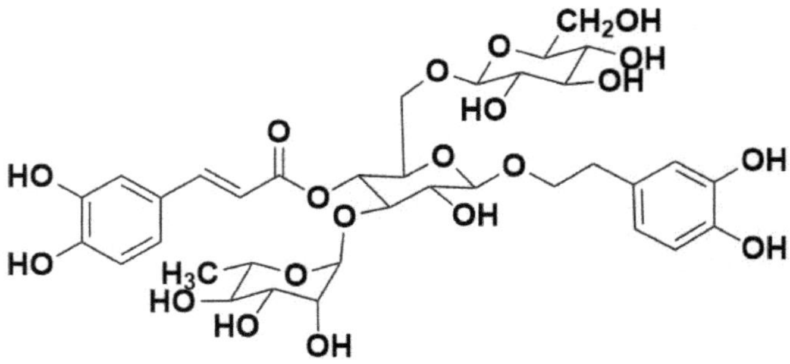

FIGURE 16.4 The immune system stimulant echinacoside.

with a daily maximum of 60 mg; this is far below the codeine dosage for pain, which is typically 240 mg/day in divided doses.[9] Care must be taken in the use of codeine, due to its sedative and respiratory depression effects. For these reasons, codeine is not recommended for use in children.[9]

Immune System Stimulants

Echinacea

Echinacea is an extract prepared from the roots of plants of the genus *Echinacea*, which are a member of the daisy family. It was widely used as a traditional medicine by American Indian Plains tribes for the treatment of respiratory symptoms such as coughs, sore throat, and pain.[10] The pharmacologically active constituent(s) of echinacea have not been identified; however, one such component is thought to be the caffeic acid derivative echinacoside.[10] Echinacea products are typically made of extracts from three or more species, with very little standardization or quality control. Little clinical evidence is available to support the claims that echinacea has immunostimulant effects.[11][12] However, there is some evidence that echinacea is effective in the treatment of respiratory infections.[13][14]

References

1. Bill J. Gurley, Peiling Wang, and Stephanie F. Gardner, "Ephedrine-Type Alkaloid Content of Nutritional Supplements Containing Ephedra Sinica (Ma-Huang) as Determined by High Performance Liquid Chromatography," *Journal of Pharmaceutical Sciences* 87, no. 12 (1998): 1547–53.

2. Peter J. Barnes, "Theophylline," *American Journal of Respiratory and Critical Care Medicine* 188, no. 8 (2013): 901–6.
3. Ashok K. Dhakad et al., "Biological, Medicinal and Toxicological Significance of Eucalyptus Leaf Essential Oil: A Review," *Journal of the Science of Food and Agriculture* 98, no. 3 (2018): 833–48.
4. Shanshan Guo et al., "The Chemical Composition of Essential Oils from *Cinnamomum camphora* and Their Insecticidal Activity Against the Stored Product Pests," *International Journal of Molecular Sciences* 17, no. 11 (2016): 1836.
5. R. Eccles, Barbara Lancashire, and N. S. Tolley, "The Effect of Aromatics on Inspiratory and Expiratory Nasal Resistance to Airflow," *Clinical Otolaryngology and Allied Sciences* 12, no. 1 (1987): 11–14.
6. Dana Bartlett, "Dangerous in Small Amounts: Ten Nondrug Substances That Cause Harm," *Journal of Emergency Nursing* 29, no. 4 (2003): 377–79.
7. Guy Paulin Poungoue Kamatou et al., "Menthol: A Simple Monoterpene with Remarkable Biological Properties," *Phytochemistry* 96 (2013): 15–25.
8. Christopher C. Presley and Craig W. Lindsley, "DARK Classics in Chemical Neuroscience: Opium, a Historical Perspective," *ACS Chemical Neuroscience* 9, no. 10 (2018): 2503–18.
9. "Drugs for Cough," *Medical Letter on Drugs and Therapeutics* 60, no. 1562 (2018): 206–8.
10. Mehdi Sharifi-Rad et al., "Echinacea Plants as Antioxidant and Antibacterial Agents: From Traditional Medicine to Biotechnological Applications," *Phytotherapy Research* 32, no. 9 (2018): 1653–63.
11. Wolfram Grimm and Hans-Helge Müller, "A Randomized Controlled Trial of the Effect of Fluid Extract of *Echinacea purpurea* on the Incidence and Severity of Colds and Respiratory Infections," *American Journal of Medicine* 106, no. 2 (1999): 138–43.
12. Ronald B. Turner, Donald K. Riker, and J. David Gangemi, "Ineffectiveness of Echinacea for Prevention of Experimental Rhinovirus Colds," *Antimicrobial Agents and Chemotherapy* 44, no. 6 (2000): 1708–9.
13. G. Frank Lindenmuth and Elise B. Lindenmuth, "The Efficacy of Echinacea Compound Herbal Tea Preparation on the Severity and Duration of Upper Respiratory and Flu Symptoms: A Randomized, Double-Blind Placebo-Controlled Study," *Journal of Alternative and Complementary Medicine* 6, no. 4 (2000): 327–34.
14. V. Goel et al., "Efficacy of a Standardized Echinacea Preparation (EchinilinTM) for the Treatment of the Common Cold: A Randomized, Double-Blind, Placebo-Controlled Trial," *Journal of Clinical Pharmacy and Therapeutics* 29, no. 1 (2004): 75–83.

Chapter 17

Natural Products Used for the Treatment of Gastrointestinal Symptoms

Keith C. Ellis, John M. Saathoff, and Jacqueline L. West

Ailments of the gastrointestinal tract can arise from a number of different causes, including infections (ulcers, diarrhea), inflammation (irritable bowel syndrome), environment (motion sickness), side effects of therapeutics (chemotherapeutics, opioids), and poor diet. While there are many traditional natural remedies that are often suggested to alleviate gastrointestinal symptoms, little clinical evidence is available to support most claims. Here we describe natural products that do have observed efficacy for gastrointestinal symptoms associated with nausea and vomiting, as well as irritable bowel syndrome.

Nausea and Vomiting

Nausea and vomiting are often experienced during ailments such as the flu and food poisoning, as well as during pregnancy and as the result of motion sickness. While many antiemetic pharmaceuticals are available and widely used, there are two natural products that are used for the treatment of nausea and vomiting: ginger and hyoscine.

Ginger

Ginger is an aromatic and pungent spice with an ancient history of use as a medicinal agent, dating back to classical Greek and Roman cultures. The ginger plant (*Zingiber officianale*) and the roots that are used as the spice are cultivated in warm tropical climates throughout the world, including Asia, Africa, India, and the Caribbean. Ginger can be isolated as both an essential oil from the rhizome and as a powder prepared from the dried rhizome.[1] The essential oil contains phenolic compounds with carbon side chains of seven or more compounds, such as 6-gingerol, that are responsible for the aromatic smell and taste.[1] When the rhizome is dried,

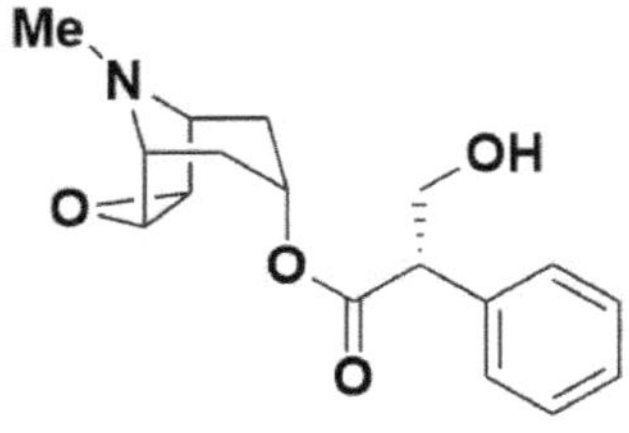

(-)-Hyoscine

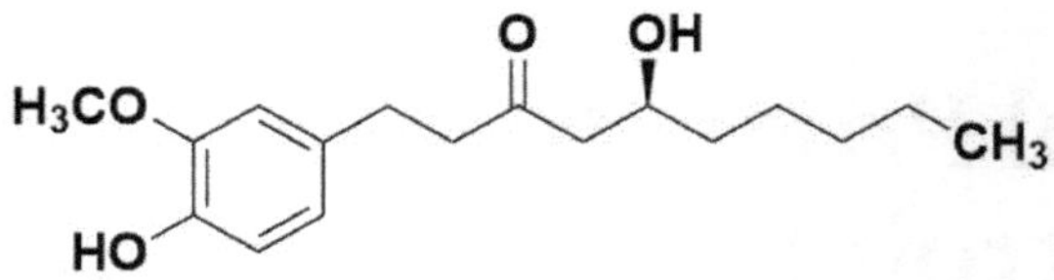

6-Gingerol

FIGURE 17.1 Hyoscine and 6-gingerol.

the gingerols are dehydrated to form shogaols, which are unsaturated carbon chains and are twice as aromatic and pungent as the gingerols.[1] This conversion of gingerols to shogaols and the increase in pungency is why ginger powder is stronger than the essential oils or fresh rhizome.[1] Ginger, especially in the form of ginger ale, is commonly suggested as a treatment for nausea and vomiting in ailments including the flu and food poisoning.[2] However, there is no clinical data to support its use under those circumstances. Three randomized clinical trials have been performed and show that ginger is an effective treatment for nausea and vomiting induced by seasickness, morning sickness, and chemotherapy.[2] However, the natural product was not effective for postoperative nausea in those three clinical trials.[2]

Hyoscine (Scopolamine)

The natural product hyoscine, also referred to as scopolamine, is a tropane alkaloid isolated from multiple species of the *Scolpolia* genus. Hyoscine is a popular remedy for motion sickness and seasickness, including for divers, and is available both as an oral dose of 400 g and as a 2 mg transdermal patch.[3] Structurally, the tropane ring system is reminiscent of cocaine, and like cocaine, hyoscine acts as a CNS agent.[4] The antiemetic effect of hyoscine results from it acting as an antagonist of the muscarinic acetylcholine M1 receptor.[3] Side effects of hyoscine include delirium, delusions, elevation in body temperature, and possibly death.[3] Hyoscine had been used for morning sickness in the past; that suggested use has been discontinued due to health concerns for both the mother and fetus. Hyoscine's pseudonym, scopolamine, is often referred to in pop culture, movies, and literature as a truth serum or abduction drug similar to rohypnol; however, there is no clinical evidence to document those effects.

Irritable Bowel Syndrome

Irritable bowel syndrome (IBS) is a functional gastrointestinal disorder characterized by pain in the lower left abdomen, with diarrhea and/or constipation not caused by any known underlying condition. While the diarrhea and constipation symptoms can be treated with antidiarrheal medications (such as loperamide) and bulk laxatives, respectively, there are few other pharmaceutical treatments for IBS. The natural product peppermint offers some relief for IBS under certain circumstances.

Peppermint

Peppermint is a naturally occurring hybrid of the species of water mint (*Mentha aquatica*) and spearmint (*Mentha spicate*) known since circa 2600 BC Egypt. Therapeutic preparations from the plant include teas brewed from the leaves and peppermint oil collected by steam distillation of the plant. Both preparations have medicinal uses, as both contain high concentrations of (-)-menthol. Caution must be taken, however, in how the natural product is administered for treatment of IBS. While (-)-menthol is an antispasmodic and can be used to treat IBS, the desired site of action is in the intestine, not the stomach. Peppermint oil ingested directly actually acts as an irritant to the stomach and does not provide relief from IBS symptoms. Enteric-coated peppermint oil capsules are effective for IBS, as they allow delivery and absorption exclusively in the intestine, bypassing irritation to the stomach. The efficacy of this formulation was tested in a placebo-controlled randomized trial, which found that 75 percent of patients in the peppermint capsule group showed a >50 percent reduction in total IBS symptoms, compared to 38 percent in the placebo group, offering evidence that the natural product is effective for IBS.[5] The antispasmodic activity of (-)-menthol has been shown to be due to its action as a Ca^{2+} antagonist.[6]

References

1. Dabo Pan et al., "Non-volatile Pungent Compounds Isolated from *Zingiber officinale* and Their Mechanisms of Action," *Food and Function* 10, no. 2 (2019): 1203–11.
2. Wolfgang Marx et al., "Ginger—Mechanism of Action in Chemotherapy-Induced Nausea and Vomiting: A Review," *Critical Reviews in Food Science and Nutrition* 57, no. 1 (2017): 141–46.
3. Ruirui Qi et al., "Anti-Cholinergics Mecamylamine and Scopolamine Alleviate Motion Sickness-Induced Gastrointestinal Symptoms Through Both Peripheral and Central Actions," *Neuropharmacology* 146 (2019): 252–63.
4. Kathrin Laura Kohnen-Johannsen and Oliver Kayser, "Tropane Alkaloids: Chemistry, Pharmacology, Biosynthesis and Production," *Molecules* 24, no. 4 (2019): 796.
5. G. Cappello et al., "Peppermint Oil (Mintoil®) in the Treatment of Irritable Bowel Syndrome: A Prospective Double Blind Placebo-Controlled Randomized Trial," *Digestive and Liver Disease* 39, no. 6 (2007): 530–36.
6. Bruno P. Chumpitazi, Gregory L. Kearns, and Robert J. Shulman, "Review Article: The Physiological Effects and Safety of Peppermint Oil and Its Efficacy in Irritable Bowel Syndrome and Other Functional Disorders," *Alimentary Pharmacology and Therapeutics* 47, no. 6 (2018): 738–52.

Chapter 18

Natural Products as CNS Stimulants

Yana Cen

Introduction

Natural products have been rich sources of biologically active small molecules. As a matter of fact, more than 45 percent of the bestselling drugs on the market these days are derived from natural products.[1][2] Many of the naturally occurring compounds target the central nervous system (CNS). Natural product stimulants can be classified into two major categories: analeptics and central stimulants. Analeptics are stimulants that primarily influence the autonomic functions of the body, including respiration, circulation, and urination.[3] Strychnine and picrotoxin are examples of analeptics. These natural products generally are not associated with abuse problems. The second major category of natural stimulants are the central stimulants or behavioral stimulants. These are molecules that primarily influence motor activity, such as cocaine, cathinone, and ephedrine. Unfortunately, most of these compounds are closely associated with drug addiction and drug abuse issues. The following discussion will focus on a selected group of central stimulants. Individual molecules, along with their plant source(s), synthetic analogs, and actions, will be introduced first, followed by a section summarizing the mechanisms of action (MOAs) of these stimulants.

Caffeine

Caffeine, or 1,3,7-trimethylxanthine, is a methylated xanthine derivative (see Figure 18.1). Caffeine is unique because it has both analeptic and mild central stimulant actions. It helps restore alertness and reduce fatigue. At the same time, caffeine can also serve as a metabolic stimulant. Many weight loss products contain high concentrations of caffeine. Addiction to caffeine and

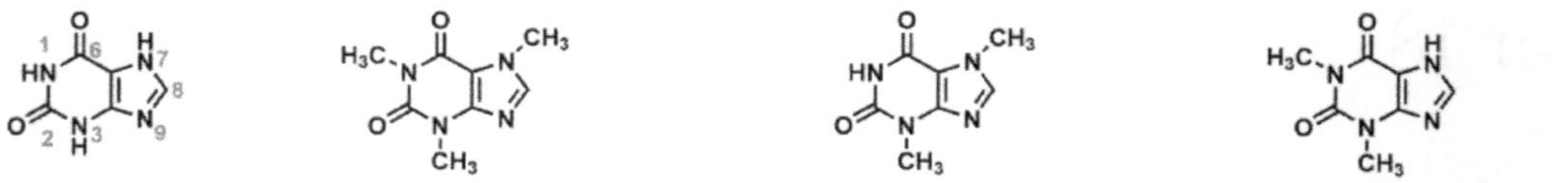

Xanthine | Caffeine (1,3,7-trimethylxanthine) | Theobromine (3,7-dimethylxanthine) | Theophylline (1,3-dimethylxanthine)

FIGURE 18.1 Chemical structures of caffeine and related compounds.

the associated withdrawal phenomena are well documented.[4][5] Caffeine is not the only naturally occurring xanthine analog. Theobromine and theophylline (see Figure 18.1) are dimethylated xanthine derivatives isolated from botanical sources, both of which are stimulants but less potent than caffeine.[6][7]

Caffeinated beverages are among the most popular beverages in the world. In the United States alone, more than 90 percent of people consume at least one caffeinated beverage on a daily basis.[8] Caffeine, therefore, is considered the most popular legal psychoactive substance in the world. Caffeine has a long and rich history in human civilization. Nearly every major civilization has had a favorite caffeine-containing drink. Coffee beans can be roasted and brewed. The leaves of coffee plants can be chewed directly to gain energy. In certain cultures, coffee beans are mixed with other ingredients to create an "energy bar" type of snack.[9] Caffeine can be isolated from coffee plants, and these plants were first discovered on the Ethiopian plateau, according to folklore.[9] The goatherds noticed that their goats became extremely energetic after eating the fruits of the coffee shrub. Later on, these plants were brought to and cultivated in other parts of the world, such as Asia and the Middle East regions. Coffee gained popularity quickly in these areas. For example, in the 1500s, there were coffeehouses on almost every corner in Istanbul, sort of like Starbucks is today. Coffee was first introduced to the United States in the 1600s but only became popular after the 1773 Boston Tea Party event.[10] This event forever changed the American drinking preference to coffee.

Caffeine and related xanthine analogs occur naturally in coffee plants (see Figure 18.2). There are more than 120 different species of coffee plants, among which *Coffea arabica* is the best known and *Coffea robusta* has a higher caffeine content.[11] Different cultivation conditions, constituents in the coffee plants, brewing methods, and flavoring ingredients greatly impact the taste and aroma of coffee. Coffee plants are rich in not only caffeine and xanthine derivatives but also more than 1,500 other chemical substances.

In addition to coffee plants, caffeine and methyl xanthine analogs can also be found in chocolate, tea, guarana, maté, and cola. The caffeine contents in different plant sources are listed in Table 18.1.

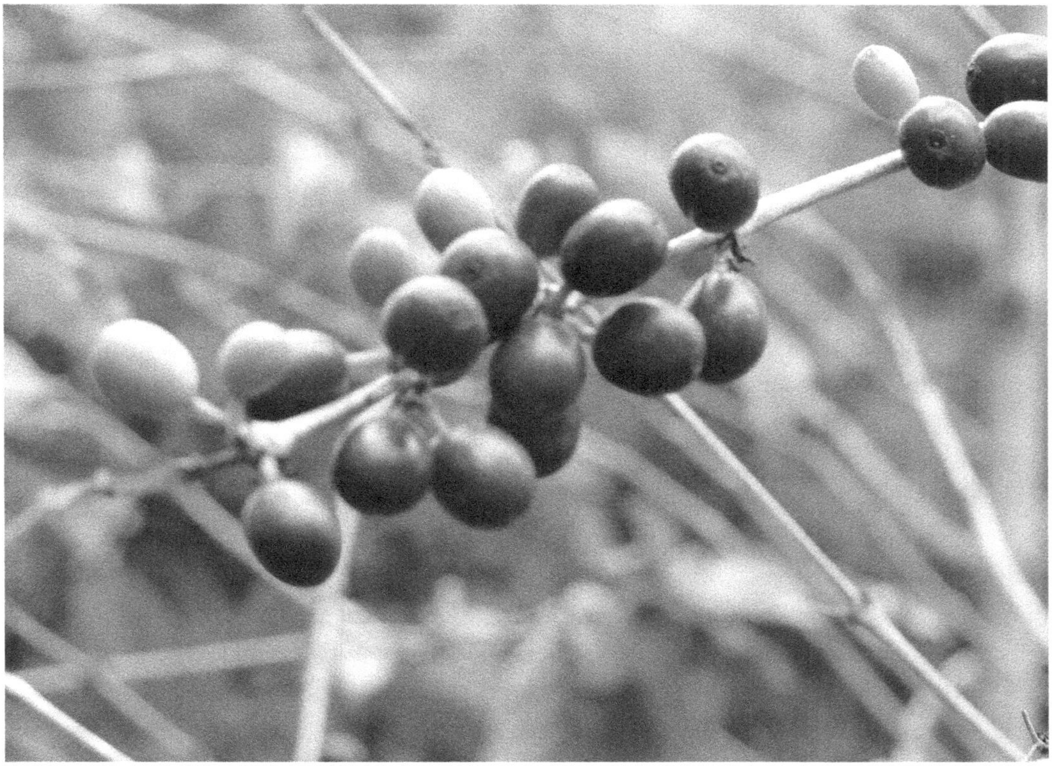

FIGURE 18.2 A close-up of *Coffea arabica*. The coffee beans are inside the plant's green and red berries.

TABLE 18.1 Comparison of Plant Caffeine Content[a]

	Approximate Caffeine % (by weight)
Coffee Bean (Arabica)	1.1
Coffee Bean (Robusta)	2.2
Tea (leaf and bud)	3.5
Cola Nut	1.5
Cacao Bean	0.03
Guarana Seed	> 4
Maté Leaf	0.7

[a]*Adapted from reference 12.*

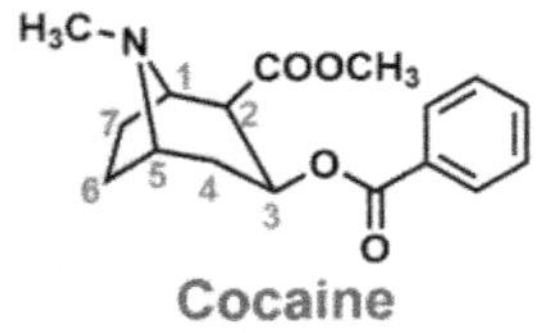

FIGURE 18.3 Chemical structure of cocaine.

Cocaine

Cocaine belongs to the alkaloid family (see Figure 18.3). The coca tree (*Erythoxylum coca*) is the major botanical source of this compound. The coca tree was once called the "divine plant of the Incas."[13] The leaves are chewed to avert hunger and fatigue. Nowadays coca leaves are still legally available in some countries, such as Bolivia and Peru. Cocaine, the active ingredient in coca leaf, was first isolated in the mid-1800s and became extremely popular right away.[14] However, it also caused a major drug abuse problem (e.g., "crack"). Cocaine is classified as a Schedule II Controlled Substance and can be used as an ocular and nasal anesthetic in clinical practice.

Ephedrine

Ephedrine is found in *Ephedra sinica*, a plant that is indigenous to China.[15] It has been used by the Chinese for more than 5,000 years as an herbal medication or home remedy for a variety of health problems, including asthma, flu, circulatory problems, and appetite control. Today, ephedrine-related synthetics are used for similar purposes and also for "recreational" purposes. Due to constriction of the blood vessels and increased heart rate leading to, in some cases, death from hypertension, the FDA issued a ruling to prohibit the sales of dietary supplements containing ephedra in 2004.[16]

The simplicity of ephedrine's chemical structure (see Figure 18.4) prompted the production of synthetic analogs such as amphetamine and methamphetamine (see Figure 18.4). Both compounds act as potent CNS stimulants to suppress appetite and induce sympathomimetic effects.[17] Ephedrine, on the other hand, has significantly reduced stimulant potency due to the presence of the hydroxyl group, which decreases its ability to cross the blood-brain barrier. Ephedrine can be used to illegally synthesize methamphetamine in one step in clandestine laboratories.[18]

Ephedrine has four possible stereoisomers: (+)/(–)-ephedrine and (+)/(–)-pseudoephedrine (see Figure 18.5). Pseudoephedrine is used as a bronchodilator but is less effective than ephedrine.[19]

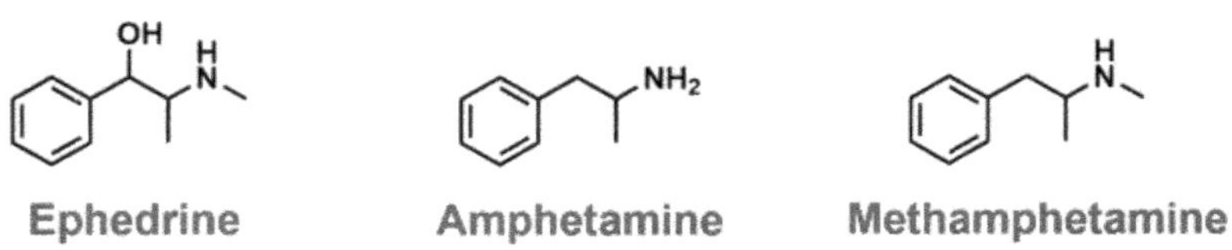

FIGURE 18.4 Chemical structures of ephedrine and related synthetic analogs.

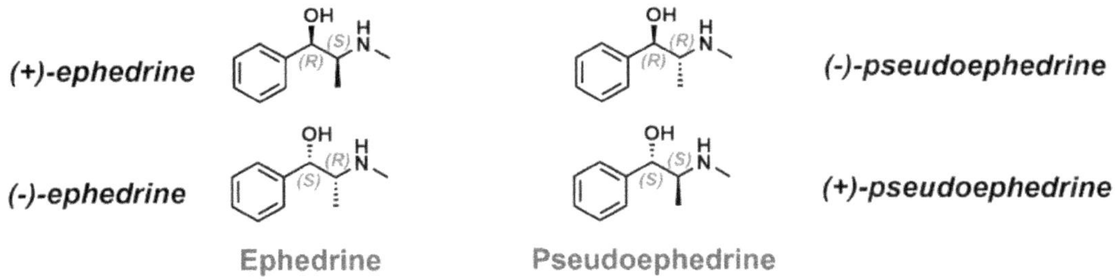

FIGURE 18.5 Stereoisomers of ephedrine.

Cathinone

Cathinone is isolated from the plant khat (*Catha edulis*), a shrub native to East Africa.[20] It is a naturally occurring aromatic ketone. Khat leaves are chewed or brewed as a tea for their stimulant action in the same way many use coffee. Aged khat leaves are less desirable, because during the aging process, cathinone can be reduced to its less potent analog, cathine (see Figure 18.6).[21] Cathinone is classified as a Schedule I Controlled Substance. Methcathinone (MCAT), methedrone, flephedrone, and mephedrone are the synthetic analogs of cathinone (see Figure 18.6). Collectively, they are called the "bath salts." These psychoactive compounds have been greatly abused as "recreational" drugs for their rewarding properties.[22]

Basics of Neurotransmission

Neurotransmission is a signal transduction process that promotes neuronal communication and interaction. In order to do so, the neurons utilize a special group of small molecules called "neurotransmitters." Examples of neurotransmitters include dopamine and serotonin. Normally the neurotransmitters are stored in the synaptic vesicles inside the presynaptic neurons

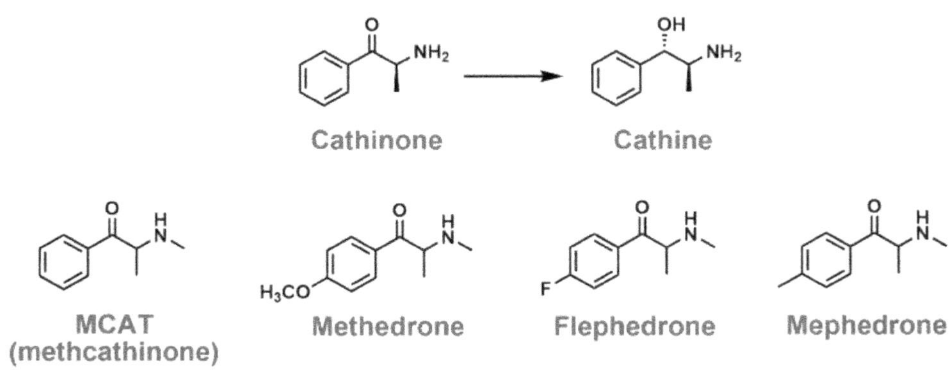

FIGURE 18.6 Chemical structures of cathinone and related compounds.

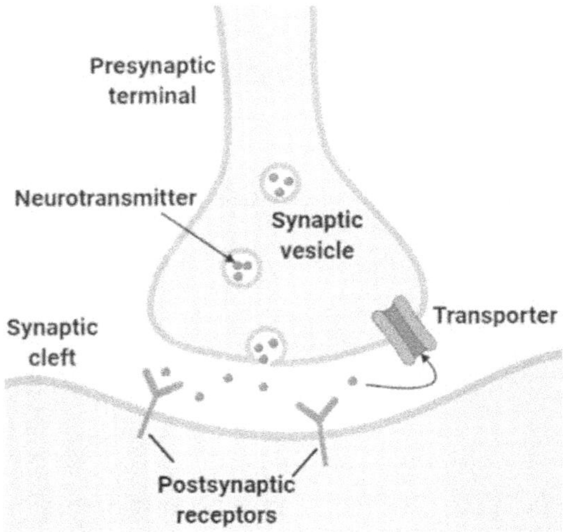

FIGURE 18.7 Schematic representation of neurotransmission.

(see Figure 18.7). When required, the neurotransmitters will be released into the synaptic cleft between the two neurons. Subsequently, they diffuse across the synaptic cleft and interact with the receptors located on the postsynaptic neurons to induce cellular responses. Similar to all the other signal transduction processes, neurotransmission needs to be properly terminated when the desired physiological response is completed. This is accomplished through the reuptake of neurotransmitters by the transporter proteins, which are normally unidirectional. The neurotransmitters can then be re-stored in the synaptic vesicles, waiting for the next round of neurotransmission events.

Mechanism of Action (MOA)

Dopamine is a neurotransmitter that plays critical roles in the regulation of locomotion, cognition, and emotion.[23] Both amphetamine and cocaine can influence dopamine transmission. Amphetamine triggers the release of dopamine into the synaptic cleft by reversing the action of dopamine transporters (see Figure 18.8, left).[24] Cocaine, on the other hand, blocks the transporters to prevent the reuptake of dopamine (see Figure 18.8, right).[25]

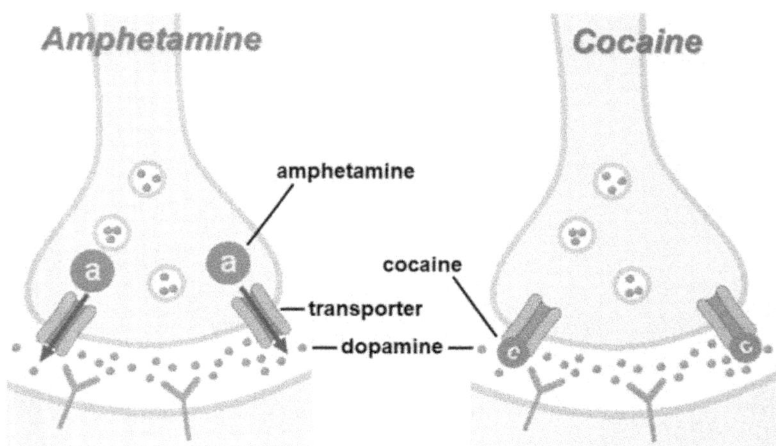

FIGURE 18.8 Mechanism of action of amphetamine (left) and cocaine (right).

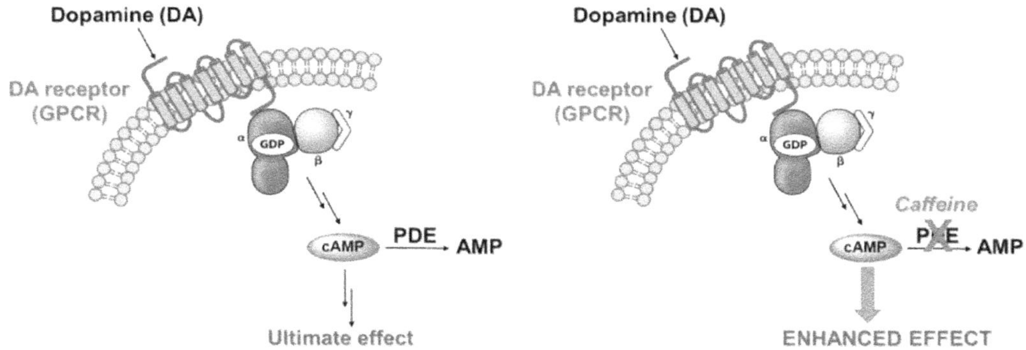

FIGURE 18.9 Caffeine is a weak PDE inhibitor. Left: Dopamine-induced signal transduction pathway. Right: Caffeine suppresses PDE activity to potentiate the physiological response.

Ultimately, amphetamine and cocaine both increase synaptic dopamine levels to activate postsynaptic dopamine receptors.

As mentioned above, dopamine in the synaptic cleft starts interacting with the dopamine receptors to initiate the downstream signaling process. Upon binding to dopamine, the dopamine receptor, which belongs to the GPCR family, will bind and activate the G protein (see Figure 18.9, left). This signal will be further amplified by several other enzymes to significantly elevate the concentration of cyclic AMP (cAMP), an important second messenger. The increased level of cAMP stimulates various cellular events to induce the ultimate physiological response. The intracellular cAMP concentration is tightly and precisely regulated by phosphodiesterase (PDE), which converts cAMP to AMP. Caffeine acts as a weak inhibitor of PDE to maintain a high level of cAMP, leading to enhanced effects (see Figure 18.9, right).[26]

cAMP participates in many signaling processes.[27] Its ability to interact and activate other cellular proteins and enzymes accounts for its widespread use as a second messenger. In dopamine signaling, cAMP is able to stimulate some downstream regulatory proteins for the ultimate effects (see Figure 18.10, left). The same set of regulatory proteins is also under the tonic inhibitory control of adenosine signaling, a process mediated by adenosine receptor A_{2A} (see Figure 18.10, right). Caffeine also serves as an A_{2A} antagonist.[28] It blocks the inhibitory effect on the regulatory proteins to potentiate the final effects. In summary, caffeine's MOA is twofold: to increase cAMP level via inhibiting PDE and to derepress the regulatory proteins via antagonizing adenosine receptor.

This chapter focuses on a selected group of naturally occurring central stimulants. These seemingly simple structures have profound CNS activities, many of which contribute to drug addiction and abuse. The chemical structures of the abovementioned natural products, their natural sources, and the botanical names are summarized in Table 18.2.

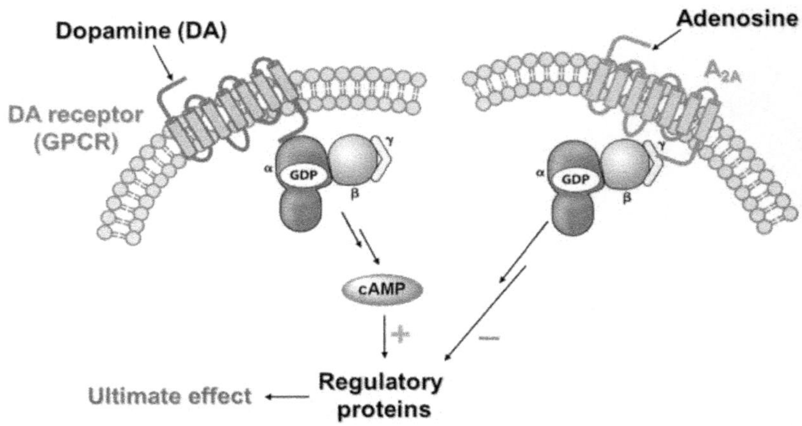

FIGURE 18.10 Dopamine- and adenosine-signaling processes target the same group of regulatory proteins. Left: Increased cAMP in dopamine pathway activates the regulatory proteins. Right: Adenosine pathway suppresses these proteins.

TABLE 18.2 Summary of the Naturally Occurring CNS Stimulants

Constituent	***Natural Source***	***Examples***	***Structure***
Caffeine	**Coffee**	***Coffea arabica***	
	Tea	***Camellia sinensis***	
	Chocolate	***Theobroma cacao***	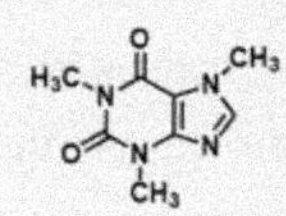
	Guarana	***Paullinia cupana***	
	Kola (Cola)	***Cola acuminate***	
	Yerba Mate	***Ilex paraguariensis***	
Cocaine	**Coca Leaf**	***Erythroxylum coca***	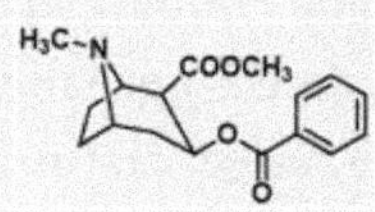
Ephedrine	**Ephedra**	***Ephedra sinica***	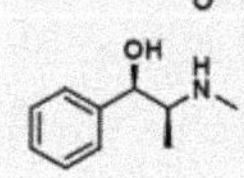
Cathinone	**Khat**	***Catha edulis***	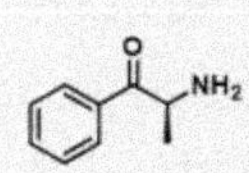

References

1. Frank E. Koehn and Guy Thomas Carter, "The Evolving Role of Natural Products in Drug Discovery," *Nature Reviews Drug Discovery* 4, no. 3 (2005): 206–20.
2. Mark S. Butler, "The Role of Natural Product Chemistry in Drug Discovery," *Journal of Natural Products* 67, no. 12 (2004): 2141–53.
3. W. Jänig, "Autonomic Nervous System," in *Human Physiology*, edited by Robert F. Schmidt and Gerhrad Thews (Berlin, Germany: Springer, 1989), 333–70.
4. Steven E. Meredith et al., "Caffeine Use Disorder: A Comprehensive Review and Research Agenda," *Journal of Caffeine Research* 3, no. 3 (2013): 114–30.
5. Suzette M. Evans and Roland R. Griffiths, "Caffeine Withdrawal: A Parametric Analysis of Caffeine Dosing Conditions," *Journal of Pharmacology and Experimental Therapy* 289, no. 1 (1999): 285–94.
6. J. Timson, "Theobromine and Theophylline," *Mutation Research* 32, no. 2 (1975): 169–78.
7. Juan A. Carrillo and Javier Benitez, "Clinically Significant Pharmacokinetic Interactions Between Dietary Caffeine and Medications," *Clinical Pharmacokinetics* 39, no. 2 (2000): 127–53.
8. Diane C. Mitchell et al., "Beverage Caffeine Intakes in the U.S.," *Food and Chemical Toxicology* 63 (2014): 136–42.
9. Antony Wild, *Coffee: A Dark History* (New York: W. W. Norton, 2005), xi.
10. James M. Volo, *The Boston Tea Party: The Foundations of Revolution* (Santa Barbara, CA: Praeger, 2012), 278.
11. Aaron P. Davis et al., "An Annotated Taxonomic Conspectus of the Genus *Coffea* (Rubiaceae)," *Botanical Journal of the Linnean Society* 152, no. 4 (2006): 465–512.
12. B. A. Weinberg and Bonnie K. Bealer, *The World of Caffeine: The Science and Culture of the World's Most Popular Drug* (New York: Routledge, 2001), xxi.
13. M. D. W. Mortimer, *Coca: Divine Plant of the Incas* (Berkeley, CA: Ronin Publishers, Inc., 2017).
14. F. Gaedcke, "Ueber das Erythroxylin, dargestellt aus den Blättern des in Südamerika cultivirten Strauches Erythroxylon Coca Lam" [About Erythroxylin, Depicted from the Leaves of the Erythroxylon Coca Lam Shrub Cultivated in South America], *Archives der Pharmazie* 132, no. 2 (1855): 141–50.
15. M. R. Lee, "The History of Ephedra (Ma-Huang)," *Journal of the Royal College of Physicians of Edinburgh* 41, no. 1 (2011): 78–84.
16. Amy M. Ling, "FDA to Ban Sales of Dietary Supplements Containing Ephedra," *Journal of Law, Medicine, and Ethics* 32, no. 1 (2004): 184–86.
17. Michela Ferrucci et al., "The Effects of Amphetamine and Methamphetamine on the Release of Norepinephrine, Dopamine and Acetylcholine from the Brainstem Reticular Formation," *Frontiers in Neuroanatomy* 13 (2019): 48.

18. Jane Carlisle Maxwell and Mary-Lynn Brecht, "Methamphetamine: Here We Go Again?" *Addictive Behaviors* 36, no. 12 (2011): 1168–73.
19. L. A. Laitinen et al., "A Comparison of the Bronchodilator Action of Pseudoephedrine and Ephedrine in Patients with Reversible Airway Obstruction," *European Journal of Clinical Pharmacology* 23, no. 2 (1982): 107–9.
20. Nezar N. Al-Hebshi and Nils Skaug, "Khat (Catha Edulis)—An Updated Review," *Addiction Biology* 10, no. 4 (2005): 299–307.
21. Steven J. Simmons et al., "DARK Classics in Chemical Neuroscience: Cathinone-Derived Psychostimulants," *ACS Chemical Neuroscience* 9, no. 10 (2018): 2379–94.
22. Michael H. Baumann, John S. Partilla, and Kurt R. Lehner, "Psychoactive 'Bath Salts': Not So Soothing," *European Journal of Pharmacology* 698, no. 1–3 (2013): 1–5.
23. Richard J. Beninger, "The Role of Dopamine in Locomotor Activity and Learning," *Brain Research Reviews* 287, no. 2 (1983): 173–96.
24. Erin S. Calipari and Mark Ferris, "Amphetamine Mechanisms and Actions at the Dopamine Terminal Revisited," *Journal of Neuroscience* 33, no. 21 (2013): 8923–25.
25. Irene Riezzo et al., "Side Effects of Cocaine Abuse: Multiorgan Toxicity and Pathological Consequences," *Current Medicinal Chemistry* 19, no. 33 (2012): 5624–46.
26. Victoria Boswell-Smith, Domenica Spina, and Clive P. Page, "Phosphodiesterase Inhibitors," *British Journal of Pharmacology* 147, no. S1 (2006): S252–57.
27. Kuo Yan et al., "The Cyclic AMP Signaling Pathway: Exploring Targets for Successful Drug Discovery (Review)," *Molecular Medicine Reports* 13, no. 5 (2016): 3715–23.
28. Rafael Franco and Gemma Navarro, "Adenosine A2A Receptor Antagonists in Neurodegenerative Diseases: Huge Potential and Huge Challenges," *Frontiers in Psychiatry* 9 (2018): 68.

Credits

Fig 18.2: Copyright © 2007 by Forest & Kim Starr, (CC BY 3.0) at https://commons.wikimedia.org/wiki/File:Starr_070617-7332_Coffea_arabica.jpg.

Part IV

Case Study

Chapter 19

Case Study Introduction

Yan Zhang

During teaching practice, in order to overcome one major challenge in covering the tremendous amount of information available on herbal medications and natural products involved in pharmacy practice within a limited credit-hour course schedule, a team-based project (number of students per team to be determined) can be implemented to allow students to study outside the topics covered by the lectures so that classes do not have to discuss all the medications/drugs in didactic lectures. This project can be finished, submitted, and evaluated as a poster presentation or a written report.

The natural/herbal product case study can be a semester-long project for the teams. The advantages of adopting this educational method include encouraging team spirit, reinforcing essential principles and concepts of the knowledge by application, training for conducting literature searches and analysis, and building skills on poster presentation and/or written report preparation. We believe that a team-based project of this nature will lead to stimulation of higher-order thinking and problem-solving. Appropriate guidance from the teachers of the course should be in place to provide support at each stage of the project. These efforts from our practice are discussed in the following chapters.

In addition, some practicum exercises can be adopted to provide hands-on experience to the students on herbal medication regulation. A protocol of herbal medication quality analysis (QA) lab is included here as an example.

Chapter 20

Quality Analysis of Herbal Product

St. John's Wort

Yan Zhang

Introduction

To get some hands-on experience and further strengthen the concepts and knowledge on the course topics, it is recommended that students work individually to conduct a quality control experiment constituting a quantitative analysis of an herbal product in the pharmacy practicum laboratory.

Grading of the wet laboratory practice based on performance in terms of quantitative analytical results may be optional. Instead, the students may be asked to finish the laboratory exercise, collect and analyze data, summarize their findings in a laboratory report, and respond to several questions related to the laboratory practice.

Key Terms and Concepts

analyte: (noun) a substance whose chemical constituents are being identified and analyzed
phytomedicinal: (adjective form) related to phytomedicine, a plant-based herb-based traditional medical practice that has both preventive and therapeutic applications; sometimes used in noun form to identify and categorize a plant or herb

Use of Herbal Products

Annual sales of herbal products in the United States now exceed $34 billion. The crude drugs involved have often been used for centuries, and lack of patentability prevents recovery even of research costs. Consequently, only a handful of herbs have been approved for use as drugs.

Most are sold as foods or food supplements. No information regarding therapeutic utility appears on their labels; however, a vast literature has built up around them, providing product "information."[1]

In order to equip PharmD students with practical knowledge of herbal medication quality control and quantity control, an herbal product quality analysis laboratory practice for the course can be adopted. This experiment may familiarize the student with quantitative fluid measurement techniques and the use of a spectrophotometer to verify the dose of an herbal product formulation. Fluid measurement techniques and spectrophotometry are often used for quantitative analyses to evaluate purity, dose, dose uniformity, dissolution characteristics, chemical stability, or other chemical characteristics. The *United States Pharmacopeia* and the Food and Drug Administration set guidelines on the acceptability of these quantitative results for drugs, before they can be used, to document the integrity of pharmaceutical products. However, herbal products are not subject to the same premarketing regulatory scrutiny as FDA-approved medications, and the route to the marketplace for natural products is much less tortuous; the Dietary Supplement Health and Education Act of 1994 permits herbs or phytomedicinals to be sold as dietary supplements provided health or therapeutic claims are not specified on their labels. A statement may appear on the label to describe the product's role in affecting "structure or function in humans."

Pharmacognosy Laboratory Practice for Chemical Analysis

In the laboratory practice associated with the pharmacognosy course, students will be asked to conduct basic analytic chemistry analysis to determine the amount of hypericin contained in one commercially available St. John's wort product. The students will conduct sample transfer, analyte extraction, purification, dilution, measurement, and finally, data collection and analysis in executing this experiment.

Grading the wet laboratory practice based on their performance in terms of quantitative analytical results may not be needed, though it is recommended at the end of the narrative. The students should at least be asked to finish the laboratory exercise, collect and analyze data, summarize their findings in a laboratory report, and respond to several questions related to laboratory practice.

The laboratory can be offered as part of a course and may provide a good opportunity for students to understand the importance of quality and quantity control of herbal medication and the potential problems and challenges thereof.

St. John's Wort: Its Composition and Use

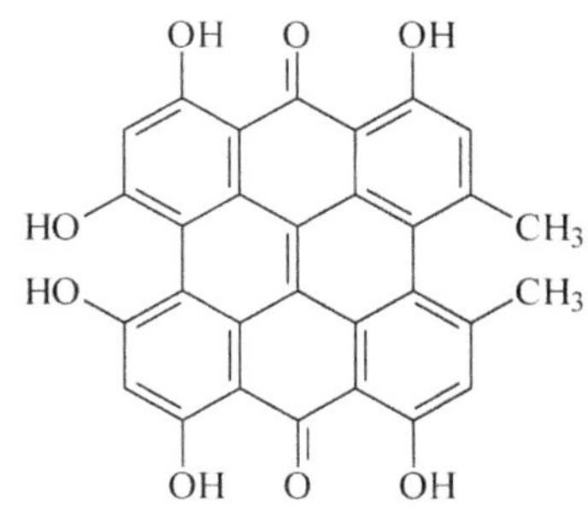

In folk medicine, St. John's wort has been used for external treatment of wounds as well as internally to treat minor depression and mood swings. In various studies, isolation of a large number of substances from different structural types and their pharmacological properties have been described. Recently, strong antiviral effects of an ingredient in St. John's wort, hypericin, have been discovered.[2] The structure of hypericin is as follows:

Hypericin has characteristic absorbances at 558 and 598 nm in water.[3] According to Beer's Law, the concentration of a substance is proportional to the absorbance of light at a given wavelength (A_λ) as follows:

$$A_\lambda = {}_\lambda bc$$

where

$_\lambda$ is molar extinction coefficient ($M^{-1} cm^{-1}$) at wavelength;

b is the path length of cell in cm; and

c is the molar concentration of the substance in solution.

Quantitative Measurement of Hypericin

Each student will finish one complete test individually.

Materials Needed

1. St. John's wort capsules (can be purchased from any local community pharmacy)
2. 15 mL screw-capped centrifuge tubes
3. 10 mL glass pipettes
4. 5 mL disposable pipettes
5. Adjustable pneumatic pipets (1 mL)
6. 1 mL pipette tips
7. Tube rack
8. Laboratory marker
9. 0.1% (w/v) ammonium phosphate buffer pH 7.0
10. Reusable spectrophotometric plastic vials for absorbance measurements with b = 1 cm
11. Weigh trays or weighing papers

12. Filter (0.45 micron)
13. 5 mL syringes
14. Spatulas

Equipment Needed

VWR Spectrophotometer UV-1600PC UV/VIS

Preparation of Samples

1. Note the brand name, batch number if available, and reported hypericin content (in % w/w) of St. John's wort bottle. Also note the amount (in mg) per capsule.
2. Label a 15 mL polypropylene centrifuge tube with your name and transfer the contents of a capsule into it. **Make sure that you do not leave any material in the capsule.** If needed, use a small spatula to remove any solid sticking to the capsule wall.
3. Add 10.0 mL of 0.1% ammonium phosphate buffer pH 7.0 to each tube and screw cap onto the tube.
4. Shake the tubes for five minutes.
5. Check to ensure that all powder is completely wetted and immersed in the buffer solution (not sticking on the wall). If any powder remains unwetted, gently tap the tube to dislodge the solid, and then shake the tube again.
6. Give your tube to the TA for centrifugation. Make sure you mark your initials on the tube.
7. Pull off the plunger of the syringe and put the microfilter onto the tip (orifice) of the barrel of the syringe tightly. Then transfer at least 3 mL of the supernatant from the centrifuge tube into the barrel. **Make sure you have a glass tube underneath the tip of the filter before collecting the filtered solution.** Carefully and slowly put the plunger back onto the top of the barrel. Slowly and steadily push the plunger down in order to filter the solution through. **Check to make sure the filtrate is clear.**
8. Withdraw 1.0 mL of the filtered clear solution from the collecting tube and transfer it to the testing cuvette. Add another 1.0 mL of 0.1% (w/v) ammonium phosphate buffer to the 1.0 mL sample in the cuvette and mix the solution by inverting two to three times.
9. Blank the spectrophotometer at 558 nm using 0.1% (w/v) ammonium phosphate buffer pH 7.0.
10. Record the absorbance of your sample at 558 nm.
11. Blank the spectrophotometer at 598 nm using 0.1% (w/v) ammonium phosphate buffer pH 7.0.
12. Record the absorbance of your sample at 598 nm.

13. Empty the tested cuvette into the sink and return the cuvette to the TA for future use.
14. Record the results of the samples of three other classmates.
15. Clean the bench and remove all trash.

Evaluation of Results and Questions

1. Calculate the concentration of hypericin in the solution for absorbance measurement (in ∫M) (b = 1 cm) using the following reported molar extinction coefficients:

$$_{558} = 10{,}000\ M^{-1}cm^{-1}$$

$$_{598} = 6{,}000\ M^{-1}cm^{-1}$$

2. Calculate the amount of hypericin (in mg) present in the sampled powder. The molecular weight of hypericin is 504. Remember to take into consideration the dilution of the hypericin solution for absorbance measurement.
3. Calculate and report the hypericin content of each capsule as determined at each wavelength using the following relationship:

(Assayed amount per sample (col. 5)/ total sample amount) × 100 = % content

4. Calculate and report the mean hypericin content at each wavelength.
5. Calculate and report the standard deviation (S) and percent coefficient of variation (COV) of measurements according to the following equations:

$$S = (((x - x_o)^2)/(n - 1))^{1/2}$$

where x = individual assayed values; x_o = assayed mean; n = number of measurements

$$COV = (S/x_o) \times 100$$

6. Is the precision of these measurements within the acceptable range that is recommended by the *United States Pharmacopeia*?
7. Do the hypericin contents determined at two wavelengths correlate with each other and with the reported content? Which measurement seems to correlate? What are the possible reasons for measured contents correlating or not correlating with the reported content?
8. Predict what would happen if the pH of the buffer were to be increased to 10? What might have to be done to assess the hypericin content of capsules under those conditions?

References

1. David M. Eisenberg et al., "Trends in Alternative Medicine Use in the United States, 1990–1997: Results of a Follow-Up National Survey," *JAMA* 280, no. 18 (1998): 1569–75.
2. Daniel Meruelo, Gad Lavie, and D. Lavie, "Therapeutic Agents with Dramatic Antiretroviral Activity and Little Toxicity at Effective Doses: Aromatic Polycyclic Diones Hypericin and Pseudohypericin," *Proceedings of the National Academy of Sciences USA* 85, no. 14 (1988): 5230–34.
3. Leonard Liebes et al., "A Method for the Quantitation of Hypericin, an Antiviral Agent, in Biological Fluids by High-Performance Liquid Chromatography," *Analytical Biochemistry* 195, no. 1 (1991): 77–85.

Herbal Product Quality—DATA SHEET

Name ______________________ Partners ______________________________________

Date __________________

Brand Name: ______________________

Amount per Capsule: ___________________________

Sample	Wavelength	Absorbance	Conc. of hypericin by Abs.	Amount of hypericin by Abs. in sample	Hypericin content of the capsule
	(nm)	(Abs. Units)	(μM)	(mg)	(%)
Blank	558				
Your capsule	558				
Your classmate's capsule	558				
Your classmate's capsule	558				
Your classmate's capsule	558				
Blank	598				
Your capsule	598				
Your classmate's capsule	598				
Your classmate's capsule	598				
Your classmate's capsule	598				

Manufacturer	Mean Hypericin Content (% w/w)		Standard Deviation		Coefficient of Variation	
	λ558	λ598	λ558	λ598	λ558	λ598

Chapter 21

Group Project Proceedings

Yan Zhang

THE CASE STUDIES OF HERBAL OR natural products and the resulting student-prepared posters or written report will serve to strengthen students' knowledge of the basic concepts and principles of pharmacognosy. Activities to conduct with the case study should include topic selection, literature review, case design, literature data collection, analysis/discussion, and final poster or report preparation and presentation. First, the team will be formed based on the class size; typically at least five team members is preferred to distribute reasonable workload. Second, each team will be asked to select one herbal medication or natural product on the market with clinical usage or with acclaimed therapeutic benefits as described in the literature. Third, each team will conduct a literature search to summarize and discuss the information and knowledge related to one major application or usage of the target medication. Fourth, the team will prepare and present their research in poster format with defined size and related characteristics that simulate those of a formal scientific conference, or a written report should be formulated with defined format and length requirements.

Team Formation

Upon the start of the course, a number of teams will be formed by random name assignment of all the students enrolled in the course. These group assignments will be made known to the class at the outset of the course. The size of each team will depend on the size of the whole class. It is highly recommended that each team be composed of five to seven students so that the workload can be distributed reasonably. It is also recommended for each team to elect a team leader to serve as a liaison and communicate with the course coordinator.

Topic Assignment

A list of herbal medications and natural products as potential topics should be provided to the students right after the team assignment. Students can also be encouraged to go beyond the list provided to identify their own topics of interest.

Faculty Support

Faculty members (course coordinator and instructors) should provide guidelines and recommendations at each stage of the project. Specific faculty input may include a seminar on how to conduct a literature search on herbal medications and natural products, a lecture on how to construct a research poster or report given by an experienced faculty member, review and approval of topics selected by each team, daily interactions between the course coordinator and each team to answer any general and/or specific questions, and/or feedback on each team's draft poster provided by the instructors.

The majority of first-year pharmacy class students do not have previous direct experience with poster presentations or have previous research exposure, and most of them have never worked in a team-based environment. Thus, the additional challenges of bringing them all up to the same or similar level with respect to quality literature research and the preparation and presentation of research posters or reports should be considered and taken care of.

Special Considerations

To prevent some student members of teams from "coasting" through the assignment without making a significant contribution, each team should be asked to distribute their duties evenly among all group members. Furthermore, each student should be asked to complete a Peer Performance Review to evaluate his or her team members' performance during the project execution. The results of the review should be counted into the final grades of the course. It has to be assured that all members of class are aware of this expectation, with periodic reminders that their performance and participation will directly influence their final course grade. Student peer evaluation may include but is not limited to the following items: quality of work, timeliness of work, task support, attendance of group meetings, responsibility, and leadership.

The benefits of these case studies include opportunities for building team spirit, reinforcement of essential principles and concepts of the course by their application, training in literature search and analysis, exploration of research philosophy, and building technical skills in poster or report preparation and presentation. For example, in order to prepare and finish the project, students will be required to cooperate with each other, coordinate their study schedules, and compromise to solve conflicts among their respective opinions. These kinds of activities help build effective team spirit. In addition, working on such a project will enable them to practically apply the knowledge learned through didactic teaching into the higher-level skills of data interpretation as related to their poster project. Because for most of them this will be their first time presenting a scientific poster or report, this will be beneficial to them in their future careers.

Grading

A series of project deadlines should be defined and relayed, while credits toward the course's final grade are awarded for meeting these deadlines. In particular, electing a team contact person (leader), defining the project topic, submitting the first and second draft of the project (in poster or report format), submitting the final version of the poster or report, and submitting the peer performance assessments within the group should be defined as goals. The final project posters or reports may be printed and presented and should be evaluated by all members of the teaching team. The evaluation criteria of the final poster should be made available at the beginning of the course so that students will be aware of their endpoint goals. A key element of the case study posters is to go through a very vigorous process of improvement and evaluation. This may include three submissions: the first draft submission evaluated by the course coordinator, with feedback to each group; the second draft submission, evaluated by teams of faculty members, with their feedback summarized by the course coordinator and provided to each team; and the final submissions, which are printed, posted, and graded by the entire faculty team, using the same detailed evaluation form for each group.

Appendix

Poster Topic Examples

(Alphabetically listed, without separation of natural products from herbal medications)

Acai, Aloe, Artemisinin, Ashwagandha, Astragalus

Bee pollen/royal jelly complex, Belladonna, Bitter melon, Black cohosh, Black cumin seed, Borage seed oil, Bromelain

Caffeine, Camphor, Cannabis, Capsaicin, Cat's claw, Cayenne, CBD oil, Chamomile, Chamomile oil, Chondroitin, Cinnamon, Coconut oil, Cranberry, Creatine, Curcumin

Devil's claw, Digitalis

Echinacea, Elderberry, Ephedra, European mistletoe, Evening primrose

Fenugreek, Feverfew, Flaxseed, Flaxseed oil, Foxglove

Garlic, Ginger, *Ginkgo biloba*, Ginseng, Glucosamine (with and without chondroitin), Grape seed extract, Green coffee extract, Green tea

Hawthorn, Honey, Hops, Horny goat weed

Indian borage

Kava, Kratom

Lavender, Lemon balm, Licorice root

Ma huang, Manuka honey, Medical marijuana, Melatonin, Milk thistle, Mistletoe, Morphine, Mugwort

Omega-3 fish oils, Opium

Paclitacel (Taxol), Penicillin, Peppermint, Peppermint oil, Peyote, Poppy, Pycnogenol

Quercetin

Raspberry ketones, Red yeast, Red yeast rice, Resveratrol

Salicylic acid, Salvia, Saw palmetto, Scopolamine, Shark cartilage, Shiitake mushroom, Snowdrop flower, St. John's wort

Taxol, Tea tree oil, Thunder god vine, Turmeric

Valerian, Valerian root

Willow bark, Witch hazel

Poster Title Examples

The Efficacy of Garlic as a Cholesterol-Lowering Agent

Efficacy of Devil's Claw in Osteoarthritis

Taxol as an Anticancer Agent

The Effect of Chondroitin Sulfate on Osteoarthritis

Effects of Capsaicin on Managing the Symptoms of Lower Back Pain

Benefits of Fish Oil (Omega-3) for Heart Health

Topical Capsaicin as an Effective Treatment for Musculoskeletal Pain

Efficacy of Echinacea in Preventing Rhinovirus Infection

Role of Turmeric in Colorectal Cancer

Effects of Green Tea Extracts on Prevention of Atherosclerosis via Reduction of LDL Oxidation

Black Cohosh and the Treatment of Menopausal Symptoms

Spasmolytic Effect of Peppermint Oil on Irritable Bowel Syndrome

Ginger and its Antiemetic Effects in Pregnant Women

Ginseng Enhances Cognitive Performance

Gamma-Linolenic Acid in Managing Rheumatoid Arthritis

Aloe Vera: Nature's Band-Aid

The Efficacy and Safety of Ephedra as an Herbal Medication for Weight Loss

An Encompassing Analysis of Kava and Its Role in Anxiety

The Efficacy of *Ginkgo biloba* for Treatment of Memory Loss

The Therapeutic Effects of Cannabis Sativa on MS, a Chronic Dilemma

Mistletoe Extract Induces Apoptosis in Tumor Cells

Camphor Toxicity and Its Clinical Implications in Children

The Effect of Melatonin in Improving the Onset of Sleep for Adults

Therapeutic Effect of Raspberry Ketone on Fat Loss

Peppermint Oil and Irritable Bowel Syndrome

Poster Evaluation Form

Poster #:

Judge's Initials:

1. **Technical** (**15 points total**)
    a. **Use of Color** (pleasing color combination, color use enhances readability and attractiveness) (3 points)
    b. **Legibility** (Space used effectively with adequate separation, adequate font size, quality of printing, etc.) (3 points)
    c. **Materials, Spelling, Grammar** (materials create a polished presentation free of spelling mistakes and grammatical and punctuation errors) (4 points)
    d. **Overall Visual Appeal** (layout of text and figures is easy to follow) (5 points)

(I) **Total technical score:** ____________

2. **Content** (**40 points total**)
    a. **Title** (effectively highlights the poster's subject matter) (2 points)
    b. **Authors** (students' names alphabetically arranged by last name; institutional affiliations listed) (1 point)
    c. **Abstract** (succinct summary of project) (5 points)
    d. **Introduction** (adequate background, given constraints of medium) (5 points)
    e. **Results and Discussion** (adequate/convincing summary of findings) (10 points)
    f. **Tables and Figures** (effectively communicate key facts) (10 points)
    g. **Conclusions** (concise and conclusive) (5 points)
    h. **References** (no more than ten, following JMC format requirement) (1 point)
    i. **Acknowledgments/Funding Attributions** (Med Chem Department must be acknowledged) (1 point)

(II) **Total content score:** ____________

TOTAL SCORE (1 + 2): /55

JUDGES: Feel free to add comments below.

Chapter 22

What Is Research Literature?

Rachel A. Koenig

RESEARCH LITERATURE IS THE PUBLISHED LITERATURE within any given field. In pharmacognosy, the research literature contains all journal articles, scholarly books, abstracts, and reports published since the field began in the early 1800s. There are three types of research literature found within pharmacognosy, as well as in biomedical literature more generally: primary, secondary, and tertiary sources. *Primary sources* present original research and are considered to be the most relevant and current sources available. Primary sources provide access to detailed information about a topic and assess the validity and applicability of reported results. Examples of primary sources include publications such as systematic reviews, basic science research articles, and controlled clinical trials. *Secondary sources* include indexing and abstracting systems that organize and provide retrieval of primary resources. Databases such as PubMed, the Cochrane Database of Systematic Reviews, and Embase are examples of secondary sources. There are a few limitations to consider when using secondary sources. First, a span of time exists between the publication of a journal article and its inclusion in a research database. Also, it is important to understand that no single database will include every journal, conference meeting, or publication and that to perform a comprehensive search, one must search in multiple research databases. Finally, *tertiary sources* condense and summarize data from the literature. Examples of tertiary sources include textbooks and some electronic databases, such as ClinicalKey's Drug Monographs and Natural Medicines. The best tertiary sources are written by experts in the field and are peer-reviewed. Tertiary sources are convenient and easy to use; therefore, they are often the first resource consulted in a professional practice setting. Similarly to secondary sources, there is a time requirement for information to be reviewed and summarized, which may cause delays in information updates within tertiary sources of information.[1]

Pharmacognosy Journal Titles:

International Journal of Pharmacognosy
Pharmacognosy Magazine
Pharmacognosy Journal
Journal of Pharmacognosy & Natural Products
Phytochemistry
Journal of Enthnopharmacology
Fitoterapia

The large majority of pharmacognosy research literature consists of publications within *scholarly journals*. A few examples of scholarly journals within the field of pharmacognosy are noted in the text box above. Scholarly journals, also commonly known as professional journals, peer-reviewed journals, academic journals, or refereed journals, publish original research *articles*. Scholarly journals are most often published monthly or quarterly, and each volume contains several articles written by experts in the field. Each article within a scholarly journal typically goes through the process of *peer review*. Researchers who want their work to be included within a scholarly journal first submit their article to a journal's editor. The editor then tasks a peer review panel, made up of scholars and experts in the field, to read through the article and determine whether it meets certain criteria. The article must be well-written, well-researched, and well-documented to pass the peer review process. Peer review ensures that articles published within scholarly journals are authoritative and that the work meets the standards of the field.

Why Is It Important to Review the Research Literature?

Reviewing the research literature is an important exercise at the beginning of any research project, whether that project involves professional clinical research, bench research, or completing a school assignment. When a researcher reviews the literature, they are essentially locating, reading, and assessing the publications relevant to their research question. Oftentimes, the researcher will summarize their findings into a review article or will include an analysis of the literature in the introduction or background sections of their report. They may additionally use research literature to contextualize the findings of their study in the discussion section. In doing so, the researcher provides the foundation for their informed decision-making and sets the stage for generated knowledge to be applied to new settings, populations, or disciplines.

Understanding the findings of research additionally has the potential to positively impact practice. When working on clinical research, conducting a review of the literature might inspire change or impact clinical decision-making through the acquisition of new knowledge. With increasing treatment options and increasing amounts of information published daily, it is best practice to incorporate emerging evidence into decision-making. Incorporating the best possible evidence can positively impact cost-effectiveness and quality of patient care.[2] Furthermore, in the laboratory, a review of recent research literature can validate current methods, tools, or instruments. A literature review can identify future trends or even motivate the researcher to rework or abandon therapies. Finally, reviewing the literature is important because it can alert the researcher to similar studies that are in progress or that have already been completed. In doing so, a review of the literature has the potential to deter the waste of resources and time and avoid duplication of the same or similar research concepts.

What Is a Research Database?

The leading scholarly journals within each field are often housed within subscription-based *research databases*. A research database is an organized collection of information, typically consisting of journal articles and other academic sources. For an overview of the relationship between articles, journals, and databases, see Figure 22.1. Some databases have a more general scope and contain information from a variety of subject areas and academic disciplines, whereas others are subject-specific and only contain relevant information for certain academic disciplines. For instance, PubMed is a database geared toward the health sciences; however, it is considered more general than Natural Medicines, which is a database specifically for those interested in researching complementary and alternative medicines, including herbs and plants. Academic libraries often subscribe to *bibliographic databases*. These research databases provide citation information for an item; however, the full text of the item is not contained within the database. A *citation* typically consists of the author name(s), article title, journal title, date of publication,

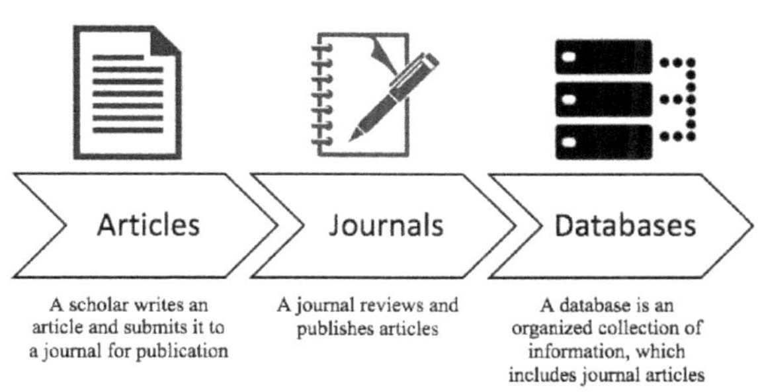

FIGURE 22.1 Articles are published within scholarly journals, which are then housed in research databases.

TABLE 22.1 Search Engines Versus Library Research Databases*

Search Engines	Library Research Databases
• Easy to use and familiar • No quality control over content • Difficult to limit a search to include only relevant results • Search engines often lead users to articles that are not freely available online • Can only be searched using keywords	• Requires a bit of instruction to use • Content must go through an editorial or peer-review process • User has a great deal of control over results (i.e., limiters and refiners) • Articles are made available through the library's paid subscription to research databases • Can be searched using keywords and controlled vocabulary

and other relevant information. PubMed is an example of a bibliographic database. Search engines (i.e., Google) are considered databases, but there is a vast difference between these tools and library research databases (Table 22.1).

Searching Techniques

It might be the researcher's first instinct to access a database and immediately enter search terms. This method may produce a few relevant results; however, the more likely outcome will be an excessively narrow search that produces only five results or an excessively broad search that produces tens of thousands of results. The researcher will subsequently assume they are missing pertinent literature related to their topic, or they may become overwhelmed and assume it will be impossible to narrow the results to a more manageable number. Therefore, it is vitally important to think thoughtfully and systematically about the words one uses in a search. The foundation for a good search that returns relevant results begins with the formation of a focused research question.

A *research question* investigates a specific component of a broader research topic. It takes time to develop a good research question. The question must not be so broad that it cannot be answered with depth and consideration, but it must also refrain from being so narrow that it is answered with a simple statistic or a "yes" or "no" answer. To develop a good research question, investigators typically begin by identifying a broader topic in which they are interested. They then complete a round of preliminary research on this topic to determine the existing literature. While scanning the literature, the researcher will discern their specific question by asking *background questions*. These questions, which are typically basic questions that can be located in current textbooks and on authoritative websites, help researchers assess what they know about a subject. Furthermore, background questions may be answered succinctly with facts, statistics, and definitions. An example of a background question may be "What is the clinical definition of nicotine dependence?"

Once a researcher is comfortable with the background of their topic, they begin the formation of *foreground questions*. Foreground questions ask for specific knowledge to inform clinical decisions or research planning. These questions are more specific and complex when compared to background questions, and they may be further categorized into one of four major types: treatment/therapy, diagnosis, prognosis, or etiology/harm. For instance, a foreground question may be "Is the combination of St. John's wort with nicotine replacement more successful in achieving smoking cessation than nicotine replacement alone?" Part of the researcher's question-building process will be to decide which foreground question to answer. They might create a list of questions to choose from and then evaluate the questions to determine which is of most interest to them and potentially to other researchers. They additionally consider if the question is appropriate for the amount of time and resources they can devote, as it is important to understand if the question is answerable for a short-term project or if it will require a year to search the literature and complete.

The components required for a well-constructed foreground question can be captured in the mnemonic *PICO*. PICO stands for Population, Intervention, Comparison, Outcome. Often in the health sciences, including the field of pharmacognosy, researchers will use PICO (or *PEO*, which stands for Population, Exposure, Outcome) to help frame their questions (see Tables 22.2a and 22.2b). PICO and PEO are most often used when framing a clinical question, but they can be used to frame research of any kind. Articulating your research

TABLE 22.2a PICO

P	Patient/Problem
I	Intervention (prognostic factor/exposure)
C	Comparison
O	Outcome

TABLE 22.2b PEO

P	Patient/Problem
E	Exposure
O	Outcome

question in this format will formulate a search strategy that retrieves information with a high degree of relevance.

To better explain how to translate PICO or PEO into a search strategy, take a look at the following example of a patient case:

> *A father comes into the pharmacy with his nine-year-old daughter. He wants to know if he can give her echinacea to reduce the severity of her common cold symptoms.*

Identify the main components of this scenario and add them to a PICO or PEO chart. First, who is the patient? Although the father is speaking with the pharmacist, the nine-year-old daughter is the patient. However, identifying the patient or population as a nine-year-old girl may be too limiting. There may not be many studies that solely examine a population of nine-year-olds. Also, limiting the search to one gender may cause issues with gaining a full picture of the clinical situation. Therefore, it may be more useful to identify children in general as the patient or population. If the search results are ultimately too broad, age and gender could be brought in to refine the results. For the intervention or exposure, echinacea is the suggested new therapy; therefore, it will be important to look at the literature to determine how this intervention affects the intended population. There are several options for the comparison component of PICO. The comparison in this case could be no comparison or simply providing the standard of care. There may also be literature available that compares echinacea to a placebo. Finally, the primary outcome to identify, based on this case, is the reduction of common cold symptoms. Once all components of PICO or PEO are identified (see Tables 22.3a and 22.3b), use them to draft a focused research question. The

TABLE 22.3a Echinacea PICO

P	Children
I	Echinacea
C	No comparison, standard of care, placebo
O	Reduce symptoms of the common cold

TABLE 22.3b Echinacea PEO

P	Children
E	Echinacea
O	Reduce symptoms of the common cold

research question for this example could be something similar to "Does echinacea reduce symptoms of the common cold in children?"

Subject Headings and Keywords

Now that we have used PICO in the above example to help develop a focused research question ("Does echinacea reduce symptoms of the common cold in children?"), it is important to identify the major concepts within that question. Identification of these concepts will guide the researcher in selection of the search terms they will use in a database. It is best practice to start with two search concepts and add a third if the results are too broad. For the above question, the researcher may start with the two concepts of "echinacea" and the "common cold." If results are too broad, a third concept of "children" could be added to the search, or an age or population search filter, which many databases contain, may be applied.

Next, the researcher will identify two types of terms to use in their search: subject headings and keywords. A *subject heading* is a single word assigned to represent a concept. Consider the ambiguity associated with the English language. For instance, a can of soda is described differently in different parts of the country. It might be referred to as soda, pop, a soft drink, Coke, or a carbonated beverage. Rather than the researcher typing each variation of the word into a search interface to retrieve all relevant articles (for instance, what if one author refers to "soda" throughout their paper but another author never mentions "soda" and instead refers to the beverage only as "pop"?), one subject heading could be searched to account for all variations. In this case, the PubMed database uses the subject heading "carbonated beverages" to account for regional dialects. Overall, subject headings help standardize synonyms and spelling variations.

Each database has its own set of subject headings. PubMed's subject headings are known as Medical Subject Headings (MeSH terms), whereas the database Embase refers to its subject headings as Emtree terms. Other databases may refer to their subject headings as controlled vocabulary, a thesaurus, descriptors, or indexes. *Keywords*, on the other hand, are everyday words researchers use to discuss their topic. "Soda" and "pop" are both keywords that may be entered into a database. When using keywords, a researcher needs to consider the many ways in which scholars refer to their topic, as well as related concepts that could pull in additional relevant results.

There are advantages and disadvantages to using subject headings and keywords. When a researcher searches with subject headings, the most relevant articles on their research topic will be located. However, there are a few limitations associated with only searching using subject headings in a search. Researchers who limit themselves to subject headings may miss out on the most recently published articles, which may not have undergone *indexing*. Indexing is completed in most databases and is a process where *indexers*, or subject experts tasked to read a number of articles, assign relevant subject headings to each citation. For instance, indexing in PubMed is semiautomated. The National Library of Medicine's automated indexing tool, Medical Text Indexer (MTI), suggests indexing recommendations based on PubMed's list of available subject headings. Human indexers then review the ranked list of recommended subject headings and determine which will be added to a particular citation.[3] Because indexing is ultimately determined by humans, it is often subjective and open to error or inconsistency. Furthermore, indexing takes time, thus articles may not yet be indexed if they were recently added to the database. It is therefore important to include keywords to account for any citations that have not yet undergone indexing. Overall, if a researcher uses the standardized terminology of subject headings, they may have less flexibility than with keyword searching, but they are more likely to find most of what the database has to offer about the topic.

With keyword searching, the researcher is able to locate the newest articles on their topic, including any articles that have never been indexed; however, keyword searching is not very sensitive. The researcher may end up with a greater number of irrelevant results, especially if the keyword is vague or broad. As previously mentioned, the researcher will also need to add in and think of synonyms, spelling variations, and related concepts on their own.

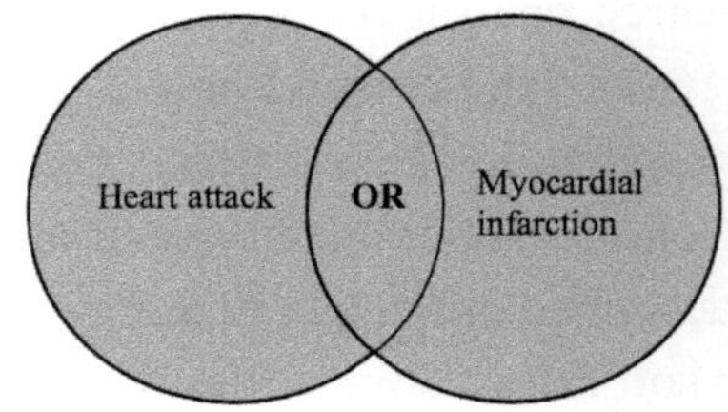

FIGURE 22.2a Example of OR operator for synonyms.

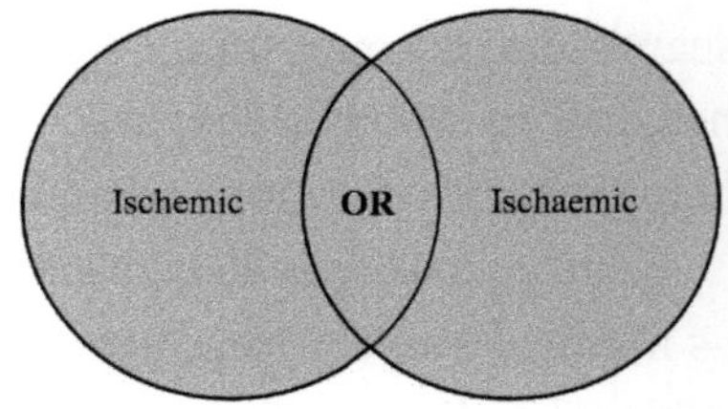

FIGURE 22.2b Example of OR operator for alternative spellings.

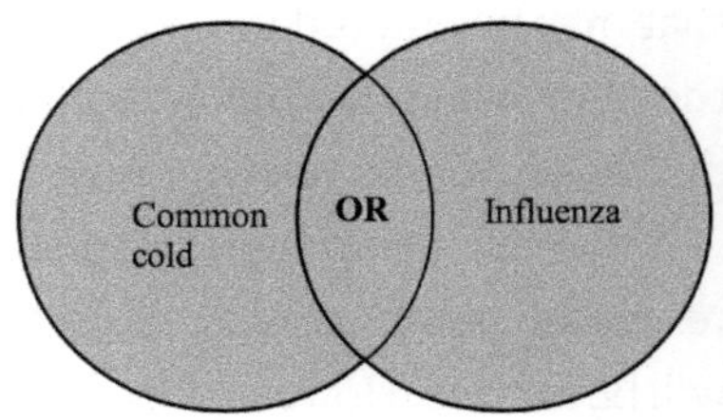

FIGURE 22.2c Example of OR operator for similar topics.

Boolean Operators

Boolean operators are another way in which researchers may be intentional about their search. Named after George Boole, a mathematician who invented the system in the nineteenth century, Boolean operators express relationships between search concepts. Without these operators, it is difficult for the database to understand the connection between terms. The Boolean operators consist of OR, AND, and NOT, and they are often seen in this capitalized format. Capitalizing the operators allows researchers to more easily visualize the different components of the search and where the Boolean operators are functioning. There are a few databases, however, that require Boolean operators to be capitalized. The Venn diagrams in Figures 22.2–22.3 define the use and meanings of the OR and AND operators.

The *OR* operator is used to retrieve results in which citations contain at least one of the entered search terms. OR allows the researcher to link various spellings of a word (i.e., *ischemic* OR *ischaemic*) or synonyms (i.e., *heart attack* OR *myocardial infarction*). The OR operator also allows the researcher to link similar topics. If a researcher is interested in the effect of echinacea on symptoms of the common cold, they may also be interested in its effect on influenza; therefore, OR could be used to link the two similar topics, even though they are not synonyms or similar spellings (i.e., *common cold* OR *influenza*). The OR operator is helpful when a researcher wants to be more inclusive with their search. They should anticipate that the search will result in an increased number of results.

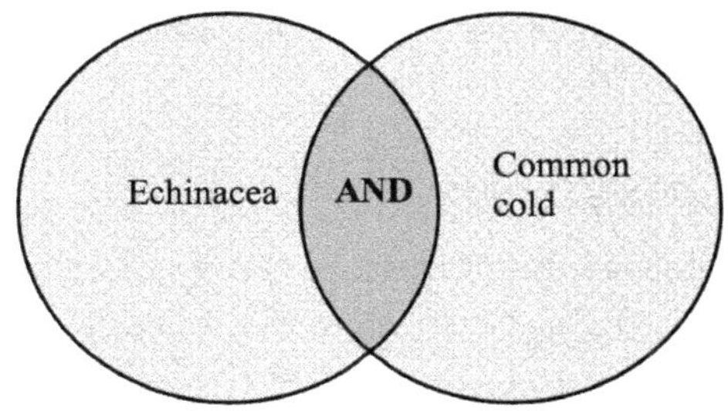

FIGURE 22.3 All results must contain both *echinacea* and *common cold*.

The *AND* operator is used to retrieve results in which each citation contains all search terms. For instance, in the above research question, "Does echinacea reduce symptoms of the common cold in children?" the researcher should use the AND operator as follows:

The researcher is essentially instructing the database to locate any citation about echinacea; however, results must also be about the common cold. AND is used to refine a search and make it more relevant. The researcher should anticipate that the search will result in a decreased number of results.

Finally, a researcher can eliminate citations through use of the **NOT** operator. Articles containing specified search terms following the NOT operator will be eliminated from the resulting list of citations. For instance, if the researcher wanted to focus only on the effects of echinacea on the common cold alone and did not want to read literature about the impact of echinacea on influenza, the NOT operator could be used as follows:

echinacea AND *common cold* NOT *influenza*

The NOT operator should be used with caution, as it has the potential to eliminate relevant citations. If a citation describes the effect of echinacea on the common cold as well as on influenza, it will be eliminated from the search; however, the researcher may want to read this citation because it contains pertinent information about the common cold. When employing the NOT operator, the researcher should anticipate that the search will result in a decreased number of citations.

Quotation Marks

Another way to be specific in searching is to use *quotation marks* around keyword phrases. Quotation marks inform the database that the researcher wants to search a specific phrase in an exact order. For example, if a researcher typed *echinacea OR common cold* into a database, they would receive more specific results if they placed *"common cold"* in quotation marks. Otherwise, the database will locate citations with *common* and *cold* somewhere within that citation, but the words will not necessarily be immediately next to each other or in the correct order, meaning that the search will be a little less specific.

Parentheses

Databases search for Boolean operators in differing orders; therefore, researchers may force the ordering of the operators by placing them within *parentheses*. This allows the searcher to group different parts of the search together. The database will process everything inside the parentheses first and everything outside second. This is very similar to the order of operations in algebra.

> To demonstrate the importance of using parentheses, take a look at the following example:

If a searcher typed *"common cold" AND echinacea OR coneflower* into a database (coneflower is a synonym of echinacea), this would essentially tell the database to first search for everything about the common cold and echinacea. Then, the database would additionally include everything about coneflower, but the articles about coneflower may not necessarily be relevant. If the searcher instead placed parentheses around echinacea and coneflower, the database would first find all results that discuss either of those search terms. It would then add the *AND "common cold"* and limit the search to only include articles that discuss the common cold and either echinacea or coneflower. The final search would be *"common cold" AND (echinacea OR coneflower)*. Overall, it is best practice to never mix Boolean operators without using parentheses. Researchers should always enclose OR or NOT statements within parentheses to keep them separated from any AND statements within the search.

How to Find Additional Resources

In addition to searching within databases, researchers employ a number of supplementary techniques to locate literature on their topic. After a researcher gathers a group of relevant articles, book chapters, or other resources, it is best practice to examine the *reference lists* of those sources. An examination of the references used within an article, especially a review article or a book chapter, may lead to undiscovered sources. It may also be useful to determine the seminal books or articles about your topic and scan those reference lists. If a researcher notices repetition among the same authors and sources, that is a good indication that those authors and sources are essential and should be included in their own review of the literature.

In scanning reference lists, the researcher is looking at literature that was published in years past. Oftentimes, those seminal articles or books can be several years old and may even contain outdated material. It may also be useful for the researcher to take that group of relevant articles, book chapters, and so on and see who has cited those resources since their publication. This tactic is called *citation chaining.* The research databases Web of Science and Google Scholar both have citation chaining capabilities. Finally, it might be useful to speak to faculty members or other scholars in a researcher's field of interest. These individuals may be able to suggest other sources to consult during the review of literature.

Overview of Content Within PubMed

For any pharmacognosy-related research, a PubMed search should be conducted. *PubMed* is a free online database that is overseen by the National Libraries of Medicine (NLM), a division of the National Institutes of Health (NIH). It contains close to 30 million citations from 7,000 journals dating back to the 1940s. PubMed is known for its coverage of core clinical, dental, nursing, biomedicine, medicine, bioethics, and life sciences journals.[4]

The name *MEDLINE* is often synonymous with PubMed; however, this is a misnomer. PubMed is one of several interfaces that can be used to search the MEDLINE database—others include EBSCO's MEDLINE Complete, Ovid MEDLINE, Medscape, ProQuest's MEDLINE with Full Text, and so on. Some of these MEDLINE interfaces require subscription access, whereas PubMed is free to search. PubMed contains both MEDLINE and non-MEDLINE citations. MEDLINE citations come from a selective set of journals called MEDLINE journals. To receive this distinction, MEDLINE journals must meet rigorous criteria set by the NIH. MEDLINE citations are also assigned Medical Subject Headings (MeSH), which, again, are the controlled vocabulary terms associated with PubMed. The MEDLINE records make up about 89 percent of PubMed's content. The other 11 percent comes from Bookshelf, a section of PubMed that provides free online access to books and other documents, and several other types of records. These records include, according to a 2019 study, "out-of-scope citations from MEDLINE journals, citations that precede the date that a journal is selected for MEDLINE, and new records submitted by publishers that have not yet been reviewed by NLM staff."[4] PubMed Central (PMC) is the final component of PubMed. PMC is a database of free full-text biomedical and life sciences journal articles. The 2008 NIH public access policy requires scientists to submit all final peer-reviewed journal manuscripts to PMC if the research was funded by certain research agencies, including the NIH.[4][5]

PubMed Search Example

At the writing of this textbook, the NLM has not yet released the newest version of PubMed. It is difficult to discern the exact ways in which the PubMed interface will function in the future. Therefore, the following paragraphs provide an overview of a successful PubMed search strategy, rather than a step-by-step guide to searching PubMed.

As mentioned above, the researcher should first begin their PubMed search by thoughtfully considering what they will type into the PubMed search box. To begin, remember the example patient case from above:

> *A father comes into the pharmacy with his nine-year-old daughter. He wants to know if he can give her echinacea to reduce the severity of common cold symptoms.*
>
> *The pharmacist remembers a 2010 study that mentioned children: Barrett et al.'s "Echinacea for Treating the Common Cold: A Randomized Trial," which was published in* Annals of Internal Medicine.

With this information in hand, the pharmacist can begin a thoughtful PubMed search. The first step is to locate the citation in PubMed. Because the pharmacist has the title of the study, they can quickly copy the title into the PubMed search box. PubMed provides the citation information for this article, including the title and abstract. The pharmacist reads through the title and abstract of the article and pulls out useful keywords or related concepts to flesh out the search. At this time, the pharmacist should also consider additional synonyms or alternative spellings to add to each concept. Remember, the major search concepts are *echinacea* and *common cold*. The pharmacist keeps each concept separate by using a table, as demonstrated in Table 22.4.

TABLE 22.4 Keywords

Echinacea	**Common Cold**
Keywords from title and abstract: • Echinacea Additional Keywords: • Coneflower	Keywords from title and abstract: • Common Cold • Upper respiratory tract infection Additional Keywords: • URI

Next, the pharmacist should build each concept one at a time. Starting with the column for "echinacea," they use the Boolean operator *OR* to combine any keywords, keyword phrases, and related concepts. They also place parentheses around the full concept to keep terms together, remembering to use quotation marks for keyword phrases:

> *(echinacea OR coneflower)*

They do the same for the "common cold" concept:

> *("common cold" OR "upper respiratory tract infection" OR URI)*

The next step is to examine the MeSH terms associated with the Barrett article. Back in PubMed, the MeSH terms are located below the citation information for the article. Remember, not every citation in PubMed will be indexed with MeSH terms, including those that are newly added to the database or that are not indexed in MEDLINE. Luckily, the Barrett article contains several relevant MeSH terms that may be added to the search. Again, the pharmacist finds it useful to keep track by creating a table, as in Table 22.5.

Next, the pharmacist adds the associated MeSH terms to each of the separate concepts. The MeSH terms can be added within the parentheses. Also, to help the database differentiate the MeSH terms from keywords, they keep the MeSH terms within quotation marks and add *MeSH* in brackets at the end of each term (see below):

> *(echinacea OR "Echinacea"[MeSH] OR "Phytotherapy"[MeSH] OR "Plant Extracts"[MeSH])*

> *("common cold" OR "Common Cold"[MeSH])*

TABLE 22.5 MeSH

Echinacea	**Common Cold**
Keywords from title and abstract: • Echinacea Additional Keywords: • Coneflower	Keywords from title and abstract: • Common Cold • Upper respiratory tract infection Additional Keywords: • URI
MeSH: • Echinacea • Phytotherapy • Plant Extracts	MeSH: • Common Cold

Finally, all three concepts are combined using the Boolean operator AND:

(echinacea OR "Echinacea"[MeSH] OR "Phytotherapy"[MeSH] OR "Plant Extracts"[MeSH])

AND

("common cold" OR "Common Cold"[MeSH])

This search retrieves several hundred results, which is a relatively large number of results to read through. As mentioned above, if the results of combining two concepts are broad and unmanageable, filters within PubMed may help researchers refine their results to a more feasible number. Because the pharmacist in the example is interested in children as a patient population, they may employ the Age filter within PubMed. PubMed defines a child as age six to 12. Once this filter is set, the number of results decreases dramatically. Now, all citations about infants, adults, or the aged are filtered out of the search results. Other limiters that might be useful to this search include the Human Species filter, the Clinical Trial Article Type filter, and the English Language filter. The pharmacist may only want to read the most recently published literature, as well; therefore, a publication date set to filter results to those published within the past five years may be useful.

Once the pharmacist has a relevant list of results, they may begin skimming through the citation titles. Useful citations may be temporarily saved by sending them to the PubMed Clipboard. They may then be sent via email to the pharmacist or exported to a citation management program. Additionally, those titles that are available via PubMed Central may be downloaded or read immediately, while other citations may be available in full text through an institution's subscription databases.

At the time of this writing, PubMed users have the option to register for a My NCBI account. Registering for an account allows researchers to customize default settings in PubMed. For instance, researchers can change their results screen from Summary Format, which provides citation information, to Abstract Format, which provides citation information, as well as the full abstract if one is available. Other customization options include the way in which results are sorted (by Most Recent, Best Match, Publication Date, etc.) or how many citations are viewed per page (5, 10, 20, 50, 100, or 200). A My NCBI account additionally allows researchers to permanently save searches and build collections. These options allow researchers to begin a search and come back to it or to certain collections of citations at a later date. For additional information on how to set up a My NCBI account or how to search PubMed more generally, see the PubMed Frequently Asked Questions and Tutorials, featured on the home screen of the PubMed interface.

Other Databases for Pharmacognosy

Pharmacognosy researchers should always make sure they are searching multiple databases. While duplication does exist, the content included within each database differs. By including multiple databases in their search, researchers will make certain they are being as comprehensive as possible in their review of the literature.

Natural Medicines

Natural Medicines, formerly known as the Natural Standard, is a database that may be of interest to pharmacognosy scholars. The resource describes itself as an "evidence-based database of information on the safety and effectiveness of natural medicines and alternative therapies,"[6] and it provides access to over 170,000 dietary supplements, natural medicines, and integrative therapies. Additionally, over 1,200 natural ingredient monographs and over 200 complementary and alternative treatment monographs are included. These resources are modeled on the standard drug monograph located within most sources of drug information. Therefore, the monographs are easy to follow for any individual already familiar with drug information.[6]

The database has a number of useful features researchers should be aware of. First, the database provides access to several patient care tools. The Interaction Checker provides information about interactions between natural medicines, including supplements and conventional medications, while the Nutrient Checker provides information about any nutrients that may be depleted while taking a certain medication. An Effectiveness Checker explains the efficacy of natural medicines for certain medical conditions, and an Adverse Effects Checker informs the reader of potential adverse effects caused by natural medicines. Finally, a Pregnancy and Lactation Checker explains which natural medicines are safe for pregnant and lactating women, as well as which to avoid. Most of the Checker tools include a rating scale (i.e., from major to moderate to insignificant) that are intended to assist the researcher or health professional in understanding the clinical significance of the medicine's nutrient depletion, effectiveness, and so on. The ratings are color coded for easy reference, as well as to assist health professionals in making swift decisions.[7]

The Natural Medicines Brand Evidence-based Rating Number (NMBER) is another useful feature of the database. According to the Natural Medicines database, "NMBER provides an objective, scientific rating for over 90,000 commercially available natural medicines and dietary supplement products."[8] The safety, effectiveness, and quality of each product are rated on a scale of one to ten, with ten being the highest. An extensive explanation of the evidence-based process involved in evaluating and rating each product is transparent on the Natural Medicines database. The highest-rated products are those that have verifiable clinical evidence to prove effectiveness for treatment or prevention of a condition and that are deemed safe. The lowest-rated products lack verifiable evidence and may have potential or documented safety and quality concerns. As with the Checker tools, NMBER gives a quick and colorful visual on overall safety, effectiveness, and quality based on each active ingredient contained in a commercial product.[8]

The information within Natural Medicines is extensively researched and cited. Hyperlinked in-text citations are provided to transport viewers to full citation information, including links to citation abstracts in PubMed. While well researched and cited, the articulation of information within the database is not verbose and is written at a level that can be understood by most health science professionals. If a patient or consumer requires information from Natural Medicines, handouts are available in English, Spanish, and French.

BIOSIS, Reaxys, and Embase

BIOSIS, Reaxys, and Embase are three other databases pharmacognosy researchers should know about. *BIOSIS* Citation Index and BIOSIS Previews index over 5,500 journals and include information about the life sciences with a focus on microbiology, biochemistry, biophysics, and medicine. BIOSIS Previews contains international meeting abstracts as well as review articles, patents, and monographs. There is some duplication between MEDLINE and BIOSIS; however, the scope of BIOSIS focuses on preclinical and experimental medicine, including pharmacognosy, proteomics, nanotechnology, and genetics.[9]

Reaxys is a database that searches compound properties and chemical reaction data, as well as patents and the research literature. It includes resources that provide information about chemical composition and bioactivity, and the database is often consulted for preclinical drug discovery work, including planning syntheses and new drug pathway discoveries.[10] Users of Reaxys can search a number of different ways, including the standard keyword search as well as a chemical structure- or reaction-based search.

Finally, *Embase* is a database that contains about 30 million citations and indexes about 8,500 journals from 1974 to present day. It provides access to a wide variety of medical research from around the world and is noteworthy for its emphasis on European content. Embase is especially helpful for research in the domains of pharmaceutics, pharmacology, general clinical medicine, genetics, biochemistry, obstetrics, gynecology, rehabilitation, and complementary alternative medicine.[11] Like PubMed, Embase also has its own set of controlled vocabulary, or subject headings. Like MeSH, Emtree terms help standardize synonyms and spelling variations to help researchers locate relevant literature.

To ensure a comprehensive review of the literature, it is important to search within multiple databases. Pharmacognosy scholars may search a number of different databases, but Natural Medicines, BIOSIS, Reaxys, and Embase are all great options and provide access to a variety of relevant content. If you are unsure of which databases to consult, medical librarians can offer valuable assistance and can additionally help navigate the different resources.

Conclusion

Understanding how to review the research literature is a vital component of education in the health sciences, including the field of pharmacognosy. A review of the literature, whether as part of a larger study or within a laboratory or clinical setting, provides context, informs methodology, and allows the researcher to join the scholarly conversation about that specific topic. To review the literature properly, you must put a great deal of thought into the literature search. Researchers should begin by asking background and foreground questions and using those questions to inform their search strategy in relevant databases. It is the hope of the author that the above considerations and recommendations improve the quality of literature reviews and that students understand the importance of a thoughtful and comprehensive literature search.

References

1. Patrick M. Malone, Meghan J. Malone, and Sharon K. Park, *Drug Information: A Guide for Pharmacists* (New York: McGraw Hill, 2018).
2. Donald R. Bordley, Mark Fagan, and David Theige, "Evidence-Based Medicine: A Powerful Educational Tool for Clerkship Education," *American Journal of Medicine* 102, no. 5 (1997): 427–32.
3. James Mork, Alan Aronson, and Dina Demner-Fushman, "12 Years On: Is the NLM Medical Text Indexer Still Useful and Relevant?" *Journal of Biomedical Semantics*. 8, no. 1 (2017): 8.
4. Matthew E. Falagas et al., "Comparison of PubMed, Scopus, Web of Science, and Google Scholar: Strengths and Weaknesses," *FASEB Journal* 22, no. 2 (2007): 338–42.
5. Peace Ossum Williamson and Christian I. J. Minter, "Exploring PubMed as a Reliable Resource for Scholarly Communications Services," *Journal of the Medical Library Association* 107, no. 1 (2019): 16–29.
6. Therapeutic Research Center, "Natural Medicines." http://trchealthcare.com/solutions/natural-medicines.

7. Therapeutic Research Center, "Explore Key Features of the Most Comprehensive Database of Its Kind," Natural Medicines. https://naturalmedicines.therapeuticresearch.com/about-us/explore-features.aspx.
8. Therapeutic Research Center, "Natural Medicines Brand Evidence-based Rating (NMBER)," Natural Medicines. https://naturalmedicines.therapeuticresearch.com/nmber.aspx.
9. Clarivate Analytics, "Web of Science All Databases Help." https://images.webofknowledge.com/images/help/WOK/hp_database.html#dsy2129-TRS_bp.
10. Elsevier, "Developing Highly Sought-after Lead Compounds for Unmet Medical Needs," Customer Stories. https://www.elsevier.com/solutions/reaxys/customer-stories/developing-lead-compounds-unmet-medical-needs.
11. Wolters Kluwer, "Embase: Excerpta Medica Database Guide." http://ospguides.ovid.com/OSPguides/embase.htm.

Credits

Fig 22.1: Copyright © 2019 Depositphotos/Rachel Koenig.
Fig 22.1a: Copyright © 2015 Depositphotos/Icon_Craft_Studio.
Fig 22.1b: Copyright © 2014 Depositphotos/lynx_v.
Fig 22.1b: Copyright © 2014 Depositphotos/soeilc.

www.ingramcontent.com/pod-product-compliance
Ingram Content Group UK Ltd.
Pitfield, Milton Keynes, MK11 3LW, UK
UKHW051453290926
15471UKWH00008B/1183